Essentials of Public Health Management

Edited by

L. Fleming Fallon, Jr., MD, DrPH, MBA
Professor of Public Health
Bowling Green State University
Bowling Green, Ohio

Eric J. Zgodzinski, MPH
Supervisor of Community Services
Toledo-Lucas County Health Department
Toledo, Ohio

JONES AND BARTLETT PUBLISHERS
Sudbury, Massachusetts
BOSTON TORONTO LONDON SINGAPORE

World Headquarters
Jones and Bartlett Publishers
40 Tall Pine Drive
Sudbury, MA 01776
978-443-5000
info@jbpub.com
www.jbpub.com

Jones and Bartlett Publishers Canada
2406 Nikanna Road
Mississauga, ON L5C 2W6
CANADA

Jones and Bartlett Publishers International
Barb House, Barb Mews
London W6 7PA
UK

Library of Congress Cataloging-in-Publication Data

Fallon, L. Fleming.
Essentials of public health management / L. Fleming Fallon, Eric J. Zgodzinski.
p. ; cm.
Includes bibliographical references and index.
ISBN 0-7637-3153-6
1. Public health administration.
[DNLM: 1. Public Health Administration—methods—United States. 2. Disaster Planning—methods—United States. 3. Personnel Management—methods—United States. 4. Public Relations—United States. WA 540 AA1 F196e 2005] I. Zgodzinski, Eric J. II. Title.
RA5.F34 2005
362.1′068—dc22

2004018716

Production Credits
Publisher: Michael Brown
Production Manager: Amy Rose
Associate Production Editor: Renée Sekerak
Editorial Assistant: Kylah McNeill
Marketing Manager: Matthew Payne
Manufacturing and Buyer: Therese Bräuer
Cover Design: Kristin E. Ohlin
Interior Design and Composition: Auburn Associates, Inc.
Printing and Binding: Malloy, Inc.
Cover Printing: Malloy, Inc.

Printed in the United States of America
08 07 06 05 04 10 9 8 7 6 5 4 3 2 1

DEDICATION

Undertaking a project such as this one requires time. Thanks, Marie, for giving me the time to complete this one.

LFF

I want to thank my parents, Ray and Judy, for their constant support and interest in this project. More importantly, I want to thank my wife Susie for her patience, devotion, understanding, and love during the last year while I worked on this book. Finally, I have to express my gratitude to my daughter Zoe for not getting too upset when the book interfered with our time together. We can now play, Zoe.

EJZ

CONTENTS

PREFACE

Management books come and go. Different theories emerge, gain popularity, and then fade as they are replaced by alternative, emerging theories. The result is that textbooks on the subject of management become ever larger.

Students, academics, practitioners, and other readers are all participants in the process of developing, presenting, sharing, and using information that is contained in books. As is often the case, these participants have different agendas. Completeness is a virtue to some but at the cost of increased length of text. Brevity is a virtue to others but at the cost of omitting some subtleties and minor points. Almost all participants agree that accessibility and utility of the information in any book is an important attribute.

Practitioners often point out that time constraints are a reality. These people may note that they once read entire textbooks but now require a briefer review of the essentials. Students often complain that teachers present too much information. The reality may lie in students' lack of experience to guide them in prioritizing the knowledge that is provided in classes. Their lack of perspective or experience hampers them from distinguishing the essentials to form a more useful picture. Teachers stress the essentials but frequently augment them with additional illustrative material.

The key word in the previous paragraph is *essentials*. This was a guiding principle during the development of this book. The senior author had previous experience teaching principles of management to resident physicians in occupational medicine. Both authors had real-world experience in situations requiring managerial expertise. In discussing this book, both agreed that a fresh approach to teaching principles of management in public health was needed. After using the word essentials a few times, part of the solution emerged.

The perspectives of practitioners are frequently evident in presentations at professional meetings. Common venues are sessions devoted to best practices. Deciding to ask practitioners to write the chapters emerged as another element of the final product.

This book is written by practitioners for practitioners. While the chapters discuss theoretical models, they are focused on day-to-day responsibilities and realities. Supplemental resources are provided at the conclusion of each chapter. Here, relevant books and journal articles are listed as well as information on Internet web sites and contact information for organizations devoted to the topic of the chapter.

People often enter their professions with highly developed technical skills. This is the case in medicine as well as public and environmental health. As people achieve success, they are promoted, often into positions of leadership. In short, they assume managerial responsibilities. Frequently, these talented people lack formal training in management. Designing a vehicle that addresses that need became another goal of this project.

Case studies enable readers to focus on a topic and provide a context for discussion. Each chapter opens with a case study. Questions for reflection are posed. The case studies are resolved at the conclusion of each chapter. The material presented within the chapter provides the basis for the suggested resolution to the case study. Case studies have been a standard item in the curriculum of business programs for many years. Students have endorsed case studies in written comments about their courses.

A potential problem with contributed volumes is variation in the vocabulary and style of writing. The authors resolved to address and minimize or eliminate this problem in the book. The senior author has written a weekly newspaper column for the past nine years. That experience has taught the importance of clearly communicating to a large audience with a variety of backgrounds and levels of education. Every chapter has been edited for consistency of grammar and presentation. The ideas and concepts of chapter contributors remain. If we have done our jobs well, the book reads as if a single person wrote it.

We want to thank all of the excellent people who contributed chapters. Their names and positions are listed elsewhere. Without their dedication and effort, there would be no reason for writing a preface. We wish to thank the fine professionals at Jones and Bartlett. Mike Brown was willing to listen and then to support this project. Kylah McNeill and Renée Sekerak have guided this project through its various stages, including a rescue of missing information.

We accept responsibility for errors that have eluded the sharp eyes of many reviewers. We also look forward to receiving any comments or suggestions about this book to improve future editions. We can be contacted at 234 Health Center, Bowling Green State University, Bowling Green, OH 43403. May the book be a useful tool for all readers.

L. Fleming Fallon, Jr.
Eric J. Zgodzinski

July, 2004

CONTRIBUTORS BIOGRAPHICAL INFORMATION

Ned E. Baker, MPH

Ned Baker has served as a Registered Sanitarian in a local department of health and the Ohio Department of Health, worked as an environmental and public health planner and Associate Executive Director of the Health Planning Association of northwest Ohio, and as the Director of the Northwest Ohio Area Health Education Center Program. He has served on the Wood County board of health from 1986 to 1999. He facilitated a community health assessment project for the Wood County Board of Health in 2001.

Mr. Baker earned an MPH degree from the University of Michigan. He was a co-founder of the National Association of Local Boards of Health. Subsequently, he has served its President (1993–1994) and Executive Director (1995–1997).

Diane Borst, MBA

Diane Borst is the owner and Senior Vice President of The Manning Organization, Inc., a New York City based health care consulting firm specializing in human resource training and operational planning in the health care field. Her experience also includes senior management level work at tertiary care medical centers in New York City. She currently devotes one day a week pro bono to a federally funded medical clinic in East Harlem, New York City.

Ms. Borst holds an MBA in economics from New York University. She teaches on the graduate faculties of Sarah Lawrence College, Bronxville, New York and St. Joseph's College, Standish, Maine.

Ronald Burger, BA

Ronald Burger has more than 30 years of experience with the Centers for Disease Control and Prevention, Atlanta, Georgia and is presently a Senior Emergency Response Coordinator. He has worked with many state and local health officials in their responses to both unintentional and intentional events which all impacted the public's health and safety. He has been the Chairman of the Rockdale County Georgia Board of Health since 1993. His other volunteer activities include serving on the Boards of the Georgia Public Health Association and the Georgia Association of Local Boards of Health. Ron is an active American Red Cross volunteer and serves on its Advisory Board. He is the President-Elect of the National Association of Local Boards of Health.

Ron received his BS degree in Education from Millersville University, Millersville, Pennsylvania.

Pamela Butler, MPH

Pamela Butler is the Director of Disaster Planning and the Health Planning Coordinator for Hospital Council of Northwest Ohio, Toledo, Ohio. She facilitates and chairs multiple committees for regional emergency preparedness through planning, coordinating, and collaborating with multiple agencies and organizations locally and statewide.

Ms. Butler received her MPH degree from the Northwest Ohio Consortium for Public Health and is a graduate of Ohio State University, Columbus, Ohio.

Virginia Cogar, PhD

Dr. Virginia Cogar has taught environmental health at Texas A&M University and Bowling Green State University, Bowling Green, Ohio. She has also worked as a Research Scientist at the Caesar Kleberg Wildlife Research Institute, Texas A&I University, Kingsville, Texas.

Dr. Cogar received her doctorate from Texas A&M University, College Station, Texas. She earned a BS in Biology from East Stroudsburg University, East Stroudsburg, Pennsylvania.

Gary Crum, PhD

Dr. Gary Crum is the District Director of Health for the Northern Kentucky Independent Health District, Covington, Kentucky. He has served as a Deputy Commissioner of Health in the Ohio Department of Health, Columbus, Ohio and as a Health Commissioner for the Jackson County Health District, Jackson, Ohio.

Dr. Crum received his doctorate from Ohio State University, Columbus, Ohio.

Joseph A. Diorio, Jr., PhD

Dr. Joseph Diorio is an industrial psychologist with extensive managerial experience. His most recent industry position was as the Manager of Human Resources for Just Born, Inc. of Bethlehem, Pennsylvania.

Dr. Diorio earned his PhD degree in Industrial Psychology from Case Western Reserve University, Cleveland, Ohio. He is currently an Assistant Professor of Psychology at LaSalle University, Philadelphia, Pennsylvania.

L. Fleming Fallon, Jr., MD, DrPH, MBA

Dr. Fleming Fallon is a Professor of Public Health at Bowling Green State University, Bowling Green, Ohio. He is also the Director of the Northwest Ohio Consortium for Public Health, an accredited MPH degree program that is offered jointly by Bowling Green State University, the Medical College of Ohio, and the University of Toledo. He has many years of experience as a management consultant and has authored more than 350 papers, chapters, and books on a variety of topics, as well as making presentations throughout the world. Dr. Fallon has written a weekly newspaper column entitled Health Thoughts continuously since 1995. He has served as both a member and president of a local board of health.

Dr. Fallon is a physician with residency training in occupational and environmental medicine. He received a DrPH degree in environmental health science from Columbia University, New York, his MD degree from St. Georges University School of Medicine, St. Georges, Grenada, and an MBA from the University of New Haven, New Haven, Connecticut. He holds a health officer license from New Jersey.

Marie M. Fallon, MHSA

Marie Fallon is the Executive Director of the National Association of Local Boards of Health that has its headquarters in Bowling Green, Ohio. She previously served as a Project Director for the same organization. Earlier in her professional career, she served as a Controller for two community hospitals. She has completed Public Health Leadership programs at the state and national levels.

Ms. Fallon earned a MHSA degree from St. Joseph's College, Standish, Maine and has a BA degree in Accounting from the State University of New York at Buffalo, Buffalo, New York.

Vonna J. Henry, MPH, RN

Vonna Henry is the Director of Public Health for Sherburne County, Minnesota. She is responsible for planning, developing, implementing, and evaluating public health programs, financial management, and community coordination. She is a current Board Member of the National Association of County and Health Officials, on the Governing Board of the American Public Health Association, and a member of the Minnesota Public Health Association and the Local Public Health Association of Minnesota.

Ms. Henry received her MPH degree from the University of Minnesota and has a BS degree in nursing from Winona State University, Winona, Minnesota. She has completed the national Public Health Leadership program.

Timothy E. Horgan, MPH

Timothy Horgan recently retired as the Health Commissioner for the Cuyahoga County Board of Health, Cleveland, Ohio. Prior to becoming a Health Commissioner, he held a number of other managerial positions in departments of health. He has lectured widely on the topic of innovating situations rather than waiting for them to occur on their own.

Mr. Horgan received his MPH degree from the University of Hawaii.

Adam Kinninger, BS

Adam Kinninger is currently a student at the Ohio University College of Osteopathic Medicine in Athens, Ohio. His contribution to this book is an outgrowth of a senior independent study project. He has a BS degree in Applied Health Science from Bowling Green State University, Bowling Green, Ohio.

Jan Larson, BA

Jan Larson is the County Editor at the Sentinel-Tribune, Bowling Green, Ohio. She has held other positions at the same newspaper. She has won several awards from the Associated Press for her journalistic efforts and an award for her coverage of public health issues. She is involved in her community as a board member for the Wood County Court Appointed Special Advocates Program and the Wood County American Cancer Society Board.

Ms. Larson has a BS degree in Journalism from Bowling Green State University, Bowling Green, Ohio.

Jay MacNeal, MPH

Jay MacNeal is the Project Director for Public Health Preparedness and Workforce Development for the National Association of Local Boards of Health, Bowling Green, Ohio. His responsibilities include helping local health departments improve their emergency preparations. He is a paramedic and teaches incident command. He has received awards for his actions in times of emergency.

Mr. MacNeal received his MPH degree from the Northwest Ohio Consortium for Public Health and a BA degree from Bowling Green State University, Bowling Green, Ohio.

Charles R. McConnell, MBA

Charles McConnell is a consultant with the VMC Group, Niagara Falls, New York. He has many years of experience in health care management and human resources. He has authored 13 books and more than 250 articles. He serves as the editor of a quarterly professional journal.

Mr. McConnell received an MBA and BS in Engineering from the State University of New York at Buffalo, Buffalo, New York.

Kip E. Miller, MBA, RN

Kip Miller began his career as a nurse primarily in the care of burn patients. He advanced to Executive Vice President of the Wood County Hospital, Bowling Green, Ohio. Currently, he is a Senior Vice President of the Fisher-Titus Medical Center, Norwalk, Ohio. Mr. Miller believes that an important key to success as a manager is knowing and understanding the employees with whom one works so that rewards can be tailored to motivate them.

Mr. Miller holds an MBA degree from Bowling Green State University, Bowling Green, Ohio. He is an adjunct faculty member at Bowling Green State University.

Kimberly Moss, MPH, RN

Kimberly Moss is the Health Commissioner for the Defiance County General Health District, Defiance, Ohio. Prior to assuming these responsibilities, she worked as a nurse for the Health District and in hospitals. She has coordinated two successful tax levies in her county.

Ms. Moss received her MPH degree from the Northwest Ohio Consortium for Public Health. She received her BSN degree from St. Francis College, Fort Wayne, Indiana.

David Pollick, MSEPH

David Pollick is currently the Health Commissioner of the Sandusky County General Health District. He was formerly the Executive Director of Northwest Ohio Health Planning, Inc., the state designated Health Service Agency for the eleven counties of Northwest Ohio. He has been active in planning, data analysis, needs assessment, and consultation with both the public health and provider communities.

Mr. Pollick completed his graduate and undergraduate degrees at the University of Toledo, Toledo, Ohio. He is also a graduate of the Health Executives Development Program through the Sloan School of Business Administration at Cornell University, Ithaca, NY.

Anthony J. Santarsiero, MBA

Tony Santarsiero is the Lead Public Health Advisor for CDC Public Health Systems Partnerships with the Division of Public Health Systems Development and Research in the Public Health Practice Program Office at the Centers for Disease Control and Prevention, Atlanta, Georgia. In this capacity, he serves as a program consultant and advocate for the planning, development, and execution of core public health infrastructure activities. He advises on special projects designed to build and strengthen the public health system and infrastructure by promoting the public health roles of assessment, policy development, and assurance. He has been integrally involved in building and strengthening the nation's terrorism preparedness and emergency response infrastructure. Prior to joining the CDC, he was a hospital administrator in the US Air Force.

Mr. Santarsiero received his MBA degree from Florida Technological University, and has a BBA from the University of Georgia, Athens, Georgia. He is a Fellow in the American College of Healthcare Executives and has completed the national Public Health Leadership program.

Peter D. Schade, MPH

Peter Schade is the Environmental Health Division Deputy Director for the Cuyahoga County Board of Health, Cleveland, Ohio. He previously worked as a Registered Sanitarian for the Ohio Department of Health and as an Inspecting Sanitarian for the Ohio Department of Agriculture. He is a Past President of the Ohio Environmental Health Association.

Mr. Schade received his MPH degree from the Northwest Ohio Consortium for Public Health and is a graduate of Ohio State University, Columbus, Ohio.

Hans Schmalzried, PhD

Dr. Hans Schmalzried is the Health Commissioner of the Fulton County Health District, Wauseon, Ohio and the Commissioner of the Henry County/Napoleon City Health District, Napoleon, Ohio. He is an Assistant Professor of Public Health, Bowling Green State University, Bowling Green, Ohio. He has been active in public health administration activities at the local and national levels through publications, presentations, and task forces.

Dr. Schmalzreid earned his doctorate at the University of Toledo, Toledo, Ohio. He is a Registered Sanitarian.

Kathy S. Silvestri, MPH

Kathy Silvestri is the Director of Health Planning for the Healthy Communities Foundation of the Hospital Council of Northwest Ohio, Toledo, Ohio. Previously, she served as a Health Information Specialist for the same organization. She also serves as a Project Coordinator for the Northwest Ohio Strategic Alliance for Tobacco Control. She is an active member of the Ohio Public Health Association.

Ms. Silvestri received her MPH degree from the Northwest Ohio Consortium for Public Health and holds a BA degree in Business Administration and Allied Health.

Mark D. Tolles, JD

Mark Tolles is an attorney in private practice in Wood County, Ohio. He is the Assistant City Prosecutor for the City of Bowling Green, Ohio. He serves as the Village Prosecutor for Weston, Ohio and Pemberville, Ohio and as the Village Solicitor for Milton Center, Ohio.

Mr. Tolles received his law degree from the University of Toledo, Toledo, Ohio. He also earned a BA in Political Science from the same institution.

Vaughn M. Upshaw, DrPH, EdD

Dr. Vaughn Upshaw is a Lecturer in Public Administration and Government where she trains local elected officials and their professional managers in governance and leadership. She previously served as a Clinical Assistant

Professor in the Department of Health Policy and Administration at the University of North Carolina at Chapel Hill's School of Public Health. From 1987–1993, she was the Executive Director of the Association for North Carolina Boards of Health. She served as President of the National Association of Local Boards of Health in 1999 and has been a member of the Public Health Foundation board, an advisory group member for Mobilizing Action through Planning and Partnerships with the National Association of City and County Health Officials, and a participant in the Center for Disease Control and Prevention's National Public Health Performance Standards Program.

Dr. Upshaw received her EdD from North Carolina State University and her DrPH degree from the University of North Carolina-Chapel Hill. She has a BA degree from Ohio Wesleyan University, Delaware, Ohio.

Harvey Wallace, PhD

Dr. Harvey Wallace is a professor of health education and head of the Department of Health, Physical Education, and Recreation at Northern Michigan University. He has been a member of the Marquette County Board of Health since 1987, president of the National Association of Local Boards of Health, and president of the Michigan Association for Local Public Health. He has presented widely and been honored by the Public Health Practice Program Office of the Centers for Disease Control and Prevention for exemplary service.

Dr. Wallace earned his doctorate from the University of Toledo, Toledo, Ohio and has a BS degree from the University of California at Los Angeles, Los Angeles, California.

Diana Wilde, BA, N6WWT

Diana Wilde is a longtime, active member of her community's emergency response program in Orinda, California. She served on the Orinda Disaster Council that established a community-wide, multi-agency emergency response program and stand-by Emergency Operations Center within the city offices and has promoted the program at the neighborhood level to ensure city-wide coordination and cross-community preparedness. Ms. Wilde volunteers time with the local fire district's emergency response team, staffing a mobile communications relay facility during area-wide major emergencies. She is a member of the Radio Amateur Civilian Emergency Services, the Mt. Diablo Amateur Radio Club, and the American Radio Relay League.

Ms. Wilde has a BA in English from the University of California. Professionally, she manages her specialized divorce mediation business.

Eric J. Zgodzinski, MPH

Eric Zgodzinski is currently a Supervisor of Community Services for the Toledo-Lucas County Health Department, Toledo, Ohio. He has previously served as a Registered Sanitarian in a large, urban department of health. He has made many presentations on the subjects of food sanitation and bioterrorism preparedness. He is a member of the Toledo-Lucas County Metro Medical Response System committee and is active in the Ohio Environmental Health Association.

Mr. Zgodzinski received his MPH degree from the Northwest Ohio Consortium for Public Health and is a graduate of Thiel College, Greenville, Pennsylvania. He is an Adjunct Assistant Professor of Public Health at Bowling Green State University, Bowling Green, Ohio.

PART I

Introduction

CHAPTER

1

Introduction

L. Fleming Fallon, Jr.
Eric Zgodzinski

Chapter Objectives

After reading this chapter, readers will:

- Appreciate the importance of management knowledge for public health practitioners.
- Understand the layout of this book.
- Know the various features of this book.

Summary

This book is about management. It introduces readers to management concepts that are essential for success in a public health career. The format and layout of the book are briefly introduced and described.

Case Study

John Simpson was so happy that he was floating on a cloud. John had just been promoted to Program Manager. He called his wife to share the good news. "Yes, that's right," he told her, "Program Manager. I'll be supervising two regular employees and an intern."

"Do you get a raise?" his wife inquired.

"Yes," beamed John, "I'll get a 9 percent raise."

"That's great honey. Congratulations," his wife said. She was thinking about new drapes for the living room.

They said goodbye and hung up. John wrote his name and new title on a piece of scratch paper. Fear started to replace joy as John realized that he had neither experience nor formal training in management. His science curriculum in college had not included any management coursework. What advice would you give to John?

INTRODUCTION

For many, the mention of public health evokes mental images of immunization clinics, food-service inspections, and school nurses performing their daily duties. However, public health is much more than a series of programs. Members of the public see only a fraction of the activities performed by public health departments and often are unaware of the planning required to offer public health programs and services. This book discusses how health departments conduct their business, how they develop new programs, what techniques they use to hire and discipline employees, the role of the media in public health, and a myriad of other issues that require an understanding of the practical knowledge required for creating and sustaining successful public health agencies.

This book contains the word *essentials* in its title. The authors of this text have chosen to include concepts that are required for managerial success in public health. The chapter authors represent a mix of those in public health practice and those in academic positions. All of the chapter authors are experts in the discipline about which they have written. All have had practical experience working in so-called "real-world" positions within public health or related disciplines.

Practical knowledge can be defined as an optimal blend of techniques learned through experience and theoretical studies. When these elements are not balanced, public health is unlikely to reach its full potential. Sound, proactive, and efficient public health programs and practices require a highly trained workforce that can cope with any issues that may arise. The contributors to this book describe the real-life experiences of those who are actively studying and making public health their careers.

Most current textbooks on management, finance, leadership, and other issues are excellent sources of theory and information on complex issues. They accomplish their set tasks, describing and providing information on the building blocks of theory. The information in this book is presented in a format that is developed for students from real-world experiences of practitioners and stewards of public health.

The original reason for writing this book was to present information on management in a public health context in a format that was accessible to people in different stages of their careers. Students of public health include university learners, public health staff, and people in positions of leadership. Stewards of public health include members of boards of health and other government officials who require sound, usable information. This book was written so that board members can gain a greater understanding of the managerial procedures and concerns regarding public health.

FORMAT OF THE BOOK

Readers will find the material in this book to be accessible. Each chapter begins with a case study related to the material that follows. The case study is resolved at the conclusion of the chapter. This book is intended to serve both teaching and reference needs. Each chapter can stand on its own, or the book can be read in its entirety to provide a unified introduction to public health management.

The book has several references to Midwestern venues. These reflect events to which the authors were personally privy. However, the book is national in scope and applicable to any pubic health jurisdiction. The chapter authors work in settings throughout the United States. The cross-section of contributors gives rise to a work that reflects many different viewpoints and areas of expertise.

Resources are provided at the conclusion of each chapter. Periodicals and books direct readers to printed materials. Web sites provide supplemental information in electronic form. Organizations link readers with others having similar interests, greater expertise, or additional resources in areas related to the topics of a given chapter. Portions of some chapters have previously appeared in a different form in *State of the Art Reviews in Occupational Health*.

CONCLUSION

This book provides a concise and readily accessible introduction to management in public health. Returning to John, the newly promoted Program Manager in the initial case study, an office colleague suggested that John read a copy of *Essentials of Public Health Management* by Fallon and Zgodzinski. The colleague had been in a similar situation six months ago. The book had gotten him off to a great start in his new job.

John took his colleague's advice. When last seen, he was enjoying success in his new job. John's wife decided to go with a burgundy color scheme for the living room.

Resources

Organizations

American Public Health Association
800 I Street, NW
Washington, DC 20001-3710
Phone: 202-777-2742
Fax: 202-777-2534
E-mail: comments@apha.org
Web site: www.apha.org/

Centers for Disease Control and Prevention
1600 Clifton Road
Atlanta, GA 30333
Phone: 404-639-3311

Public Inquiries: 404-639-3534 or 800-311-3435
E-mail: www.cdc.gov/netinfo.htm (e-mail form)
Web site: www.cdc.gov/

National Association of County and City Health Officials
1100 17th Street, Second Floor
Washington, DC 20036
Phone: 202-783-5550
Fax: 202-783-1583
E-mail: naccho@naccho.org
Web site: www.naccho.org

National Association of Local Boards of Health
1840 East Gypsy Lane Road
Bowling Green, OH 43402
Phone: 419-353-7714
Fax: 419-352-6278
E-mail: nalboh@nalboh.org
Web site: www.nalboh.org/

National Environmental Health Association
720 S. Colorado Blvd., Suite 970-S
Denver, CO 80246-1925
Phone: 303-756-9090
Fax: 303-691-9490
E-mail: staff@neha.org
Web site: www.neha.org/

Public Health Foundation
1220 L Street, NW, Suite 350
Washington, DC 20005
Phone: 202-898-5600
Fax: 202-898-5609
E-mail: info@phf.org
Web site: www.phf.org/

CHAPTER

2

The History of Public Health

Eric Zgodzinski
L. Fleming Fallon, Jr.

Chapter Objectives

After reading this chapter, readers will:

- Appreciate the depth of the history of public health.
- Know the chronology of events that have shaped public health from prerecorded history to the present.
- Learn of public health in ancient civilizations.
- Recognize the emergence of public health as a scientific discipline.
- Know of health-related events in modern times.
- Recognize possible future directions of public health.

Chapter Summary

The history of public health predates the rise of communities. Public health began among bands of hunter-gatherers. Diseases of animals become diseases of humans as animals were domesticated.

Public health and medical knowledge have not accumulated at a steady rate. Major advances have often been driven by health calamities such as epidemics, natural disasters, and warfare. Recent events affecting public health are incompletely understood: AIDS, SARS, and bioterrorism provide convenient examples. Public health continues to evolve.

Case Study

A group of public health students were sharing an adult beverage after their first introductory class. "That anthrax scare really got people moving," said one student. "It sure seemed to catch people by surprise," added another. "I'm glad that my nursing training included some lectures on hand washing," added a third, "the people in public health could benefit from some of that thinking."

The students were meeting each other for the first time. They were discussing their undergraduate programs and recent graduations. One older student simply listened to his younger colleagues.

"What should we call you, Doctor or Peter?" asked the first student.

"Pete is fine," was the reply.

They turned to him with expectant eyes, "What do you think about dealing with anthrax, Pete?" "And hand washing?" added the young nurse.

Doctor Peter just smiled before he replied.

How do you think Peter replied to his very young colleagues?

INTRODUCTION

The word *history* conjures up many different thoughts. For many people, history is synonymous with a high school teacher lecturing on some important event of the past that lacks any relevance to the present. Others link history with one or more specific points in time. Many can recall exactly what they were doing when they learned that President John F. Kennedy or Dr. Martin Luther King, Jr. was assassinated. Younger people may recall watching the space shuttle Challenger explode or the World Trade Center buildings as they fell on 9-11. The images associated with different historical events are less important than the actual message of history. If people do not learn from history, society is very likely to repeat mistakes. Public health is not exempt from this rule. This is the reason for the present chapter.

The events of history are sprinkled with surprises that affect health in general and public health in particular. The Black Death in the Middle Ages and the worldwide eradication of smallpox in the twentieth century provide dramatic examples. Advances in public health, namely draining swamps, enabled the Panama Canal to be constructed. The results of major and minor events have shaped public health in its present configuration. Through the efforts of public health practitioners, people in many regions of the world now enjoy long lives that are largely free from many of the diseases that affected communities in the past. These benefits are not universal. Reviewing the history of public health provides perspective on the past and demarcates a starting point for the future. The future of public health will be contained in chapters yet to be written.

THE BEGINNING

The origins of public health are hidden in the events of prerecorded history. One member of a hunter-gatherer community may have watched one person eat a red fruit (tomato) and another eat the leaves from the same plant. The leaf-eater would have been lucky to only become sick. Observers would connect an action with an illness and know not repeat the action. Thus, prevention was born. Similar connections were undoubtedly made before any written records were kept.

The history of man and the history of disease go together. Hunter-gatherer peoples had few diseases or disabilities other than trauma. The successful ones ate reasonable diets and reproduced. Constant movement simultaneously kept them fit and wore them out. An early invention that supported the development of communities was agriculture. The advent of agriculture promoted the eventual development of cities. Because of agriculture, communities could not only grow in size, but could also support a limited number of persons who did not directly produce food. Healers were among the first such people to be supported by communities.

The development of agriculture was followed by the domestication of animals. Having animals conveniently available improved human diets by making protein more readily available. This resulted in faster population growth. Domestication also brought humans into prolonged and intimate contact with animals. An unanticipated side effect of animal domestication was a shift in disease infectivity and the transfer of infectious diseases to humans. For example, chickens were the original reservoir for pneumonia. Influenza jumped from swine to humans. Cattle delivered tuberculosis in their milk. Encephalitis originally came from horses. Crowding led to the spread of lice, pinworms, and syphilis among humans. Intestinal parasites infected humans who ate improperly cooked beef, pork, and fish. Other than tuberculosis, which was essentially eliminated from American dairy herds by 1920 due to the continual testing of herds, these diseases continue to pose health problems for humans.

Living in communities improved the quality of pregnancies and increased infant survival by improving nutrition, permitting some planning for the timing of pregnancies and allowing people to acquire specialized skills related to delivery and childbirth. This caused populations to increase. Communities also made epidemics possible. Smallpox, influenza, measles, and chickenpox are diseases that are spread from person to person. Living in close proximity allows them to spread in a short time span. Other diseases, such as tuberculosis and leprosy, are also spread by prolonged contact.

Archaeological data have provided evidence of occupational diseases that date from ancient times. People who worked with lead and mercury developed shakes or tremors. Smelters of lead and mercury ores and people who made pottery were among the most often affected. Mercury was used in the felt for hats. Lewis Carroll's character of the Mad Hatter was based on people who developed tremors after inhaling mercury vapor generated during the steam pressing of hats in the 1800s. Dust from mining or glassmaking caused lung disorders. Dust from the processing of cotton also caused lung diseases. Public health efforts have had an impact on reducing the incidence of occupational diseases. Much work remains to be done.

Public health has often been stressed through religion or beliefs. Many religions had rites and rituals that improved public health. Religious prohibitions on eating swine protected followers from pig tapeworm and trichinosis. Prohibitions on eating shellfish also served a protective purpose. Clams, mussels, and oysters from sewage-contaminated waters can carry hepatitis or other diseases.

PUBLIC HEALTH IN ANCIENT CIVILIZATIONS

The civilization on the island of Minos built temples for healing and worshiped Hygeia, the Greek goddess of health. Drugs were used by Mesopotamian healers. In the New World, people practiced *trephining,* making holes in skulls to treat abnormal behavior. Even though this activity occurred more than 3,500 years ago, the recipients recovered. (Modern surgeons use a similar procedure to drill holes in skulls to relieve pressure on the brain from internal bleeding.)

Greece and Rome

During the Greco-Roman era, public health was relatively advanced. The Greeks developed the Hippocratic Oath. Galen developed and wrote about a system of health based on four humors. His medicinal theories persisted for over 1,500 years. The Romans built great engineering systems to bring water to Rome from distant sources and to remove sewage from the city. Unfortunately, they lined their aqueducts with lead. In the opinion of many scholars, this caused mild lead poisoning among Rome's citizenry and contributed to the city's eventual downfall (Rosen, 1993).

The Middle Ages

During the Middle Ages, public health declined to low levels. Many of the earlier advances in health were ignored or forgotten. The advent of secular warfare initiated this decline. Disease and lack of sanitation were the hallmarks of cities during the Middle Ages. Community and personal sanitation were virtually nonexistent. The pursuit of learning was forgotten in most cities of Western Europe. A handful of universities in Spain nourished learning, maintaining knowledge for reawakening in the future. Health and medical knowledge was sustained in this manner.

During the Middle Ages, trade started to link cities throughout the known world. Rats and other carriers of disease also traveled with traders. The first major episode of bubonic plague (also called the Black Death) swept through Europe between 1349 and 1354, killing approximately one-third of the population. More than a century would be required to replace the number of people lost in the epidemic. People who lived in rural areas and people who fled from cities often survived the epidemic. The concept of quarantine was developed near the end of the first Black Death epidemic. Quarantines were imposed in subsequent waves of the plague, which swept through Europe approximately every 25 years over the next two centuries. This public health lesson was not lost. The utility of quarantines continues to the present day.

Near the end of the Middle Ages, leaders initiated a number of advances in health care. The first hospitals were organized. The goals of those hospitals were not much different from those of contemporary health care institutions. However, resources and knowledge were so limited that disease was more likely to be spread among patients in a hospital than among those who stayed at home. Until the 1800s, hospitals were places for dying rather than healing.

Rudimentary food-safety guidelines were developed during the Middle Ages. And, as people kept their food clean, they became sick less often. In cities, streets were periodically washed or swept clean of debris and animal waste. Epidemics continued to occur, but their virulence slowly diminished. This allowed the populations of communities to slowly increase after centuries of devastating epidemics.

■ THE EMERGENCE OF PUBLIC HEALTH

The Renaissance

During the Renaissance, lost knowledge reemerged in Western Europe. The quest for accurate medical knowledge led to the systematic study of anatomy in Italy. Dissection was the new means for obtaining knowledge of the human body. Through dissection, William Harvey discovered that blood circulated through the vessels of the body. The first systematic classification of diseases was undertaken. Paracelsus described diseases related to occupations. All of this knowledge is still in use today.

The Enlightenment

The Enlightenment gave rise to several concepts that improved the public's health. Individuals began to clamor for more freedom, and governments began to appreciate the economic and political benefits associated with a healthy populace. Demographic data had initially been collected via periodic censuses largely to support military adventures and international expeditions of the monarch. John Graunt (1662) assembled the first modern data on mortality and morbidity. The first systematic surveys seeking information related to diseases and health in general were developed and administered during this era. Jenner's observation that milkmaids who had cowpox did not contract smallpox led to the invention of variolation. This provided such better protection against smallpox that General George Washington ordered all of the soldiers in the Continental Army to be inoculated.

At the start of the industrial revolution, engineering advances such as the installation of pipes to transport water increased people's comfort. The installation of pipes also helped to reduce the incidence of some diseases, such as typhoid fever. However, many of the comforts such as steam power to ease work in mines, smelting to produce iron that was used in bridges, and the combination of both in the development of railroads provided by the industrial revolution also caused water and air pollution. During the industrial revolution, the personal health of miners, industrial workers, and people living in industrial areas declined.

The Sanitary Movement

The sanitary movement, a time of increased awareness about the importance of regular bathing, clean water, and controlled disposal of human wastes encompassed a half-century, beginning in approximately 1830. It was a by-product of the industrial revolution. Throughout the world, populations in cities dramatically increased. The western portion of the United States was opened to settlement. First canals and then railroads connected cities, establishing communities along rights of way in their wake. At the beginning of the industrial revolution, clean water was abundant in rivers and lakes. However, as the industrial revolution advanced, pollution began to destroy these resources. Another consequence of industrialization was the substandard living conditions for many people, including the urban poor and many new immigrants.

New York City constructed one of the first municipal water systems during this period. The motivation behind the water system was not improved health, but fire protection. A series of fires in the early years of the 1800s had destroyed large groups of buildings. However, the clean water provided by the system positively impacted public health. By the end of the nineteenth century, municipal water systems were common throughout cites in the United States. Ironically, the availability of clean water set the stage for the emergence of a major public health problem—polio.

The first attempt by the federal government to protect surface water was the River and Harbor Act of 1899. The act sought to limit dumping of debris into waterways as a means to enhance commerce by reducing accidents. This provided the legal basis for the federal government to assume jurisdiction over a body of water. It was later used as the basis for protecting waterways from pollution via discharge into rivers.

During the middle and late portions of the 1800s, Louis Pasteur in France (1860s to 1870s) and Edward Koch in Germany (1880s to 1890s) developed the germ theory of disease. This linkage between pathogen and disease led to rapid advances in public health. Improved sanitation resulted in decreases in the incidence of diseases. In Boston, Edwin Chadwick worked to improve living and working conditions in that city. Epidemics still occurred, but the number of victims began to decrease.

In 1854, a cholera epidemic broke out in London. John Snow, a local general practitioner began to think about the outbreak. He made a map that noted the residences of persons who had cholera. He mapped other data. One map that caught his attention was a map of the water sources used by different cholera victims. All of the people with cholera had drawn water from the same pump. Snow had no knowledge of microbiology, but he did have the intuitive sense to remove the handle from what appeared to be the offending pump. After that action, no additional cases of cholera were reported. Snow had initiated the study of epidemiology.

Then, as in the present day, developments in engineering and science were occurring at a steadily accelerating pace. The causal connections first established by Pasteur and Koch were extended and amplified in the work of others. Remembering the work of Paracelsus, connections between occupational conditions and adverse health consequences began to be made.

The Age of Bacteria

In the late 1800s, scientists realized that bacteria and viruses caused diseases. Pasteur had earlier noted that heating killed the microorganisms that were responsible for tainting wine. In particular, Pasteur noted that heating milk greatly increased its safety by killing microorganisms that were found in raw milk. This heating process is used today and is called Pasteurization. In an effort to preserve food for armies and scientific expeditions, Pasteur applied the heating concept to food. He succeeded in developing a method of preserving food for long periods of time. Because he used tin cans, the term *canning* became associated with the process. He applied the process to a variety of foods and eliminated many milk-borne diseases. Preservation by canning also enabled many exploratory voyages to hostile regions of the earth to succeed by ensuring a supply of food. In the United States, the process of pasteurization is applied to all milk that is transported from the dairy in which it is produced. This is a requirement of the Pure Food and Drug Act. Pasteurization is not required for milk that is purchased directly from the dairy where it is initially produced.

From the perspective of their ability to cause serious human diseases, important species of bacteria were isolated and identified during this the second half of the 1800s and first decades of the 1900s. The scientific method was successfully applied in this effort. Early isolates included *Escherichia coli* and *Staphylococcus*. These pathogens continue to cause disease in humans. *Vectors* are organisms that spread the pathogens that actually cause diseases. Vectors were identified for many diseases. The importance of these discoveries to public health was significant. Controlling disease vectors meant stopping the spread of disease. In this way, many diseases were controlled through vector control before the cures for the diseases were discovered. Elements of the immune system were being studied and described. This knowledge enabled more accurate means of diagnosis to be developed. These developments justified the creation of regional laboratories dedicated to disease research.

Once proper drinking water and wastewater sewage treatment plants were installed, mortality from typhoid fever decreased. Improved sanitation prolonged the lives of children and reduced infant mortality. Mandatory school attendance laws resulted in the education of large numbers of children. Improved sanitation and access to education probably contributed more to improving the health of children than did laws prohibiting child labor.

MODERN TIMES

The opening years of the twentieth century were characterized by growing attention to sanitation. Environmental interventions such as draining swamps led to a decline in the incidence of many mosquito-borne diseases. The First World War raged from 1914 to 1918. Poison gas was used as a weapon. Political refugees posed significant political as well as public health problems. In 1919, a worldwide influenza epidemic killed an estimated 30 million people. This was more than had died during the war. All of the previous examples of events affected the health and lives of many people. Each involved health in some manner.

During the 1920s, the League of Nations was established. The first antibiotics were put onto the market. An international depression engulfed the world, slowing, but not totally stopping, advances in public health. Alexander Fleming discovered penicillin in 1928. During the Second World War, political refugees again became a public health issue. Another 30 million or more people lost their lives. The majority of these were civilians. For the first time in military history, efforts were made to protect the health of soldiers. The result—more soldiers died from battle injuries than died from infections. This was in part due to the use of penicillin, which became commercially available in 1944.

During the post-war period, from 1945 to 1950, the United Nations emerged from the legacy of the League of Nations. The World Health Organization was founded in 1948. The next generation of antibiotics were synthesized and brought to market. In 1954, Salk succeeded in creating a vaccine for polio, solving the public health problem that improved water supplies had created 50 years earlier. In 1957, Sabin created an oral preparation of the vaccine, moving the polio vaccine from a syringe to a sugar cube.

Many colonies gained independence from their European masters during the 1960s. During this decade, a gap began to appear between the developed and undeveloped worlds. During the 1970s, this gap continued to widen. In the industrialized countries, nongovernmental organizations began to emerge to provide assistance to developing countries. The Rockefeller Foundation funded research into rice production in Mexico. The research was so successful that it came to be called the *green revolution*. In 1976, the first report of a frightening new disease called Ebola was received from Africa. In 1978, the World Health Organization declared that smallpox had been eradicated. In 1979, the first report of another new disease, which would eventually be called Acquired Immune Deficiency Syndrome, was published.

In the 1980s, poison gas returned as a weapon of war. AIDS became an everyday reality. The U.S. Food and Drug Administration created a program to provide economic incentives for US pharmaceutical firms to develop new drugs having limited marketing potential in this country. The result has become known as the orphan drug program. Ivermectin was developed under this program. After only a few years of use in treating river blindness (onchocerciasis), the disease almost disappeared. Before Invermectin, onchocerciasis was the leading cause of blindness in the world, robbing the sight of more than 1 million people each year.

During the 1990s, polio was eliminated from the Americas. Polio is still a problem in countries in Asia and Africa. The size of tropical rain forests is shrinking while the size of the Sahara desert is increasing. The health consequences of these environmental changes have not been fully appreciated. Severe Acute Respiratory Syndrome (SARS); bovine spongiform encephalitis (BSE), or mad cow disease; and a preoccupation with terrorism have accompanied the beginning of the twenty-first century. These are elements of the current history of public health.

■ THE FUTURE

What will be the future of public health? Recent terrorist attacks have returned public health to a central position in the political world. Greater opportunities and increased responsibilities accompany the renewed recognition of public health. Readers of this book will help to determine the future of public health.

Doctor Peter, the older public health student, had the perspective of working in the medical field for over 30 years. He also knew that much of the history of medicine was intimately linked with the history of public health. Concepts such as quarantine and hand washing were developed in public health rather than strictly medical contexts. From observing many other young people just entering the field of public health, Peter knew that they would learn and appreciate the rich heritage that is associated with public health. He found it ironic that public health had a high probability of being asked to solve the same problem twice. Smallpox had been eradicated in the 1970s. Its possible return as a weapon of terror meant that a second eradication effort might be needed. Peter appreciated the value of prevention. He also understood that prevention efforts mirrored the history of public health. Adequate prevention was often low key and did not involve much high-tech equipment. Many citizens do not fully comprehend the activities or the achievements of public health. That insight was reasonable for Peter. Like the wine he was sipping, the achievements of public health increased in value with each passing year.

References

Graunt, J. 1662. *National and political observations mentioned in a following index and made upon the bills of mortality. With reference to the government, religion, trade, growth, ayre, diseases and the several changes of the said city*. London. [This is reproduced in William Petty, *The Economic Writings of Sir W. Petty*, vol. 2, ed. C.H. Hull (New York: Augustus M. Kelley, 1964):314–431. A portion is reproduced in Tufte, E. 2003, *The Cognitive Style of PowerPoint*. Cheshire, CT: Graphics Press.]

Rosen, G. 1993. *A History of Public Health*. Baltimore, MD: Johns Hopkins University Press.

Resources

Periodicals

Abel, E. K. 2003. From exclusion to expulsion: Mexicans and tuberculosis in Los Angeles, 1914–1940. *Bulletin of the History of Medicine* 77(4):823–849.

Barry, J. M. 2004. The site of origin of the 1918 influenza pandemic and its public health implications. *Journal of Translational Medicine* 2(1):3–8.

Black, J. 2003. Intussusception and the great smog of London, December 1952. *Archives of Diseases of Children* 88(12):1040–1042.

Horowitz, B.Z. 2003. Polar poisons: Did Botulism doom the Franklin expedition? *Clinical Toxicology* 41(6):841–847.

Larsen, C.S. 2003. Animal source foods and human health during evolution. *Journal of Nutrition* 133(11, Suppl 2):3893S–3897S.

Litsios, S. 2003. Charles Dickens and the movement for sanitary reform. *Perspectives in Biology and Medicine* 46(2):183–199.

Books

Bashford A. 2004. *Imperial Hygiene: A Critical History of Colonialism, Nationalism, and Public Health*. New York: Palgrave Macmillan.

Duffy, J. 1994. *Sanitarians: A History of American Public Health*. Champaign-Urbana, IL: University of Illinois Press.

Porter, D. 1999. *Political History of Public Health*. London: Routledge.

Rothstein, W.G. 2003. *Public Health and the Risk Factor: A History of an Uneven Medical Revolution*. Rochester, NY: Boydell & Brewer.

Walzer-Leavitt, J.W., and Numbers, R.L. 1993. *Sickness and Health in America: Readings in the History of Medicine and Public Health*, 3d ed. Madison, WI: University of Wisconsin Press.

Web Sites

- History of the Health Sciences World Wide Web Links: www.mla-hhss.org/histlink.htm
- National Library of Medicine: www.nlm.nih.gov/exhibition/phs_history/80.html
- National Museum of Health and Medicine: nmhm.washingtondc.museum/
- Ten Great Public Health Achievements in the 20th Century: www.cdc.gov/od/oc/media/tengpha.htm
- The Germ Theory Calendar: germtheorycalendar.com
- United States Public Health Service: www.surgeongeneral.gov/phs200/

Organizations

American Association for the History of Medicine
P.O. Box 529
Canton, MA 02021-0529
Web site: www.histmed.org/

American Public Health Association
800 I Street, NW
Washington, D.C. 20001-3710
Phone: 202-777-2742
Fax: 202-777-2534
E-mail: comments@apha.org
Web site: www.apha.org/

Center for the History and Ethics of Public Health
722 W. 168th Street, 9th Floor
New York, NY 10032
Phone: 212-305-0092
Fax: 212-342-1986
E-mail: hphm@columbia.edu
Web site: 156.145.78.54/heph/

Pan American Health Organization
525 23rd St., NW
Washington, D.C. 20037
Phone: 202-974-3000
Fax: 202-974-3663
Web site: www.paho.org/

PART

II

Department of Health Operations

CHAPTER

3

The Legal Basis for Local Departments of Health

Mark D. Tolles

Chapter Objectives

After reading this chapter, readers will:

- Understand how the American legal system has developed over time.
- Know the Constitutional and statutory provisions that establish the basis for local departments of health.
- Understand the legal basis under which local boards and departments of health operate.
- Know the legal responsibilities that have been placed on boards of health.
- Appreciate some of the issues that have arisen due to the legal requirements of the public health system.

Chapter Summary

The American legal system is largely based on common law. The Founding Fathers borrowed the common law system from the British, largely because they were familiar with it. This was the system used in the colonies prior to the American Revolution.

The common law system has several defining features. First, the common law system is an adversarial system; parties or their representatives (generally lawyers) present evidence and argue their positions before a judge or other impartial magistrate who has no stake in the outcome. The judge acts as a referee between the parties and issues decisions.

Second, the system generally allows some form of appeal. Such an action may be made to an appeals (or appellate) court, to a legislative body, or to the executive branch of the government.

The most important feature of the common law system is its reliance on precedent. The concept of precedence means that prior decisions of either the court in which the proceeding is being held or of any higher (appellate) tribunal in that jurisdiction are given the force of law and can be used to influence the outcome of any subsequent cases. This saves the trial court from having to start over every time a similar issue is presented. The precedent in effect defines the situation and can be used to interpret either terms not specifically defined in a statute or terms in general usage that are not specifically covered by a statute. The parties can present prior rulings to the court during a proceeding and argue whether the conclusions of those rulings should be followed based on the particular facts of the pending case.

Case Study

How should local public health agencies address the issue of public smoking? In the past few years, various issues have been raised about smoking in public places. Several methods to limit exposure to smoke in public places have been proposed. These range from establishing separate smoking and nonsmoking areas to total bans on smoking. Sealed-off smoking areas have been established, as in some airports. For several years, a total ban of smoking on domestic airline flights has been in place. These measures have been implemented through federal legislation in conjunction with local ordinances due to the high degree of federal regulation of the aviation industry. Smoking bans have been imposed by local health departments, city or village councils, and through referendum petitions by citizens of a community. A significant number of these local regulations and ordinances have been tested before the courts. The results have been varied. How would people in your community respond to an antismoking ordinance?

INTRODUCTION

When the colonies became independent of England, they kept the judicial system with which they were familiar. As a result, a decision in a 200-year-old case can still be considered to be good law, if it has not been overruled. A decision can be overturned by a higher court, by the same court making a new decision, by a legislative enactment, or by a constitutional amendment.

This common law system is the basis of most state legal systems, with the notable exception of Louisiana. That state's system is based on the Napoleonic Code, which is a variety of the continental legal system more often followed on the European continent (Presser and Zainaldin, 2003).

CONSTITUTIONAL AND STATUTORY PROVISIONS

In addition to the common law system, the Founding Fathers developed a federal system. Under this system, government consists of two distinct layers: the national, sometimes referred to as the federal, and the state. Prior to the adoption of the U.S. Constitution, the states were totally sovereign. That system proved to be inadequate for the situation in which the newly independent states found themselves. As a result, the states adopted and ratified the Constitution.

The Constitution called for a system of federal courts. Today, the federal court system is composed of district courts, the circuit courts of appeals, and the Supreme Court. To be heard in one of these courts, a case must involve a federal issue or fall within a limited class of situations that have been granted jurisdiction by either the Constitution or an act of Congress. A federal issue is one that involves the interpretation of a Constitutional or a statutory right. Federal courts can review state laws if there is an issue relative to a federal right.

Each state has its own court system. In most states, trial courts are generally referred to as courts of common pleas or district courts. Above the trial courts are intermediate appellate courts, generally called courts of appeals or circuit courts. A state's highest court is usually called the supreme court. New York is the major exception to the nomenclature applied to courts. Initial trials are held in the Supreme Court, Trial Division. The intermediate appeals court is called the Supreme Court, Appellate Division. Its highest court is called the Court of Appeals.

Because of the way issues may be raised, it is possible for a case to start in a state system and then move into the federal system. It is also possible for a case to begin in the federal system and move to the state system, but this is not common.

Under the Constitution, the states gave certain powers to the national government and retained other powers for themselves. The Constitution does not have any provisions that directly give the national government any power of authority over public health issues. However, several provisions and amendments address this subject in one way or another. The apparent intent of those framing the Constitution was to delegate issues of health to the responsibility of individual states.

The writers of the Constitution believed that the new national government would be able to provide for the general welfare of the states. There were no provisions that required the national government to provide specific services at the time the Constitution was drafted but the door was left open should such services be required in the future. This was due to the Founding Fathers' belief that the states were to remain sovereign. Each state would handle its own affairs, with only certain powers granted to the federal government.

> No person shall . . . be deprived of life, liberty or property, without due process of law; nor shall private property be taken for public use without just compensation.—Fifth Amendment to the Constitution
>
> The powers not delegated to the United States by the Constitution, nor prohibited by it to the States, are reserved to the States, respectively, or to the people.—Tenth Amendment to the Constitution

The Fifth and Tenth Amendments of the Bill of Rights imposed further limitations on the national government. The Fifth Amendment indicated that the new national government would not be able to deprive any person of life, liberty, or property without following appropriate legal procedures. Further, property could not be not be taken for public use without just compensation, the value of which would ultimately be determined by the legal system. The Tenth Amendment indicated that individual states could exercise power over those areas not preempted by the federal government. Further, the people themselves could retain powers as well. The power of the national and state governments ultimately comes from the people.

> . . . No State shall make or enforce any law which shall abridge the privileges or immunities of Citizens of the United States; nor shall any State deprive any person of life, liberty, or property without due process of law; nor deny to any person within its jurisdiction the equal protection of the laws.—Fourteenth Amendment to the Constitution

The Fourteenth Amendment applied some of the Fifth Amendment prohibitions to the states, who became subject to the due process and equal protection requirements that had been previously applied only to the federal government. State constitutions could grant these rights to the citizens before the Fourteenth Amendment was ratified, but the states did not *have* to provide these protections. After ratification of the Fourteenth Amendment, states had to provide these protections to the persons or citizens within their borders. Protecting the public's health occasionally requires imposition of quarantine and some police power to enforce such actions. These needs conflict with the basic freedoms guaranteed by the Constitution. The amendments noted were steps used to legalize the activities of local health departments.

In addition to Constitutional provisions that impact public health, federal statutes have more directly addressed the topic. Federal legislation has created federal programs such as the Food and Drug Administration (FDA) and the Centers for Disease Control and Prevention (CDC). Other statutes have been concerned with local boards of health. These statutes tend to either establish procedures for local agencies, provide funding for them, or both.

BASIS FOR LOCAL BOARDS AND DEPARTMENTS OF HEALTH

Other than federal guidelines for handling certain health issues, the states have been left fairly free to determine their own approaches to public health. States can use legal sources such as state constitutional provisions, statutes, administrative regulations, or a combination of these to empower local boards of health located within their own jurisdictions. Because state constitutions establish a framework for a system of state government, there are few references in them specifically directed at public health issues. The general rule is that state constitutions empower either the state legislature or the executive branch to address public health issues. Often, a state board or department of public health is established by statute, regulation, or executive order.

Ohio, for instance, has no more direct provision for public health in its state constitution than does the U.S. Constitution. Ohio has statutory system of a dual tier of agencies for addressing public health issues. It has established a State Department of Health, consisting of a Director of Health and a Public Health Council. The Public Health Council consists of seven members: three physicians, one pharmacist, a registered nurse, a sanitarian, and one person at least 60 years of age who is not associated with or financially interested in the practice of medicine, nursing, pharmacy, or environmental health. All of the professionals on the Council must be licensed to practice in Ohio. The Director of Health prepares sanitary and health regulations for the Public Health Council to consider and submits recommendations for new legislation to the Council.

LEGAL RESPONSIBILITIES OF LOCAL BOARDS OF HEALTH

A statutory system has also been developed for local boards of health in many states. In Ohio, a local board of health may serve a city or a general health district may serve parts of a county that are not in a city. In other states, notably Massachusetts and New Jersey, the jurisdiction of boards may be limited to a particular municipality. In states such as Montana, Wyoming, and Idaho, a local board of health may encompass several counties. In states such as California, the state acts as a local board of health for all citizens. Rhode Island does not have any local boards of health.

Local boards of health in Ohio and most other states are granted powers to abate nuisances and determine the locations, construction, and repair of water closets, privies, cesspools, sinks, drains and plumbing. Throughout the country, local boards may impose a quarantine on vessels, railroads, or public or private vehicles during a time of an actual or threatened epidemic or when a dangerous communicative disease is present. Boards may quarantine houses or localities where an infectious or communicable disease has been located. Health departments are required to provide care, and, if necessary, food and other necessities to quarantined persons. Other duties include periodic inspections of schools, recording diseases reported to the health commissioner, and inspecting county institutions. Most local boards have the power to hire people to remove waste and establish and designate hospitals for cases of communicable disease. Some local boards have the power to levy taxes to support a health department. Some departments must seek the permission of voters to levy taxes. This topic is discussed in Chapter 32.

LEGAL ISSUES

In recent years, several concerns have brought public health issues into the spotlight. Because local public health agencies have focused on preventing communicable diseases and epidemics, health departments are generally given significant powers to further these ends. Quarantine severely limits the ability of detainees to exercise other rights, such as freedoms of association and travel, both of which are protected by the Constitution (*NAACP*, 1958; *Shapiro*, 1969).

Potential epidemics from diseases such as HIV/AIDS have raised concerns about the powers granted to local health departments and boards to place persons or locations under quarantine. On one hand, HIV/AIDS is communicable and is spread from person to person. It is also fatal. On the other hand, the method of communication is different from diseases such as bubonic plague, measles, and influenza. These two factors demonstrate that there is room for discussion about the various means used to address different communicable diseases.

CONCLUSION: FUTURE LEGAL ACTIVITY FOR LOCAL PUBLIC HEALTH AGENCIES

Because of the growing public awareness about new hazards to public health, local public health agencies will likely receive pressure to take on additional tasks. They will be asked to create rules governing various health issues. In urban areas, local public health agencies will be under pressure to achieve the goals mandated by federal and state public health agencies. These goals are likely to be addressed through the exercise of municipal police powers. Agencies serving rural areas will probably be slower to act. Public opinion and legal theory do not appear to support allowing local public health agencies to determine what behaviors will be allowed or prohibited.

Health departments can inform members of the public about what environmental or physical conditions are deemed to be adverse to the health of people and address situations such as health emergencies or disease outbreaks that have already occurred. Local health departments usually cannot engage in active rule making. This probably stems from the fact that public health administrators are not elected. Members of the public will not support agency proposals in the same way they would support proposals from their elected representatives. Given the derivation of government power in the United States, this seems unlikely to change in the future.

Returning to the issue of smoking bans raised in the initial case study, an interesting situation involved the city of Toledo, Ohio. On May 24, 2001, the Lucas County Regional Health District, which has jurisdiction over all of Lucas County, Ohio, adopted a regulation that prohibited smoking in all public areas. The regulation defined public places as "every enclosed, indoor area to which members of the general public are invited or in which members of the general public are normally permitted." The regulation also prohibited smoking within 20 feet of any entrance or open window of any public area, as well as on all public transportation vehicles. The net result of the regulation was to prevent smoking in all bars, restaurants, bowling alleys, public areas in places of employment, stores and tobacco shops. The only indoor places that remained available for smoking were "private residences, private cars and private clubs" (*D.A.B.E.*, 2002). The regulation was to take effect on July 8, 2001.

On June 28, 2001, a group of 27 business owners filed a complaint in the common pleas court of Lucas County, the state trial court. The complaint requested a judgment from the court that declared the regulation to be invalid. The suit alleged that the Lucas County Board of Health had acted beyond its scope of authority granted under Ohio statute. In short, the legislation was alleged to be illegal. The plaintiffs also alleged that a federal constitutional violation in the regulation amounted to a taking of the plaintiff's property without just compensation. Based on the federal claim, the defendants asked that the case be transferred to the federal district court.

The plaintiffs moved for a temporary restraining order and preliminary injunction to prevent the enforcement of the new law. On July 6, 2001, the federal district court granted the preliminary injunction, preventing the enforcement of the regulation until the claims of the plaintiffs could be heard at trial. In an opinion, the district court stated that jurisdiction should be transferred to the federal court system, but that the judges should refer certain issues of Ohio law to the Ohio Supreme Court for their opinion. There were four issues: (1) Did the Ohio Revised Code authorize a board of health to prohibit smoking in all public places? (2) If the answer is yes, does delegation by the state legislature violate the Ohio Constitution? (3) Does such regulation conflict with other provisions of the Ohio Revised Code that already govern smoking in public places? (4) In a conflict, which should take precedence, a regulation of a local board of health or an ordinance of a home-rule city?

In addressing these questions, the Ohio Supreme Court began by looking at the statute that created some authority for action by the health district. The following is the pertinent part of the law:

> The board of health of a general health district may make such orders and regulations as are necessary for its own government, for the public health, the prevention or restriction of disease, and the prevention, abatement, or suppression of nuisances.—Ohio Revised Code §3709.21

The court then indicated that although this provision seemed to grant the board authority to make the regulation, it would also be necessary to look at other provisions that had been enacted by the legislature that granted or limited the power of a local board of health. In reviewing other provisions of the Ohio Revised Code, the court found that several provisions had been enacted that granted specific powers to boards of health. These would not have been necessary had the intention of the legislature been to provide a full and complete grant of plenary (legislative) power to local boards. By granting specific powers, the legislature indicated that it did not mean to grant full power to regulate any matter related to public health. In short, the court held that only those powers that were specifically indicated, either in the statute under review or in another statute, were to be delegated to local authorities.

In reaching this determination, the court relied on the outcome of an earlier verdict (*Johnson's Markets,* 1991). In that case, a supermarket was remodeled. The local health department did not approve changes in the meat cutting area because the changes did not meet the requirements of a regulation that had been enacted before the remodeling. The local board of health ordered the store to cease operations in the meat-cutting area until it complied with the regulation. The store argued that legislation providing for Department of Agriculture regulation in a food-processing area preempted the local board's regulation.

The trial court agreed with the store, but the court of appeals reversed the decision. The Supreme Court of Ohio affirmed the court of appeals, holding that there were some provisions in the Revised Code that allowed local boards to regulate the manufacture of foodstuffs and some that gave authority to the Department of Agriculture. No provision gave the Department of Agriculture sole authority over food processing.

In the smoking ban case, the Ohio Supreme Court ruled that because there was no specific grant of power, the local health board could not enact a regulation such as the smoking ban. The court did not need to address the other questions. Based on this interpretation, the regulation was dropped. However, that was not the end of smoking bans in Lucas County, Ohio.

In 2003, the City Council of Toledo passed a citywide public indoor smoking ban. This ordinance did allow for smoking in certain areas, provided that businesses made provisions to keep smoke out of the smoke-free areas. While some bar owners did opt to create smoking zones in their establishments, others decided to use the legal system to fight the new ordinance.

The first step was a petition drive to have a referendum to overturn the ordinance passed by city council placed on the ballot. After the petitions were turned in, the Lucas County Board of Elections compared the signatures on the petitions against the Board's list of registered voters. Not enough valid signatures of registered voters were gathered to place the referendum on the ballot. Bar owners apparently overlooked several things. First, many referendum and initiative petition drives fail because some of the people who sign them are not registered voters. Second, having petitions in bars for patrons to sign probably spurred many patrons to show their interest by signing more than one petition. Multiple signatures are as invalid as the signatures of unregistered voters.

A group of the owners then filed an action in the federal district court, seeking a temporary restraining order, a preliminary injunction, and a permanent injunction against enforcement of the ordinance. The district court denied their request, first overruling the motion for a temporary restraining order, then denying the rest of the requested relief.

The owners next decided the way around the ban would be to transform their bars into private clubs. This can be accomplished by requiring payment of a special cover charge to enter. They established an organization called "Taverns for Tots" that they labeled a nonprofit charity. To belong to the Taverns for Tots organization, bar owners had to agree to pay 1% of their profits to the organization. By belonging to Taverns for Tots and charging each patron the special cover charge, bar owners thought that they would be able to allow their patrons to smoke.

The City of Toledo challenged the plan and obtained a judgment that the scheme was illegal. The basis for the action was that Taverns for Tots was created as a sham to circumvent the smoking ban.

In addition to the problem of not being a legal charitable organization, the owners failed to consider that, as a charity, they had to give away or use the collected proceeds. They could give the money to other charities or make distributions as an entity. The latter course of action could become an administrative problem, because they did not desire to have a full time staff. They offered donations to several agencies who were serving needs of children. Their offers were turned down, with comments by the agencies that they did not care to have so-called blood money.

After spending much time in the courts and paying legal fees, the City of Toledo and the bar owners now have a smoking ban, whether they like it or not. This may not be so much a sign of the failure of bar owners to act as it is an indication public perceptions of smoking have changed.

Some of this is a result of fewer people smoking today than 20 to 50 years ago. Much is due to nonsmokers intolerance of smoking and smokers.

During some of the later legal proceedings, and after the Toledo ordinance went into effect, other cities in Ohio began to consider similar bans. To prevent lengthy legal battles, smoking bans could be implemented in other ways. An initiative petition offers citizens the right to directly propose legislation and then vote on it. This can be effective when there is reluctance on the part of the legislative branch to propose a law or to vote in favor of one.

In a city approximately 20 miles from Toledo, a citizen began an initiative drive to ban smoking in most public places. Once the petitions were filed and the requisite number of signatures validated, a vigorous debate of the issue began. Meetings were held, letters to the editor noting both the pros and the cons of the proposal were printed in the local newspaper, and an election was held. As a result, Bowling Green, Ohio, bans smoking in most public places. Bars were exempted, but smoking is now prohibited in most other public places.

References

Presser, S.B., and Zainaldin, J.S. 2003. *Law and American History,* 5th ed. Eagan, MN: Thompson West.

NAACP v. Alabama, 357 U.S. 449, 78 S.Ct. 1163, 2 L.Ed2d 1488 (1958).

Shapiro v. Thompson, 394 U.S. 618, 89 S.Ct. 1322, 22 L.Ed2d 600 (1969).

D.A.B.E., Inc., d.b.a. Arnie's Saloon, et al., v. Toledo-Lucas County Board of Health, et al., 96 Ohio St.3d 250, at 251 (2002).

Johnson's Markets, Inc., v. New Carlisle Dept. of Health, 58 Ohio St.3d 28 (1991).

Resources

Periodicals

Health Law Digest
American Health Lawyers Association
1025 Connecticut Avenue NW, Suite 600
Washington, D.C. 20036-5405

Journal of Public Health Management and Practice
Aspen Publishers Incorporated
7201 McKinney Circle
Frederick, MD 21704

Journal of Public Health Policy
208 Meadowood Drive
South Burlington, VT 05403

State Capitals Newsletters, Public Health
Wakeman Walworth Incorporated
P.O. Box 7376
Alexandria, VA 22307

Books

Goodman, R.A., Rothstein, M.A., Hoffman, R.E., Lopez, W., and Matthews, G.W. 2002. *Law in Public Health Practice.* New York: Oxford.

Gostin, L.O. 2001. *Public Health Law: Power, Duty, Restraint.* Sacramento, CA: University of California Press.

Gunther, G., and Sullivan, K.M. 2003. *Sullivan and Gunther's Constitutional Law,* 14th Set. Eagan, MN: Thompson West.

Mandelker, D.R. 2003. *State and Local Government in a Federal System*, 5th Ed. New York: Lexis Law Publishing.

Web Sites

- American Health Lawyers Association: www.healthlawyers.org
- American Lung Association: www.lungusa.org
- Center for Law and the Public's Health: www.publichealthlaw.net
- U.S. Environmental Health Agency, Indoor Air/Second-hand Smoke: www.epa.gov/smokefree/pubs/etsbro.html

Organizations

American Cancer Society
1599 Clifton Road, NE
Atlanta, GA 30329-4251
Phone: 800-227-2345
Web site: www.cancer.org

American Health Lawyers Association
1025 Connecticut Avenue NW, Suite 600
Washington, D.C. 20036-5405
Phone: 202-833-1100
Fax: 202-833-1105
Web site: www.healthlawyers.org

National Center for Chronic Disease Prevention and Health Promotion
Centers for Disease Control and Prevention
1600 Clifton Road
Atlanta, GA 30333
Phone: 404-639-3311
Public Inquiries: 404-639-3534 or 800-311-3435
E-mail: www.cdc.gov/netinfo.htm (Web form)
Web site: www.cdc.gov/

The Center for Law and the Public's Health at
Georgetown & Johns Hopkins Universities
Georgetown University Law Center
600 New Jersey Avenue NW
Washington, D.C. 20001
Phone: 202-662-9373
Fax: 202-662-9408
Web site: www.publicheathlaw.net

Johns Hopkins University
Bloomberg School of Public Health
615 N. Wolfe St.
Baltimore, MD 21205
Phone: 410-955-7624
Fax: 410-614-9055
Web site: www.publichealthlaw.net

CHAPTER

4

Assessing Community Health

Ned E. Baker

Chapter Objectives

After reading this chapter, readers will:

- Appreciate the importance of a community health assessment.
- Know how to conduct a community health assessment.
- Know how to select an assessment facilitator.
- Be able to identify and assemble members for project committees and subcommittees.
- Know how to involve persons and groups from the community.
- Know the tools available for conducting a community health assessment.
- Be able to report findings to appropriate groups and organizations in the community.
- Find ways to involve members of the media in disseminating the results of the public health assessment.
- Understand how to begin the process of implementing recommendations.

Chapter Summary

This chapter defines the importance and value of a community health assessment as a function of a local public health agency. It highlights the purpose, process, organization, implementation, reporting, and follow up when conducting an assessment. Step-by-step guidance for conducting a community health assessment is included. Information is provided on the various tools available to assist in conducting a community health assessment.

Case Study

The newly appointed members of a local board of health were attending their first regular meeting. After introductions, one asked when the next needs assessment would be conducted in the community. The older board members looked puzzled. "We have never done that," said one. Another added, "We have been functioning quite well for a long time." A third asked, "What is a needs assessment?" How should the new health board member respond to the comments of the older, existing members?

COMMUNITY HEALTH ASSESSMENT: A CORE PUBLIC HEALTH FUNCTION

The Institute of Medicine (1987) identified assessing the health status and the health needs of a community as a core function of public health. The Institute's report recommended that every public health agency regularly and systematically assemble, analyze, and make available information on the health of its community. The report further stated that each public health agency bears the responsibility for seeing that this core function is fulfilled. This responsibility cannot be delegated.

Because public health is a community affair, it is important that the public health agency engage the community in its health assessment. This begins with the public health agency and the board of health jointly acknowledging the need for a health assessment. This acknowledgment should include the purpose of the assessment, a commitment of resources, and a request for the community's involvement.

Typically, the board of health passes a resolution authorizing the health officer or health commissioner and the health department to engage members of the community in a health-assessment process. This resolution should be widely disseminated through all available media outlets in the community. The resolution should include the following components: one or more purposes, a definition of priority, assurance of adequate resources, seeking support from one or more community partners and delineating a venue for presenting final results to members of the public.

The purposes of a community health assessment include analyzing a population's current health status, determining the strengths and weaknesses of the community's health system, identifying a community's health needs, developing recommendations to meet the identified needs, identifying existing or needed resources to meet the identified needs, and prioritizing the identified needs. A health department must establish the community health assessment as a priority activity. This entails authorizing staff time and ensuring adequate financial support. Members of the community must participate in the assessment process by establishing partnerships with community members and representatives of community groups and organizations and seeking formal commitments from other health agencies, organizations, and groups.

After the board and the department of health have established the need and commitment to a community health assessment, the community must build a coalition to conduct the assessment. The board of health members, in cooperation with the health officer or health commissioner, should arrange to visit with other potential resources within the community to enlist their support and obtain a commitment to be involved in the process. These visits should include board members and staff from other health agencies and organizations, academic experts, and health practitioners in the community. It is equally important to gain the support of elected officials. The needed commitment may include donated staff time, service on committees, sharing of data, and/or financial support. Prior to meeting with these groups, the board and the health officer or health commissioner should have established a probable length of time for the process, staffing needs, and a budget for the project. These can then be used as guides when soliciting commitment and any necessary financial support.

Additional financial support may be needed to employ a facilitator for the project, fund outside consultants to conduct surveys, develop a community health assessment Web site, and produce and print the final community health assessment report.

IMPLEMENTING THE HEALTH ASSESSMENT PROCESS

After the board of health and the health department, in conjunction with the community partners, make the initial commitment to conduct a community health assessment, it is important to identify the person or persons who will facilitate and coordinate the community health assessment. Designating a facilitator or coordinator is important to the success of the assessment. This person will have several key responsibilities:

- Identify possible assessment tools to be used
- Establish a process plan and timetable
- Identify staffing needs and coordinate project personnel
- Assist in identifying community participants for the process
- Assign community members to subcommittees
- Ensure that the committee members are provided with adequate and timely notices as well as any materials that they may request
- Provide staff assistance and facilitation for committee meetings
- Identify and assemble needed data
- Ensure that minutes of meetings are kept and distributed
- Provide information to the public in a timely manner
- Coordinate the publication and distribution of the committee's final report and recommendations

When selecting a facilitator or coordinator, it is important to realize that the responsibilities of this position will be time intensive for at least two years. Therefore, the person should not be expected to carry out other staff duties during this period. The facilitator or coordinator should have skills in community organization, group dynamics, and communication. Although working under the direction of the health officer, this individual should be acceptable to the other community partners.

ASSEMBLING PROJECT TEAM PERSONNEL

Once the facilitator is selected, the health officer and the facilitator should begin to assemble the project staff team. Members of the team may come from the health department staff, other health agencies, or be community volunteers.

The next important step is the selection of a project steering committee. This committee will be expected to provide oversight for the community health assessment process. The steering committee should represent the various health stakeholder partners and the community. Committee members could be chosen to include representation from elected officials, the boards of health and education, the county extension service, any hospitals and other health care providers, experts from academia, representatives of special populations (minorities, ethnic, elderly, youth and universities), representatives of businesses or manufacturers, the chamber of commerce, and other governmental agencies concerned with health (departments of jobs and family services, parks, police, alcohol, drug and mental health, law enforcement, fire and emergency responder groups). The size of this committee should be kept manageable so that it can provide effective guidance. Other individuals from the community can be involved and serve on the various committees that will be formed throughout the assessment process.

TOOLS

A variety of tools are available to guide or assist communities in conducting a health assessment. These tools include the following:

- **Assessment Protocol for Excellence in Public Health (APEX PH).** This is an older health department and community health assessment instrument.
- **Mobilizing for Action through Planning and Partnership (MAPP).** This is a community-wide strategic planning tool for involving members of a community in a partnership with public health officials to improve the health and quality of life in the community.
- **National Public Health Performance Standards Program (NPHPSP).** This tool is designed to assist public health agencies and the com-

munity in measuring how well the public health system is providing essential public health services, including governance at the local and state levels.

- **Planned Approach to Community Health (PATCH).** This is a flexible tool that communities can use to identify, prioritize, and address health problems.
- **Healthy People 2010.** This is a set of national health objectives that can be used for establishing community objectives or evaluating a community.
- **Protocol for Accessing Community Excellence in Environmental Health (PACE-EH).** This tool is used to evaluate a community's environmental health status.

These tools should be reviewed by the health department facilitator and discussed with members of the project steering committee. All members of the group should have a role in determining which tools will be utilized in the assessment process. The tools are designed to be used in their entirety. However, the tools may be used in combination or modified to meet the needs of local communities.

Web sites for each of the tools are provided at the end of this chapter. Additional information on these and other aids for conducting a community health assessment is generally available from several national public health organizations. Contact information for these organizations is also provided at the end of this chapter.

DATA

Collecting, assembling, and analyzing data are essential steps in the community health assessment process. Data are not usually available in a single location or from a single source. National, state, regional, or local sources may be called upon to provide needed data. Federal data sources include the Centers of Disease Control and Prevention (CDC), the U.S. Health Resources and Services Administration, the U.S. Census Bureau, and other federal agencies. State departments or agencies of health, human services, safety, environmental protection, mental health, and alcohol abuse are useful resources. Regional resources include hospital councils, councils of government, disaster service groups, and the like. The local health department; hospitals; mental health, human services, alcohol counseling agencies; school systems; police and emergency management agencies; and planning bodies are useful sources for local data. This list is not meant to be all inclusive. Any previous specific health assessments conducted for the community should be collected, reviewed, and considered. Once data are assembled, it must be organized into a readable form for use by the committees involved in the assessment. Additional discussion of sources for data is contained in Chapter 7.

INVOLVING THE COMMUNITY

When the steering committee, the facilitator, and the staff are in place and the basic health data have been assembled, the next task is to reach out and involve members of the community. During this process, the community's perceptions of health strengths and weaknesses are evaluated. A community health perception survey should provide some insight on how the citizens feel about the community's health and their own personal health. The CDC and most state health departments have guides for such surveys.

Information related to perceptions of health might include the factors citizens believe would improve their quality of life, identifying the factors that have the greatest impact on the community's health, reviewing the incidence of individual behaviors that have the greatest impact on health, and noting important local environmental factors. Citizens should be asked to rate the health of the community and their own health. Finally, they should be asked how they pay for health care services.

Responders should be asked to supply basic demographic information. Such data usually include gender, age, marital status, ethnicity, education, and income. This information can be valuable in pinpointing particular health concerns and disparities.

The desired information can be obtained in at least three ways. The first way is through a formal random phone survey. A second way is by organizing citizens into focus groups and conducting interviews. A third way of obtaining input is through a printed survey form to be used in a variety of locations such as a county fair, grocery stores, libraries, or senior centers. Surveys can be included in mailings of pay checks, utility bills, or distributed by meals on wheels programs. People can be encouraged to complete surveys by offering them an incentive such as a bottle of ice water or having grocery stores donate a food basket or cash award to be distributed through a random drawing of all people who complete a survey.

Keeping the public informed and involved throughout the process is very important. Project staff members should meet regularly with representatives of the news media and provide them with updated information. Members of the media should be encouraged not only to attend committee meetings, but also to actively participate.

To maximize the community's involvement and ownership in the health assessment process, the facilitator and the steering committee should identify others in the community who are interested in becoming more deeply involved in the process. These persons may constitute an advisory committee that can become involved in reviewing and studying the data that have been generated. This group should be diversified and represent as many local interests as possible. In addition to representing health organizations, health professionals, elected officials and governmental agencies, it should include representatives from labor groups, farm interests, senior citizens, students from all levels, ethnic and minority groups, and religious groups. It is also important to ensure geographic representation from all sectors of the community.

The steering committee should identify enough residents for the advisory committee so that four or five subcommittees can be formed to address specific areas of community health. As an example, the MAPP process suggests forming four groups. Each studies a separate aspect of a community's health. The four groups' areas of responsibility include the following: community themes and strengths, the local public health system, the community's health status, and forces of change.

In the beginning, the steering and advisory committees should meet as a single group for the purpose of meeting each other and the staff who will be involved. They should be presented with information about the process, including time lines and expectations for members of the advisory committee. Prior to this meeting, it is helpful for staff members to assemble a manual containing necessary and pertinent information and data for all participants. At this first meeting, consideration should be given to conducting a nominal group process for the purpose of determining how the committee perceives the health of the community. This also provides a means of generating enthusiasm for participating in the process. Some areas that potentially may be addressed in this nominal group process include family issues, health services, mental health, substance abuse, neighborhoods, physical health, and the socioeconomic status and environmental health of the community. When planning for a lengthy meeting, experienced facilitators suggest providing healthy snacks and drinks for the participants throughout the meeting.

The second meeting of the advisory committee should be devoted to organizing and beginning the work. Steering committee members should also be invited and encouraged to participate in this and future meetings of the advisory committee or subcommittees. At the second meeting, the results of the nominal group process and the community health perception surveys should be presented, compared, and discussed. This organizational meeting also provides an opportunity for organizing the smaller subcommittee groups. Subcommittee chairs can be selected, subcommittee charges made, and future meeting dates set.

As an alternative to the MAPP method of utilizing subgroups, some communities have chosen to focus more on specific topics. These topical areas encompass people from all ages and groups from within the community. Examples of organizational topics include community health infrastructure, community and population health throughout the life span, community and population health promotion, and environmental health protection. Community health infrastructure involves reviewing a community's health establishment as it relates to health care, public health, behavioral health, dental health, school health, emergency preparedness, long-term care, chronic care, and transportation. Community and population health throughout the life span encompasses studying health through the various stages of life (reproductive health, infant, child, youth, adult, and older adult). Community and population health promotion includes studying general health status and evaluating the effectiveness of remedial health promotion programs. Environmental health protection includes various environmental issues, including problems related to emerging pathogens and land use. The PACE-EH tool can provide useful guidance for this subcommittee. It is important that one or more resource staff persons be assigned to each subcommittee for the purpose of keeping minutes, arranging for meeting notices, and securing other resources as needed.

At a minimum, the subcommittees can expect to meet at least twice each month for a six-month period. During this time, they will be studying the data, the results of the nominal group process, and the community health perception survey as it relates to their particular subcommittee topic. They will probably want to identify and call on other resources in order to help them to identify strengths and weaknesses, determine needs, rank order needs, and develop recommendations to meet identified needs.

The work of the subcommittees is the core of the community health assessment process. It is in this environment where questions can be raised and information can be discussed, dissected, and analyzed. Interaction between members of the subcommittee helps to build an understanding of the issues that the community must ultimately address. The intense involvement of subcommittee members during this phase of the process is where community ownership of the health assessment is developed and solidified.

Because each subcommittee may be addressing different but related aspects of the community's health, it is important to develop linkages among the subcommittees. Throughout this phase of the evaluation process, it is necessary for the facilitator and the staff members of each subcommittee to meet regularly and share the progress and findings being analyzed by their respective groups. Such sharing can often identify common issues and bring salient facts to the attention of others.

■ REPORTING FINDINGS

Once each of the subcommittees has made its evaluations and decisions, recommendations should be developed to address each identified need. A final report should be prepared by each subcommittee and submitted to the project steering committee. During this phase, the staff of the health department may be asked to organize and prepare the final report. It is important that the staff serve only as recorders and organizers of the report. Some important elements to include in a subcommittee report include the names of those serving on the subcommittee, the purpose (focus) of the subcommittee and the processes used, definitions of the health areas considered, descriptions as to how these areas were evaluated, and a summary of the resources that were used for the evaluation. Other elements of the report include a description of the community's current health status, identification of actual needs, and recommendations for addressing those needs. Finally, the committee has an ethical responsibility to rank order the priority of the needs and provide supporting material to justify the needs and recommendations. This last piece of information is often summarized in the report with more complete detail provided in technical appendices.

Each subcommittee should present its report at a meeting of the steering committee or health assessment oversight body. The presentation should be made by the chair or a designated person from the subcommittee. This is important because it reinforces the community's ownership of the project. After discussion, the oversight steering committee should either approve the report as submitted or suggest amendments that the entire group can agree and support. The steering committee may decide to further prioritize needs and recommendations for developing objectives and action plans. At this point in time, it is valuable to keep the community informed by inviting the media to this meeting. Often a preliminary or follow-up meeting between the news media, the chair of the steering committee, and each of the advisory body's subcommittee chairs can be beneficial. Such a meeting enhances the media's understanding of the issues and enhances the process of informing the public.

Producing a final report from the diverse subcommittee reports and recommendations is a challenge to both the steering committee and its associated staff. It should be clearly noted that a community health assessment report is not an implementation plan. Its purpose is to identify the community's strengths and needs in the realm of health. The report is a guide for future health program and resource development for organizations and individuals in the community.

In some community health assessments, establishing priorities can be embedded in the assessment process. In some situations, the assessment process may stand alone, allowing another body, individual agencies, or organizations to establish their own priorities. Once priorities are established, goals, objectives, and action plans for programs should be developed to address the identified priorities. The priority-setting process is important for determining program and resource needs. Agency and organization strategic plans should consider the identified needs and recommendations contained in the community health assessment.

Drafting the final report is usually the responsibility of the facilitator, with assistance from identified staff members from the health department. An important task of the facilitator is to gather input from the steering committee throughout the drafting process. Once the document is complete, the entire steering committee must formally adopt it.

After the steering committee adopts the final report, two tasks remain: releasing the final report to the public and recognizing the efforts of all participants. Because the board of health authorized the assessment, it is appropriate for it to call a public meeting for the purpose of officially accepting the report. At the same time, the report can be presented to appropriate elected officials and to members of the community. Everyone who worked on the assessment should receive special invitations to the meeting. Elected officials and members of health agencies and organizations should also be invited. It is vital that representatives from the news media be invited.

At the meeting, the chair of the steering committee or a designated member of the committee should review the highlights of the report. A question-and-answer period should follow this presentation. The written report should then be formally presented to the president of the board of health. Copies of the report should be available for all in attendance.

At this point it is appropriate for the president of the board to acknowledge official acceptance and indicate how the board will act on the assessment. The health officer or health commissioner and the board president should also express their thanks and appreciation to all who gave of their time and talent for the preparation of the community health assessment.

Printed copies of the completed report should be given to all persons and organizations who participated in the evaluation process. All agencies, organizations, boards, and others who will have a responsibility for implementing recommendations should also receive copies. A copy of the report should be made available on an Internet Web site. Health departments and libraries frequently have the needed facilities and will provide such assistance as a community service. It also is advisable to prepare a shortened, printed version of the report to share with members of the general public. A local newspaper may publish the abbreviated report as a public service.

■ CONCLUSION

Conducting a community health assessment that involves diverse representatives from the local community is important when developing a vision for health for an entire community. Agreeing on the health needs and resources to meet the community's health vision is an important component of the process. Conducting a community health assessment also provides for a better-educated community whose citizens understand the health of their community and how their local health department delivers essential public and personal health services. A formal assessment will also demonstrate how well the community is prepared to provide needed and desired services.

The community health assessment report will provide guidance to health agencies and organizations in developing strategic plans and programs for a community. All in all, conducting a health assessment is a positive experience for the entire community. In providing for a community health assessment, the leadership of a public health agency fulfills one of its core functions. It also provides an entire community the opportunity to unite in a partnership for health.

The new members of the local board of health mentioned in the initial case study gathered information and support from the Institute of Medicine's *The Future of Public Health*. Ultimately, they prevailed. The health board and department conducted a needs assessment. The final actions of the steering committee were to establish goals for evaluation and to set a tentative date for the next community needs assessment.

Reference

Institute of Medicine. 1988. *The Future of Public Health*. Washington, D.C.: National Academy Press.

Resources

Periodicals

Clark, M.J., Cary, S., Diemert, G., Ceballos, R., Sifuentes, M., Atteberry, I., Vue, F., and Trieu, S. 2003. Involving communities in community assessment. *Public Health Nursing* 20(6):456–463.

Feldman, P.H., and Oberlink, M.R. 2003. Developing community indicators to promote the health and well-being of older people. *Family and Community Health* 26(4):268–274.

Heft, M.W., Gilbert, G.H., Shelton, B.J., and Duncan, R.P. 2003. Relationship of dental status, sociodemographic status, and oral symptoms to perceived need for dental care. *Community Dentistry and Oral Epidemiology* 31(5):351–360.

Hwang, S.W., Martin, R.E., Tolomiczenko, G.S., and Hulchanski, J.D. 2003. The relationship between housing conditions and health status of rooming house residents in Toronto. *Canadian Journal of Public Health* 94(6):436–440.

Misra, R., and Ballard, D. 2003. Community needs and strengths assessments as an active learning project. *Journal of School Health* 73(7):269–271.

Sharma, R.K. 2003. Putting the community back in community health assessment: A process and outcome approach with a review of some major issues for public health professionals. *Journal of Health and Social Policy* 16(3):19–33.

Books

Institute of Medicine. 2003. *The Future of the Public's Health in the 21st Century*. Washington, D.C.: National Academy Press.

Kemm, J., Parry, J., and Palmer, S. 2004. *Health Impact Assessment: Concepts, Theory, Techniques and Applications*. London: Oxford University Press.

Nardi, D.A., and Petr, J. M. 2003. *Community Health and Wellness Needs Assessment: A Step-by-Step Guide.* Albany, NY: Delmar.

Peterson, D.J., and Alexander, G.R. 2001. *Needs Assessment in Public Health: A Practical Guide for Students and Professionals.* Hingham, MA: Kluwer Academic Publishers.

Web Sites

- Assessment Protocol for Excellence in Public Health (APEX PH): www.naccho.org/project47.cfm
- Mobilizing for Action through Planning and Partnership (MAPP): www.naccho.org/project77.cfm
- National Public Health Performance Standards Program (NPHPSP): www.phppo.cdc.gov/nphpsp/
- Ohio Department of Health: www.odh.state.oh.us/resources/reports/oh_plan/phpcont.htm
- Planned Approach to Community Health (PATCH): www.cdc.gov/nccdphp/patch/00binaries/00patch.pdf
- Healthy People 2010: www.healthypeople.gov/
- Protocol for Accessing Community Excellence in Environmental Health (PACE-EH): www.cdc.gov/nceh/ehs/PIB/PACE.htm

Organizations

National Environmental Health Association
720 S. Colorado Blvd., Suite 970-S
Denver, CO 80246-1925
Phone: 303-756-9090
Fax: 303-691-9490
E-mail: staff@neha.org
Web site: www.neha.org/

Centers for Disease Control and Prevention
1600 Clifton Road
Atlanta, GA 30333
Phone: 404-639-3311
Public Inquiries: 404-639-3534 or 800-311-3435
E-mail: www.cdc.gov/netinfo.htm (Web form)
Web site: www.cdc.gov/

National Association of County and City Health Officials
1100 17th Street, Second Floor
Washington, D.C. 20036
Phone: 202-783-5550
Fax: 202-783-1583
E-mail: naccho@naccho.org
Web site: www.naccho.org

National Association of Local Boards of Health
1840 East Gypsy Lane Road
Bowling Green, OH 43402
Phone: 419-353-7714
Fax: 419-352-6278
E-mail: nalboh@nalboh.org
Web site: www.nalboh.org/

Public Health Foundation
1220 L Street, N.W., Suite 350
Washington, D.C. 20005
Phone: 202-898-5600
Fax: 202-898-5609
E-mail: info@phf.org
Web site: www.phf.org/

CHAPTER

5

Configuring the Department

Timothy Horgan
Eric Zgodzinski

Chapter Objectives

After reading this chapter, readers will:

- Understand the organizational requirements of a public health department.
- Appreciate the roles and duties of employees at all levels of a public health department.
- Know that growth requires creativity and patience.
- Be able to structure a health department for optimal productivity.

Chapter Summary

The structure of an organization often evolves. Growth often occurs in reaction to increased demands from the population being served. Growth is desirable for a health department. Realizing growth requires funding. Justifying such increases in funding may require creative thinking and effort by top health department leaders. The senior administrative officer of a successful health department summarized the contents of this chapter in a succinct manner: Plan for departmental and individual growth, manage for it, and require it.

Case Study

The health commissioner of a large county health district was faced with the difficulty of trying to address ever-increasing demands for programming and services without being provided any resources for new personnel. In short, the capacity of the department was limited. The commissioner was convinced that the problem was due to the limited tax or general fund allocations made available to the health district. Over the years, budget-cutting requirements had led to a department with a commissioner, two directors, and a large number of young and inexperienced staff who were essentially paid entry-level salaries.

This is a typical problem for many public agencies and a very difficult one to remedy. Dramatic increases in funding for tax-supported agencies were unlikely. After years of tight budgets, the capacity for a dramatic reorganization was limited at best. What advice would you give to this health commissioner?

INTRODUCTION

Public health rarely gets sufficient funding from nonlocal sources, such as state and federal governments, to adequately handle local demands for service. Consequently, local health districts usually stretch budgets to the breaking point and hold salaries or wages to a minimum. Obviously, budget constraints must be addressed on an annual basis. This leads to an institutionalized mind-set that the budget will be constrained every year. There is never enough money in the budget to accomplish all of the tasks at hand. Therefore, long-term plans and goals must be handled in a proactive rather than reactive manner.

No organization can expect success if it is not properly configured. Organizational structure provides the backbone of any health department. Several different structures are used by various organizations. Civil service requirements normally require public agencies to demonstrate a line of authority from top to bottom. Line organizations can be very responsive if properly structured. However, they are not very successful if they do not provide adequate levels of staff or if they do not maintain separate sections or divisions for different classes of tasks.

This discussion of configuring an organization will describe how to establish a line organization and review some of the additional configurations that are useful for addressing unique tasks or special challenges.

ORGANIZATIONAL REQUIREMENTS

Mind-set

Configuring a health department is important on many levels. Most importantly, a departmental configuration provides not only a structure, but also a mind-set that must be carried out with the utmost determination. If the department is configured properly, several of the pitfalls that agencies often encounter can be avoided. The working environment will promote productivity, and staff will be motivated to advance public health within a community. Most importantly, public health program delivery and customer service will increase with the proper organizational configuration.

Board Governance

The configuration of public health departments usually mirrors the statutes under which they operate. Governing bodies are most commonly of either a board-authority or a city-council format. For most departments, the board is made up of individuals residing within the community who can either be elected or assigned to the board. Operational authority is vested in the board. A council governing board is usually associated with a city-run local health department. The board is advisory in nature with operational authority remaining within the city council to which the board reports or advises. With this structure, a mayor is usually the president, and council members also serve as board of health members. The board's authority is derived from a governing council that elects the members of the board. In some instances, additional board members may be appointed. The board is the entity to which the health commissioner reports and that grants power to the commissioner. In addition, the board, by vote, oversees such items as large purchases, budgets, salaries, contracts, and other issues. Oversight by the board has a large impact on the configuration of a health department.

Directorate

Local health departments often have many different levels. Each level has a specific function. The highest level is the executive office or the directorate. The directorate provides and maintains guidance for the overarching tasks of an organization that must always be present. The directorate sets the tone for the entire organization and is ultimately responsible for its success or failure. It is responsible for organizational uniformity, fiscal success, and the accomplishment of the organization's mission.

The directorate is headed by a chief executive officer who usually carries the title of commissioner, director, or health officer. This individual reports directly to the governing board.

Reporting to the chief executive officer are the department heads of the directorate. There are several common organizational functions or functional areas whose department heads usually constitute the directorate or senior management team. The first is budget and fiscal management. Human resources comprises the second area. Human resources handles personnel, payroll, benefits, and some reporting to the federal government. Administration is the portion of the directorate that is responsible for reporting information related to programs and some operations. Another functional area is legal services. For some departments, the workload is sufficient to justify a full-time legal employee. In smaller departments, a municipal prosecutor or external counsel provides legal services on a part-time basis.

A medical director is required by some departments that are not headed by a medical doctor. In such a situation, the medical director provides advice and is available to address medical questions as needed.

Divisions

Organizational divisions comprise the next structural level of a local health department. Divisions are usually organized along major professional or programmatic areas. Areas are subdivided to provide concentrated expertise. In addition, they are developed to establish promotional opportunities and career paths, not simply jobs. Divisions ensure that qualified professionals are managed and directed by people with similar or more extensive professional backgrounds. Divisions also provide a career ladder for promotion in separate professional areas. An important function of divisions is to prevent budget mixing and competition among programs and professions. For example, home health care programs and food-protection programs would be housed in two separate divisions. Similarly, registered sanitarians and licensed nurses would be in two separate divisions.

Divisional Breakdown

The number and scope of divisions depends on an organization's size. Smaller organizations have fewer organizational levels. Larger organizations typically have more divisions than smaller ones. Smaller organizations have less diversity of professions, and hence may only have two or three divisions. Large organizations may have many divisions based on the number and distribution of professions. Examples of some typical organizational charts are shown in **Figures 5-1** through **5-4. Figure 5.1** depicts a relatively small department (20 to 50 employees). **Figure 5-2** shows a medium-sized department (40 to 100 employees). **Figure 5-3**

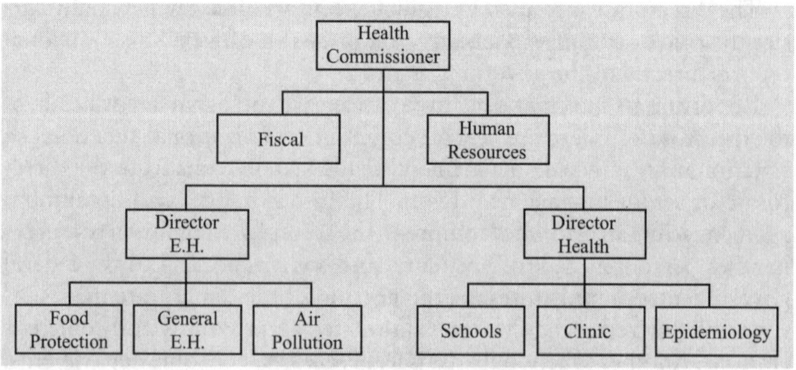

Figure 5-1 Organization of a small department (20 to 50 employees).

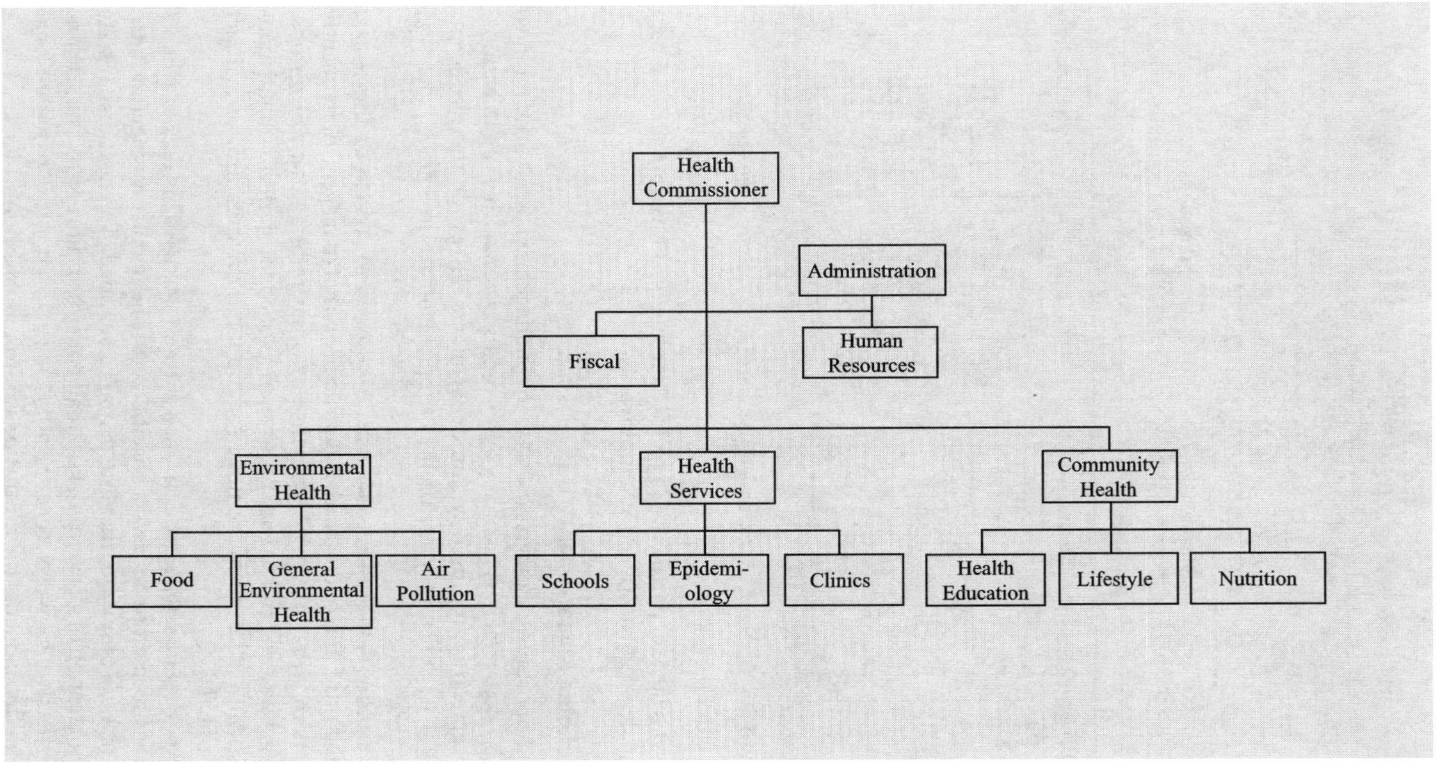

Figure 5-2 Organization of a medium-sized department (40 to 100 employees).

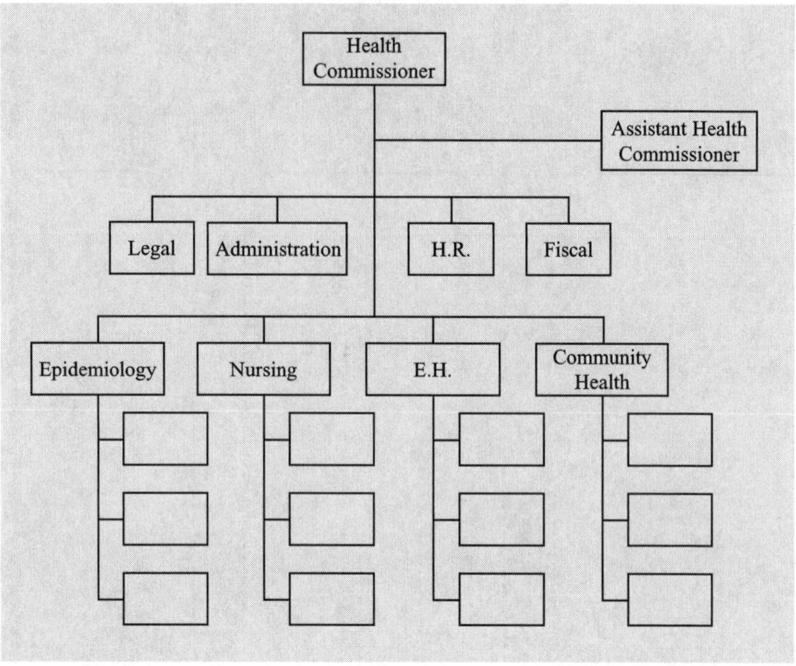

Figure 5-3 Organization of a large department (75 to 150 employees).

shows a large department (75 to 150 employees). **Figure 5-4** shows a very large department (over 150 employees).

Conflicted Management

It is important to understand that the management structure of a local health department is normally a line organization. Other organizational concepts are often used within departments. However, these concepts only work when they are used as supplements to the line organization structure.

Situational management is used to respond to current or short-term conditions. The concern with this structure is that management frequently reacts to situations at the expense of other public health programs. Budgeting and productivity become areas of concern. If situational management is allowed to continue for too long, the organization will get out of balance.

Another management approach is to use teams. This occurs when a team is formed to address a specific task. The team stays together until the task is completed, then the team is disbanded. The next task results in the creation of a new team. For small projects or short-term issues, teams are effective. However, they are not efficient or appropriate within local health departments for routine or day-to-day operations.

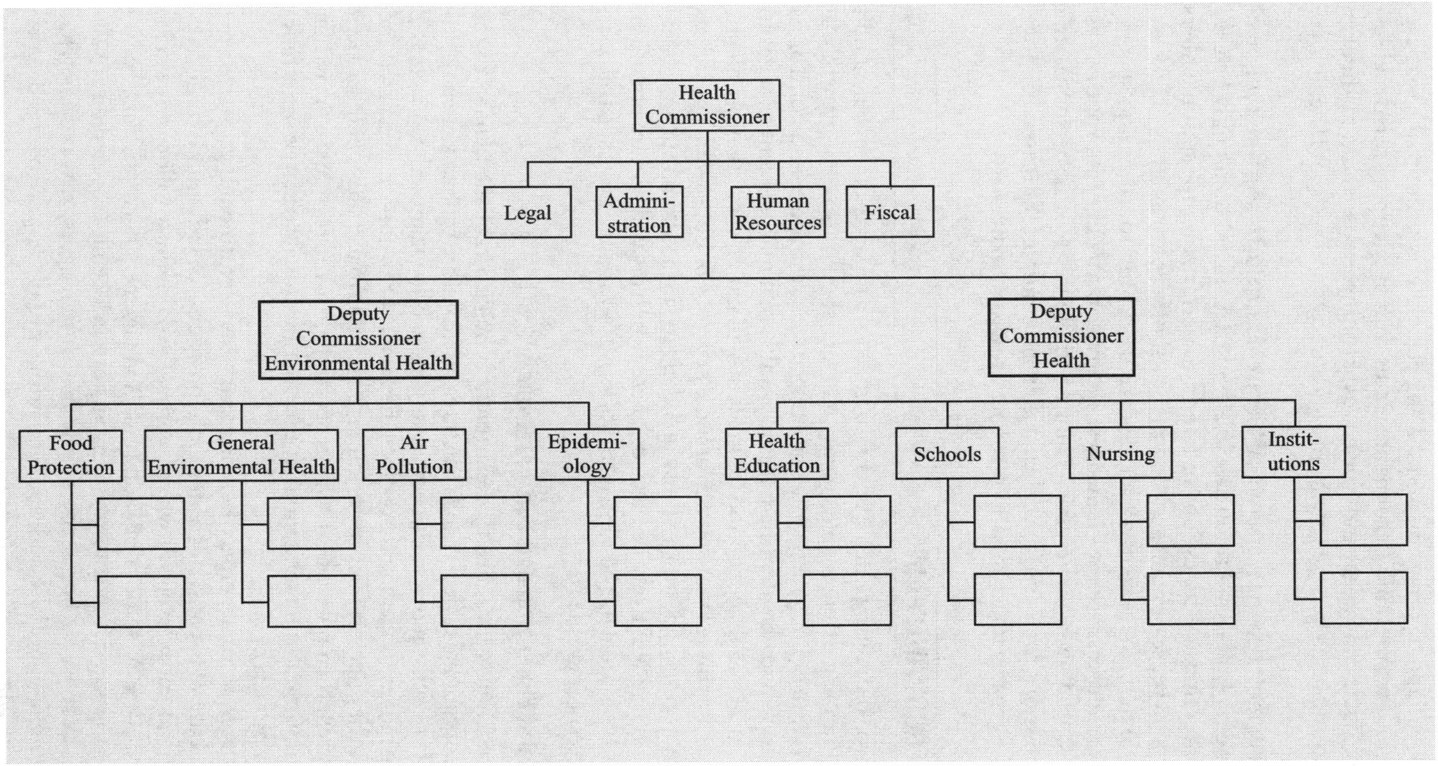

Figure 5-4 Organization of a very large department (over 150 employees).

Overlapping programs and sharing personnel is an approach that uses bubble groups. Bubble groups are teams with overlapping personnel rosters. While convenient and efficient over short periods, over time they can create nightmares when trying to allocate costs and account for employee time.

For most departments, typical hierarchal structures work best for managing programs and resources. Different structures should only be used to meet unusual conditions or to add some variation for staff members at the expense of managers and the fiscal officer.

Novel management structures are useful for coordinating specific tasks, addressing new challenges, or invigorating existing routine systems. It allows an energetic group of employees to mix personnel and professions for a unique challenge. The most important reason for novel management structure is to promote growth and diversity.

GROWING PAINS

When configuring a department for growth, a separate management unit within the existing management structure should focus on growth opportunities. Budgetary and reporting issues to sustain and control its function must be identified. It is inevitable that management changes to encourage and accommodate growth will cause personnel problems. Some employees may have to assume new jobs or duties. Staff problems such as resistance and jealousy are likely to surface. Finally, a great deal of training will likely be needed. These problems will require attention, but they should not be allowed to stifle organizational or personal growth or to suppress ideas.

Lateral Expansion and Vertical Growth

Unless a new local health department is being established, many of the organizational concepts and structures discussed are probably already partially or fully in place. Understanding these organizational concepts will help readers understand how local health departments are structured and how they operate. The more important goal is to use active management to strengthen public health by generating growth. To achieve growth, it is important to understand that the organizational structure must function properly.

Lateral expansion is often necessary for departmental growth to occur. Lateral expansion creates more positions for individuals to fill, typically at entry levels. However, vertical growth must follow any lateral expansion. At some point, additional management positions must be created to successfully implement program work being delivered due to lateral expansion. For many public health managers, this is somewhat frightening, because additional positions usually require board authorization. Managers have to justify that the proposed organizational changes are necessary. A presentation to the health board or municipal council can demonstrate how additional lateral growth requires an additional person in management because of the additional resources at risk. Cost studies and comparisons of the resources being controlled by existing levels of management across the organization can be powerful tools for demonstrating need. A supervisor and program manager who each control $700,000 worth of resources but are paid at different levels constitutes an unbalanced structure. The health commissioner can often use this fact and approach the board to reevaluate the program manager position, hopefully receiving authority for a new supervisor.

Lateral expansion contributes to vertical growth. Without vertical growth, there is no incentive for advancement or additional monies for individuals. Without this incentive, lateral growth is unlikely to be efficient or successful or achieve its full potential.

RESOURCE STRUCTURING

Many unknowns must be identified before a department is restructured. Planned program budgeting should be used to properly understand the nature of any resources and/or assets. When planning for growth, it also is important to know what resources a department has or will have in the future for creating growth. Once planned program budgeting is accomplished, the required resources can be allocated.

Before positions in a department can be allocated, it must be determined what resources each position will be responsible for. For example, a sanitarian in training is normally responsible for about $30,000 in resources. Senior sanitarians may be responsible for $75,000 in resources and must complete their own workloads as well as supervise sanitarians in training. Entry-level management positions may be responsible for $100,000 to $200,000 in personnel and programs. Middle management may control $250,000 to $500,000 in resources and require expertise to understand the various programs. Upper managers may control $750,000 to $2,000,000. Top management may be responsible for $2,000,000 to $10,000,000 in resources. The amount of resources controlled is a factor when determining the compensation for each position and when rating jobs. Additional information on position descriptions and compensation are provided in Chapters 12 and 14.

The number of personnel may vary in different organizations, but the principle that management levels are directly related to the resources managed certainly helps to identify the numbers and types of management positions that are necessary for an effectively functioning organization.

Top Management Growth

Vertical growth is needed when lateral expansion begins to overwhelm a single manager with too much responsibility and too great a workload.

Experienced senior managers recommend the following guidelines. If there is 30 to 50 percent growth in workload, additional personnel are necessary. For a 50 to 100 percent growth in workload, a new management unit is needed. As an organization adds new management units, the span of control for the health commissioner increases. When the work or administrative load becomes too large for a single person to be effective, an assistant may be needed to help with the larger workload. An assistant health commissioner is usually not a line position. Such a position does not have supervisory responsibility unless specifically allocated by the health commissioner. Assistants generally are at the disposal of the health commissioner to alleviate some of the responsibility and generate avenues for further departmental growth and response.

Continued growth across an organization leads to the addition of deputy positions, which usually have line authority. Multiple divisions then report through deputy commissioners.

Middle Management

Individuals with true programmatic expertise normally occupy middle management positions. This is where the day-to-day management of personnel and programs occurs. In tight budget situations, some agencies attempt to flatten the organization and eliminate middle management positions as a cost-saving measure. Ultimately, this eliminates the necessary control and expertise that makes programs and personnel successful. Additionally, it impairs or destroys career tracks in a professional organization.

Nursing

Lateral expansion, as with most management issues, is limited by the resources that a public health department has or can envision having in the future. Additionally, the number of full-time employees varies, including the number of nurses. Several formulas for determining nursing staff numbers are available that are based on the number of immunizations administered, clinic duties, or the number of health education classes taught. Additional factors include the number of school nurses, home health care providers, and other types of nursing-related personnel offered by a health department.

Sanitarians

The number of sanitarian or environmental health specialist positions is usually related to the population being served within a jurisdiction. Smaller health departments may have one sanitarian per 10,000 people. In larger departments, one sanitarian may be employed for every 15,000 to 20,000 people. These guidelines will vary with the type and extent of services being offered.

Workloads for sanitarians also vary from department to department. One important factor in determining the number of sanitarians needed is the number of food-service operations a sanitarian can inspect in a given year. A competent sanitarian can conduct between 500 and 600 thorough inspections in a year. Sanitarians often have other duties in addition to inspecting restaurants. These include conducting investigations of food-borne outbreaks, providing in-service education for facility owners and employees, and other tasks required by departmental or community leaders.

Educators and Others

The number of health educators and other employee positions is determined much like determining the number of nursing positions. It is dependent on the programs and services offered by a health department. However, for lateral expansion to be possible, educators, epidemiologists, information workers, clerical, and support employees are important contributors to the growth of departments and in providing important services.

CONCLUSION

It is relatively easy for departments to find small amounts of money for new activities. However, transforming new funds into sustained, reliable growth is difficult. The difficulty arises not only from the resources that are needed, but also from the necessity of upper management having to calculate risks needed to advance public health. Risks can be financial, organizational or programmatic in nature. They are similar to the risks incurred by any leader who is attempting to expand the scope, size or influence of an organization. This is easier for larger departments, because there is usually a greater pool of experienced management experts to draw from compared with smaller departments. However, there are always options, however remote, that any department can draw upon for growth. Creative and innovative managers can usually expand the scope of their organizations, despite apparent fiscal limitations. For continued growth to occur, employees must perceive that vertical movement is possible.

When configuring an organization, an adequate directorate is needed to coordinate tasks across the entire organization. Divisions must be defined by major professional areas. These must support middle management to ensure programmatic success. Additionally, most individuals assume that public health entered the twenty-first century with inadequate staffing and funding levels. Programs should be established and expected to grow. Plan on lateral expansion with moderate success and provide opportunities vertical growth to achieve organizational success.

Consider the public health department described in the case study at the start of this chapter. The best way to work out this department's problems is to set the organization in a growth mode. The very limited numbers of people in management positions were unable to provide effective leadership, money, training, the proper working environment, or the program expertise to maintain a successful department. The organization did not have the human resources to handle any kind of challenge, nor did the staff see any viable opportunities for moving up through the organization through hard work and commitment. Middle management had been eliminated due to budget woes. The organization is doomed unless it is rebuilt.

The health commissioner should seek out or create opportunities for lateral expansion and vertical growth. Grant funding is a logical source for support. Creative partnerships with other key stakeholders are logical next steps. The goal of the health department is to create value for the people and organizations being served within the jurisdiction. To be successful, the process will require time and creativity.

Resources

Periodicals

Christianson, J.B., and Trude, S. 2003. Managing costs, managing benefits: Employer decisions in local health care markets. *Health Services Research* 38(1 Pt 2):357–373.

Hyland, P., Davison, G., and Sloan, T. 2003. Linking team competences to organizational capacities in health care. *Journal of Health Organizational Management* 17(3):150–163.

Kernick, D. 2002. The demise of linearity in managing health services: A call for post-normal health care. *Health Service Research and Policy* 7(2):121–124.

Succi-Lopez, M., Lee, S.Y., and Alexander, J.A. 2003. The effects of relative resource configuration, organizational legitimacy, and integration on divestiture decisions among health systems. *Health Care Management Review* 28(4): 307–318.

Books

Beaty, C.A., and Barker, B. 2004. *Building High-Performance Teams: A Facilitator's Guide.* San Francisco, CA: Sage Publications.

Burton, R.M., and Obel, B. 2004. *Strategic Organizational Diagnosis and Design: The Dynamics of Fit.* New York: Kluwer Academic.

Donalddson, L. 2001. *For Positivist Organization Theory.* San Francisco, CA: Sage Publications.

Harvey, T.R., and Drolet, B. 2004. *Building Teams, Building People: Expanding the Fifth Resource.* Lanham, MD: Rowman & Littlefield.

Web sites

- California Department of Health Services: www.dhs.ca.gov/

- Federal Commons:
  www.cfda.gov/federalcommons/health.html
- National Assembly of Health and Human Service Organizations:
  www.nassembly.org/nassembly/
- New York Medical College:
  www.complab.nymc.edu/Curriculum/ComPrevMed/OrgFunctionPubHlthSys.htm

Organizations

American College of Healthcare Executives
One North Franklin Street, Suite 1700
Chicago, IL 60606-4425
Phone: 312-424-2800
Fax: 312-424-0023
E-mail: ache@ache.org
Web site: www.ache.org/

American Management Association
1601 Broadway
New York, NY 10019
Phone: 212-586-8100
Fax: 212-903-8168
Web site: www.amanet.org/index.htm

Center For Health Administration Studies
University of Chicago
969 E. 60th St.
Chicago, IL 60637
Phone: 773-702-7104
Fax: 773-702-7222
Web site: www.chas.uchicago.edu/index.html

Public Health Foundation
1220 L Street, NW, Suite 350
Washington, D.C. 20005
Phone: 202-898-5600
Fax: 202-898-5609
E-mail: info@phf.org
Web site: www.phf.org/

U.S. Office of Personnel Management
1900 E Street NW
Washington, D.C. 20415-1000
Phone: 202-606-1800
E-mail: er@opm.gov
Web site: www.opm.gov/er/poor/ceapp.asp

CHAPTER

6

Local Public Health Operations

Harvey Wallace

Chapter Objectives

After reading this chapter, readers will:

- Understand the role of local public health agencies in communities.
- Know the main responsibilities of a chief health officer.
- Appreciate the value of CDC Health Alerts.
- Comprehend the main operational activities of a local public health agency.
- Understand the role of environmental health specialists.
- Comprehend the role of a local board of health.
- Discuss the types of local boards of health.

Chapter Summary

Local public health agencies have well-defined and important responsibilities in communities. The chief administrative person in a local public health agency is a chief health officer or health commissioner. This person is hired, evaluated, and discharged by a local board of health. Local health departments work closely with state and federal agencies. Important functional elements of health agencies include environmental health, clinical and personal health services, and community health promotion. Effective local boards of health have defined characteristics.

Case Study

The local health agency has engaged the services of a new health officer. The local board of health has governance powers as defined by the state constitution. The new health officer has extensive experience as a sanitary inspector in another state. The community she serves has an industrial base that dates to the early 1900s. She is contemplating the goals for the first year in her new position. What advice would you offer to her?

INTRODUCTION

State laws often mandate contemporary local public health agencies to provide specific services to preserve, promote, and protect the health of local communities. In addition to those mandated services, a local public health agency often provides additional services and programs supported by a combination of grants and local funding sources to further enhance its operations.

This chapter will describe operations found in a typical local public health agency. While keeping in mind the often-heard adage: "Once you've seen one health department, you've seen one health department," readers must also remember that the more than 2,900 local public health agencies do have many characteristics in common.

In 2001, the National Association of County and City Health Officials released a report that described local public health agencies as follows:

- 60 percent of local public health agencies are county based
- 69 percent serve jurisdictions with fewer than 50,000 individuals
- The median annual expenditure was $621,100 (range: zero to $836 million)
- Composition of total budgets:
    - Local government: 44 percent
    - State government: 30 percent
    - Fees-for-services: 19 percent
    - Grants and other sources: 7 percent

This report also found that the most common programs and services provided by local public health agencies include the following: adult and child immunizations, community assessment, community outreach and education, environmental health services, epidemiology and surveillance, food safety, health education, restaurant inspections, and tuberculosis testing (National Association of County and City Health Officials, 2001). Many other services, such as oral health care, mental health services, and treatment services for specific illnesses such as AIDS or diabetes, may be offered by those local public health agencies that have identified both specific needs and funding sources.

All of the previously listed activities and programs may be grouped into four categories: clinical services, environmental health services, community health promotion services, and administration. This chapter will expand on each of these categories. On a day-to-day basis, each program may operate independently with relatively little interaction with other programs within the same local public health agency. For example, local public health agency programs typically organize and conduct immunization clinics for children about to enter school, review plumbing and ventilation plans for new restaurants, provide child car seat education for new parents, or meet with local governing bodies to discuss new initiatives.

At other times, particularly when there is a threat to the community's health and well-being, the entire local public health agency will act in a unified manner to provide a coordinated agency-wide response to the perceived threat. Ever since the first agencies were established (around the time of the founding of the United States), local public health agencies have expended time and monetary resources preparing to respond to public health emergencies. More recently, the federal government has begun providing the states with billions of dollars to help local public health agencies prepare a coordinated response to the threats of nuclear, biological, chemical, and terrorist attacks. Emergency preparedness planning has, therefore, become a mandated operation at all levels of government and has had a very significant impact on every local public health agency. The services described in this chapter are all affected. When appropriate, these effects will be described. The specifics of new mandates regarding nuclear, biological, chemical, and terrorist attacks are discussed in Chapters 26 through 29.

The term *local public health agency* is used in this chapter. However, this entity goes by different names in different states. Many local jurisdictions are organized into *local departments of health*. The term *local health commission* is occasionally encountered.

ADMINISTRATIVE SERVICES

Chief Health Officer

The chief health officer is the organizational head of a local public health agency. The title varies from state to state. The titles health commissioner, health officer, health director, and executive director are also used. This individual often holds an advanced degree in public health, health administration, or a related field. The health officer may be trained in a medical field, such as a physician, a dentist, or a veterinarian, with additional training in public health. As in all business operations, the top public health official must satisfy the needs of many customers or constituent groups. These include the agency's employees, individuals served by the agency, and the agency's funding sources—local, state, and federal governmental agencies and charitable and philanthropic groups.

This need to satisfy so many individuals and constituents requires that public health officials have a thorough understanding of the enormous responsibilities inherent to their positions. In addition to the chief health officer, and depending on the size of the local public health agency, other administrative specialists may be present. These include people with training and certification in other professional disciplines as well as budget and finance personnel and support staff.

A governing board, typically the local board of health, the county commission, or a district health board, usually supervises the chief health officer. Working with the governing board, the chief health officer ensures that an ongoing community health assessment and improvement process is in place. This process serves to inform the community and the governing board of what is going well and what requires improvement and is required under Essential Service #1 (Monitor health status to identify community problems; see below). Other performance standards within the **Essential Services** guide the actions of the chief health officer.

Essential Public Health Services

1. Monitor health status to identify community health problems.
2. Diagnose and investigate health problems and health hazards in the community.
3. Enforce laws and regulations that protect health and ensure safety.
4. Inform, educate, and empower people about health issues.
5. Mobilize community partnerships to identify and solve health problems.
6. (a) Link people to needed personal health services and (b) assure the provision of health care when otherwise unavailable.
7. Evaluate effectiveness, accessibility, and quality of personal and population-based health services.
8. Assure a competent public health and personal health care workforce.
9. Develop policies and plans that support individual and community health efforts.
10. Research for new insights and innovative solutions to health problems.

Source: Public Health Foundation, 1996: Essential Public Health Services Work Group of the Public Health Functions Steering Committee.

Communication

The chief health officer is usually the spokesperson when the public needs to know what is happening in a local public health agency. Recently, the public has required facts regarding its risk of being infected by newly emerging communicable diseases such as West Nile Virus, Sudden Acute Respiratory Syndrome (SARS), and monkeypox. Health officers stay well informed by maintaining regular contact with their state health departments and the Centers for Disease Control and Prevention (CDC). To make this process easier, a system has been developed called the Health Alert Network, or HAN (CDC, 2003a). The Health Alert Network links personnel from all levels of public health agencies and public officials involved in emergency preparedness and response. The CDC operates this important network, which provides three categories of alert messages:

- **Health Alert.** Conveys the highest level of importance that warrants immediate action or attention.
- **Health Advisory.** Provides important information for a specific incident or situation that may not require immediate action.
- **Health Update.** Provides updated information regarding an incident or situation that is unlikely to require immediate action.

A Health Alert would be released in the unlikely event of the discovery of a single case of smallpox found anywhere in the world. On July 2, 2003, a Health Advisory was released to report a "Probable Source of Monkeypox Virus Associated with U.S. Outbreak Traced to Rodents Imported from Ghana." On September 10, 2003, a Health Update was released to report a "New Probable Case" of SARS in Singapore.

If the chief public health officer decides that a message from the Health Alert Network contains information needed by the community, then a preplanned system of communication is activated. Receipt of a Health Alert may be associated with a full-blown response requiring coordination of the entire local public health system, including the media, police and fire departments, emergency medical services, hospitals, local government, and many others. In the case of an outbreak of a dangerous contagious disease, the chief health officer should be the chief spokesperson. In the case of a Health Advisory or Health Update, health officers may simply communicate the information to their staff.

In addition to relaying urgent communications of the Health Alert Network, members of a local community must be made aware of the long-term strategic plans of its local public health agency. Strategic planning is part of the community health improvement process. It involves a process in which the chief health officer and the governing board use data from the annual local community public health report to establish funding and programmatic priorities. Periodically, the governing board ought to convene a forum to gather citizen input on public health issues. Following such a data-gathering process, the data should be used to revise plans and programs for the future. These elements are components of the evaluation process that assesses the effectiveness, accessibility, and quality of both the personal and population-based health services described in Essential Services #9.

Operations

The responsibility for maintaining a balanced budget is at times the most difficult task for public health officials who are responsible for maintaining services during times of both increasing and decreasing funding levels. Therefore, a health officer must work with staff members to develop a workable plan that ensures the delivery of local public health services aimed at fulfilling the goals, as adopted by the governing entity, of healthy people and health communities.

Essential Service #5 requires that a local public health agency and its governing body develop policies and plans that support individual and community health efforts. To accomplish this goal, the health officer must maintain a system of financial management that provides information necessary for planning, budgeting, and reporting of all local public health operations. The governing body requires accurate information to develop policies designed to help the local public health agency achieve its goals.

An example of where good policy development might prevent significant financial distress involves the development and implementation of a new public health service, such as opening a dental clinic or providing home health services. When new operations are contingent on significant external funding, policies that address the possibility of future losses of funding must be developed. Prudent local public health agencies begin planning for such a possibility far in advance. Such plans may include the development of additional funding sources to replace the original source. Alternatively, a plan to curtail or eliminate the newly established services might be necessary to prevent a budget deficit. Clearly, an automated information management system that provides up-to-date budgetary data is essential for effective policy development and operational planning. Finally, a well-trained billing staff that is familiar with the myriad details associated with insurance claims and Medicaid/Medicare rules and procedures will ensure that reimbursements for services are received in a timely manner. Prompt reimbursement is vitally important for the continued operation of local public health agency operations.

Other areas of administrative responsibility require the establishment of accessible and available public health services for people living in the community. Concepts such as maintaining adequate facilities, being open for service during hours convenient to the public, locating facilities in convenient areas, and providing adequate parking are all responses to reducing potential barriers to service that the administration might have to address as problem areas become known.

Legal Considerations

Essential Service #6 ensures that a local public health agency enforces laws and regulations that protect health and ensure safety. Every health official is required to comply with all federal, state, and local public health laws. Public health laws present health officials with a wide range of statutory authority. This ranges from simply requiring the presentation of information to imposing fines. It also includes the classical public health measures of arrest and quarantine for individuals who present a serious health hazard to the public.

An example of providing information as a first step is embedded in most local tobacco regulations. Something as simple as posting a "No Smoking" sign in a specific location may be required by a regulation. If the health officials are informed that signs have not been posted or should they observe the absence of required warning signs, they typically provide the sign and inform the business of the requirements under the regulation. When permits that are required by the public health code, such as those for food service establishments and on-site sewage systems, are not obtained as needed, fines are often imposed.

When individuals who are contagious with serious communicable diseases such as syphilis, typhoid fever, or HIV behave in an irresponsible manner and, as a result, put other people at risk of contracting their disease, the health officer has the legal authority to bring such persons into the criminal justice system for the purpose of isolating them from the community. Fortunately, this is an uncommon occurrence.

In addition to enforcing public health laws, Essential Service #6 also requires a local public health agency and its governing body to periodically review and evaluate laws, regulations, and ordinances. The single greatest cause of unnecessary death and disease in America is the use of tobacco products, primarily cigarette smoking. With this knowledge, several states have passed strong public health laws forbidding the smoking of tobacco products in public places. Notable examples of such states are California, New York, Delaware, and Connecticut. Some individual cities such as St. Louis, Missouri, and Toledo, Ohio, have enacted statutes banning smoking in public places.

Local public health agencies in many regions of the country have tried to achieve their goals of improving individual and community health by proposing similar ordinances and regulations. Their success has been varied. Some states, such as Michigan, have included a preemption clause in their tobacco-control laws. These clauses prevent communities from passing local clean air regulations that go beyond or are more restrictive than state requirements. With the weight of evidence against tobacco steadily increasing and the ever-rising costs of health care, it is likely that many more states will follow the lead of the states where smoking currently is prohibited in all places open to the public.

Workforce

Essential Service #8 recommends that a local public health agency ensure that a competent public and personal health care workforce is available and fully trained. The Office of Workforce Policy and Planning was established at the CDC in 2000. The primary goal of the **Office of Workforce**

Policy and Planning is to implement Essential Service #8, namely, to improve the ability of public health workers throughout the nation to perform the essential services of public health and to prepare the workforce to respond to current and emerging health threats (Centers for Disease Control and Prevention, 2003b).

It is important that a public health agency's chief health officer employ qualified personnel. This can be accomplished either directly or by contract. The professional staff members of a local public health agency are expected to engage in life-long learning through continuing education, training, and mentoring. The Public Health Foundation supports the work of the Council on Linkages between Academia and Public Health Practice. The latter organization is composed of a group of national public health leaders representing academic institutions and the public health practice community. The Council has developed a consensus set of core competencies. This set of competencies describes the skills and knowledge public health officials must have to effectively complete their jobs. Using this set of core competencies, institutions that provide training in public health will be able to develop curricula and continuing education materials to prepare today's public health workforce for the future (Public Health Foundation, 2003).

BOARDS OF HEALTH

Role of a Local Board of Health

Toby Citrin (2001), an expert in public health policy, has delineated eight characteristics of well-functioning boards of health. Local boards of health *link* with staff members of a local public health agency through the chief health officer or health commissioner. The linkage also involves elected officials and local citizens in restoring a sense of community. In this role, local boards of health can be a *mediating* structure that connects government with its citizenry. In the process of restoring confidence in government, local boards of health can *explain* and promote an understanding of public health and the role of a public health department among elected officials as well as members of the general public. Board of health members are *advocates* for public health support. They usually perform this function without being cast in the role of government bureaucrats.

Local boards of health are often cast in the role of being an *ombudsperson* for members of the community when they investigate health department problems identified by citizens or employees of a local public health agency. A local board of health can be the *liaison* between a local public health agency and other elements of a local health infrastructure. A local board of health can provide continuing *stability* by imparting long-term political support for health department operations when the elected administrative officials undergo cyclical changes in party or leadership. Finally, a local board of health can be an effective force that *reminds* citizens, leaders, and health professionals of the importance of community and the strong commitment to the health of all that is a fundamental tenet of public health.

Types of Boards

Three types of boards of health oversee the operations of local public health agencies: advisory, governing, and policy making. Almost two-thirds of the 3,186 boards profiled by National Association of Local Boards of Health (NALBOH, 1997) indicated that they perform a combination of these three functions. About 15 percent indicated that they performed just one of these functions.

Advisory boards report back to their county, city, or township commissions, conveying information about how the local public health agency is affecting the health of the community and how the community is responding to the actions of its health agency. Commissions then act on that information to establish policies and budgets for public health operations. Advisory boards also serve as the voices of their communities. In this manner, they assist governing commissions to understand community needs and concerns.

Governing boards have the authority to establish local ordinances and regulations that promote community health. Members of these boards are often elected officials who use their authority to establish fees for services, permits, and licenses. Governing boards also have the authority to hire and fire the chief health officer.

Policy-making boards have been given their authority by local governing units. They guide the management of the local public health agency, setting goals and priorities through data collection, strategic planning efforts, and policy development. Members of these boards must be sensitive to the needs of the citizens they serve as well as the local public health agency.

Clearly, members of local boards of health must understand and support the total operations of their local public health agencies. The majority of individuals who serve on local boards of health are citizen volunteers. Very few board members are trained public health professionals. Most members (70 percent) (NALBOH, 1997) are appointed to their local board of health by a local governing unit, usually a county or municipal government body, or by a nominating commission created by elected officials. The other 30 percent (NALBOH, 1997) are elected to their boards by direct citizen vote. To assist local board of health members understand their roles and responsibilities within the public health system, NALBOH, working in cooperation with the CDC and its public health partners, developed a National Public Health Performance

Standards Governance document (NALBOH, 2003a). The National Public Health Performance Standards Governance document was organized to mirror the 10 essential public health services. It was intended to serve as a tool to help communities identify and establish goals to improve the health of their citizens and communities. These standards reflect the central mission of public health.

ENVIRONMENTAL HEALTH

NALBOH published a *National Profile of Local Boards of Health* in 1997. This document was based on a large sample of the 3,186 local boards of health in the United States. Four out of five (80.2 percent) of local boards indicated that they had authority for environmental health programs. However, as noted earlier, not all local public health agencies provide the same scope of services. The National Association of County and City Health Officials addressed this issue in a subsequent publication (National Association of County and City Health Officials, 2001). The four most common environmental health services that are provided by local public health agencies include food safety (85 percent), sewage disposal (74 percent), and lead abatement and screening (74 percent). A more complete listing is provided in **Table 6-1**. Local public health agencies are often required to provide a system that monitors the environment, permits inspections, provides interventions, and ensures that enforcement activities occur. These activities are designed to reduce or eliminate exposure and risk from environmental threats and communicable diseases.

Food Safety

Food-safety programs are designed to monitor all aspects of the storage, preparation, and delivery of prepared foods within permanent and tem-

Table 6-1 Environmental Health Services Provided by Local Public Health Agencies

Program	Percentage (%)
Food safety	85
Sewage disposal	74
Lead abatement and screening	74
Private drinking water safety	72
Vectors	61
Emergency response	61
Indoor air quality	44
Surface water pollution	43

NALBOH has also published a *Local Board of Health Environmental Health Primer* (2003b). This document was designed to provide members of local boards of health with an overview of 12 environmental health topic areas, including those mentioned previously. A brief description of environmental programs most often found in local public health agencies will help illustrate their importance to communities.

porary food establishments. A license is normally required before any food-serving facility, which is usually a restaurant, but could be a county fair or church kitchen, can open for business. By requiring establishments to apply for a license, it is understood that regular inspections of the facility will occur. Inspections are conducted by sanitarians who are environmental health specialists knowledgeable in the state statutes and local ordinances related to environmental health in general and food handling in particular. Inspections may include a review of building plans, which ensures compliance with local and national standards and codes. Once the facility is open, regular, periodic food-safety inspections are conducted by sanitarians. Food-safety inspections should occur at least twice a year and must adhere to the standards established in the U.S. Food and Drug Administration (FDA) 2001 Food Code.

An illustrative example is provided by the Michigan Department of Agriculture Sanitarian Training Program. A sanitarian may perform one or more of the following official job duties:

- Serve as an official representative of a local public health agency
- Conduct investigations related to complaints and food-borne illness
- Communicate information about food safety to others
- Review construction blueprints, documents, license applications, and operating plans and specifications
- Collect samples and specimens for laboratory analysis
- Perform routine field tests
- Collaborate and cooperate with personnel in other agencies
- Work productively with other local public health agency staff members

This listing indicates that education is an important aspect of a sanitarian's job. Not only must sanitarians keep up-to-date on the latest scientific findings in food safety, but they must also teach the food-establishment operators the importance of remaining in compliance with the food code. Further, they must educate members of the public on measures they can take to protect themselves from food-borne illnesses.

Sewage Disposal, Wastewater, and Drinking Water

Local public health agencies have the primary responsibility for enforcing regulations related to the operation of on-site wastewater treatment systems and for inspecting the installation and maintenance of personal or nonpublic water supplies. Large community sewage systems are regulated by other municipal agencies. All local regulations controlling the disposal of wastewater are designed to protect the public, specifically neighbors living in close proximity to the wastewater treatment facility. A poorly constructed or failed system can easily contaminate area wells used for drinking water. Therefore, environmental health specialists are employed by local public health agencies to evaluate all parcels of land on which new or replacement on-site sewage treatment systems are proposed for installation.

The classic on-site system consists of a septic tank that collects wastewater from an attached home or business. The septic tank allows for the separation of solids from water. Discharge water draining from a septic tank flows through a series of pipes buried in a shallow trench. This wastewater then percolates through several layers of soil, which allows bacteria to act on particles suspended in the wastewater and soil to filter the sewage. The result is to generate purified water that enters an aquifer. Before wells are drilled or wastewater disposal systems are installed, a local public health agency requires permits, sets of approved plans, and on-site soil inspections. Final inspections of construction sites and a review of the well driller's log are required before any systems are approved for use.

The protection of water supplies from contamination and water-borne disease extends to municipal water supplies as well. Although a local public health agency usually does not participate in the construction and operation of municipal water plants, any time that there is a threat to public health due to contaminated drinking water, an environmental health specialist has a responsibility to investigate and help to eliminate the threat.

Lead Abatement

The National Center for Environmental Health located within the CDC provides funding to state and local health departments to reduce or remove the possibility of lead exposure. Funding through grants may be provided for research, education, or lead remediation. The objectives of this program include the following:

- Determine the extent of childhood lead poisoning
- Screen children for elevated blood lead levels
- Help to ensure that lead-poisoned infants and children receive medical and environmental follow-up
- Develop neighborhood-based efforts to prevent childhood lead poisoning

Local public health agency environmental health specialists are skilled at finding the sources of lead contamination in and around homes and buildings. A team effort is often required to identify the problem, to screen individuals who may be exposed or poisoned, to refer exposed individuals to treatment programs, and to educate the public regarding the extent of the problem and how to avoid lead poisoning in the future. Lead abatement is only one of the many programs in which almost all of the staff members of a local public health agency play a role.

The importance of environmental health specialists and sanitarians was recognized as early as 1850 in Massachusetts. It was confirmed by the work of Drs. Louis Pasteur and Robert Koch in the 1860s and 1870s with the discovery that bacteria cause many diseases. Time has not diminished the importance of their discovery. As long as communicable diseases are spread by contaminated food and water, by airborne sources and by vectors such as rats and mosquitoes, the need for environmental health specialists will remain both in America and around the world.

CLINICAL AND PERSONAL HEALTH SERVICES

Communicable Disease Control

Essential Service #2 requires local public health agencies to diagnose and investigate health problems and health hazards in their communities. To fulfill this requirement, methods for identification and surveillance of health threats must be in place as well as plans for responding to public health emergencies. These plans must consider methods to educate, examine, and treat both individuals as well as the public. Plans must also recognize the need to enforce applicable laws. Another important aspect of communicable disease control is to ensure that accurate and timely reports of surveillance and investigation activities be sent to state health agencies. These requirements are at the core of public health practice.

To control the spread of communicable diseases, a local health agency employs both new and old strategies. Isolation and quarantine have been used for centuries as a method to control the spread of diseases such as plague and tuberculosis. Identifying and treating with antibiotics those infected with bacterial diseases such as gonorrhea and other sexually transmitted diseases have greatly reduced their occurrence. Over the past century, control by immunization has dramatically reduced the incidence of most childhood diseases as well as eliminated smallpox.

Doctors and public health nurses responsible for communicable disease control work closely with epidemiologists who are trained in the science of disease surveillance. Together, these professionals are often the first to detect any unusual occurrence or cluster of people with uncommon diseases. An example of such a finding occurred in San Francisco in 1983 when a group of previously healthy young men developed a rare form of cancer, Kaposi's sarcoma, that eventually was recognized as one of the opportunistic diseases related to HIV infection.

With the recently recognized need for emergency preparedness related to possible attacks with biological weapons, a single case of smallpox found anywhere in the world would trigger an automatic response to isolate those infected and to immunize anyone with whom they had had contact. This would likely involve mass immunization efforts, isolation of the sick, and the possible isolation of entire communities. Local health departments must have a plan in place and must practice their response to an attack before such an event occurs. This topic is discussed in greater detail in Chapter 29.

Personal Health Services

Essential Service #7 requires each local health agency to link people to needed personal health services and to ensure the provision of health care when it is otherwise unavailable. Many local health departments provide some personal health services plus appropriate referrals. Other agencies may operate health clinics offering all the services one would expect to find in a family practice or primary health care setting. Many of the personal health services involve women and children. Immunization services, particularly for children, are almost universal in their occurrence. Family planning; prenatal care; Women, Infants and Children (WIC) services; and well-child care are often provided. Oral health clinic services may also be found in many urban and a few rural health departments. This topic is covered in greater detail in Chapter 34.

Population-Based Health Services

Other services designed to screen populations for targeted diseases may include breast and cervical cancer screening, colo-rectal cancer screening, or other cancer-specific clinics. Many chronic disease conditions have responded well to population-based detection, referral, and treatment efforts. The early detection of individuals with diabetes, coupled with intense follow up with education for management of the disease, has been a proven approach for reducing the public health burden of diabetes. Other chronic conditions, such as asthma, other respiratory diseases, hypertension, cardiovascular disease, and renal disease, have also responded well to intensified efforts at detection, treatment, and management that offers education. Some local health departments are also responsible for behavioral health and mental health services, such as substance abuse prevention and treatment, depression screening, suicide and crisis intervention, and other serious mental illness services.

A recent expansion of services to children and adolescents has joined the local health departments and local school systems. The introduction of school-based health clinics in many larger urban school systems has resulted in the provision of health care to populations of underserved children. This is more than simply having a school nurse available to check immunization records, hand out medications, and call parents to come pick up their sick child. School-based clinics use a multidisciplinary team that provides a full range of primary and secondary health care services, including nursing, social work, and nutrition-based interventions. Children with both acute illnesses and those with chronic conditions are able to receive free and timely treatment. As a result, they are less likely to be absent from school and more likely to be better, healthier students.

■ COMMUNITY HEALTH PROMOTION

Essential Service #3 asks local health departments to inform, educate, and empower people about health issues. This is primarily the responsibility of public health educators employed by health departments. The scope for this work was presented in the framework for *Healthy People 2010: Healthy People in Healthy Communities* (CDC, 2004). Its goals are to increase the quality and years of life and eliminate health disparities between racial and ethnic groups in communities. Improvement in personal health status requires a team effort between individuals, their families, their personal physicians, and all the members of the health system. However, there is much individuals can do for themselves. Community health promotion specialists are skilled at empowering people regarding changes in their personal health behavior.

Several health risk behaviors have been identified that individuals can change or modify to improve their health. These include the use of tobacco, alcohol, and other drugs; unsafe sexual practices; injury and violence prevention; dietary behaviors and obesity prevention; and physical activity and fitness. *Healthy People 2010* has provided public health educators with national objectives dedicated to reduce health-risk behaviors. Those objectives along with a local Community Health Profile, which is a snapshot of a community's health status, health risks, and health resources, help to define the needs and directions for public health promotion. The community health profile is a requirement within Essential Service #1, which directs local health agencies to monitor health status to identify community health problems. Conducting a community health needs assessment is discussed in Chapter 4.

To increase the chances for community health improvement, Essential Service #4 requires local health departments to mobilize community partnerships to identify and solve health problems. This requires collaboration between members of the local health system with the goal of forming community partnerships to solve local health problems. Throughout the nation, efforts at collaboration have resulted in improved access to medical care for the uninsured; improved access to adult oral health services; head-injury prevention programs providing free bicycle helmets; tobacco-free work sites; and, many, many other efforts to improve community health. Being skilled at methods of informing, educating, and empowering people, public health educators are important members of these coalitions.

■ CONCLUSION

Returning to the initial case study, the new health officer decided to concentrate the efforts of her department on basic programs. She assigned two registered sanitarians to conduct food and waste inspections. A portion of their time was spent in lead abatement activities. The community health educator conducted informational programs on the hazards of exposure to lead. At the end of the year, the number of people identified to receive treatment for lead exposure had doubled. Violations of the food-safety code had decreased. The health officer received a new contract for a three-year period.

References

Centers for Disease Control and Prevention. 2003a. Health Alert Network. Available at www.phppo.cdc.gov/han/. Accessed on March 24, 2004.

Centers for Disease Control and Prevention. 2003b. Workgroups: Office of Workforce Policy and Planning. Available at www.phppo.cdc.gov/owpp/mtgwrkgrp091201.asp. Accessed on March 24, 2004.

Centers for Disease Control and Prevention. 2004. *Healthy People 2010: Healthy People in Healthy Communities*. Washington, D.C.: US Government Printing Office. Available at www.healthypeople.gov/Publications/.

Citrin, T. 2001. Enhancing public health research and learning through community–academic partnerships: The Michigan experience. *Public Health Reports* 116(1):74–78.

National Association of County and City Health Officials. 2001. *Local Public Health Agency Infrastructure: A Chartbook*. Bowling Green, Ohio: National Association of County and City Health Officials.

National Association of Local Boards of Health. 2003a. National Public Health Performance Standards Program. Available at www.nalboh.org/perfstds/nphpsp.htm. Accessed March 21, 2004.

National Association of Local Boards of Health. 2003b. *Local Board of Health Environmental Health Primer*. Bowling Green, Ohio: National Association of Local Boards of Health.

National Association of Local Boards of Health. 1997. *National Profile of Local Boards of Health*. Bowling Green, Ohio: National Association of Local Boards of Health.

Public Health Foundation. 2003. Council on Linkages Competencies Project. Available at www.trainingfinder.org/competencies/background.htm. Accessed March 23, 2004.

Public Health Foundation, Essential Public Health Services Work Group of the Public Health Functions Steering Committee. 1996. Available at: http://www.phf.org/essential.htm. Accessed June 23, 2004.

Resources

Periodicals

Gaffield, S.J., Goo, R.L., Richards, L.A., and Jackson, R.J. 2003. Public health effects of inadequately managed stormwater runoff. *American Journal of Public Health* 93(9):1527–1533.

Griffith, J. 2003. Establishing a dental practice in a rural, low-income county health department. *Journal of Public Health Management and Practice* 9(6):538–541.

Kemper, A.R., Fant, K.E., Bruckman, D., and Clark, S.J. 2004. Hearing and vision screening program for school-aged children. *American Journal of Preventive Medicine* 26(2):141–146.
McClellan, M.B. 2003. Mission: Promoting, protecting the public health. *Food and Drug Administration Consumer* 37(2):12–17.

Books

Bassett, W.H. 2002. *Environmental Health Procedures,* 6th Ed. London: Routledge.
Centers for Disease Control and Prevention. 2001. *Public Health's Infrastructure: Every Health Department Fully Prepared; Every Community Better Protected: A Status Report.* Prepared for the Appropriations Committee of the U.S. Senate. Washington, D.C.: U.S. Government Printing Office.
Department of Health and Human Services. 2000. *Healthy People 2010, Vol. I: A Systematic Approach to Health Improvement.* Washington, D.C.: U.S. Government Printing Office.
Institute of Medicine. 2003. *The Future of the Public's Health in the 21st Century.* Washington, D.C.: National Academy Press.
Washington State Department of Health. 2001. *Standards for Public Health in Washington State: A Collaborative Effort by State and Local Health Officials.* Olympia, WA: State of Washington Superintendent of Documents.

Web Sites

- Academy for Healthcare Management: www.academyforhealthcare.com/
- American Health Information Management Association: www.ahima.org/
- Council on Linkages between Academia and Public Health Practice: www.phf.org/Link.htm
- Governance Institute: www.governanceinstitute.com/home.aspx
- Management Sciences for Health: www.msh.org/

Organizations

Association of State and Territorial Health Officers
1275 K Street NW, Suite 800
Washington, D.C. 20005-4006
Phone: 202-371-9090
Fax: 202-371-9797
Web site: www.astho.org/

National Association of County and City Health Officials
1100 17th Street, Second Floor
Washington, D.C. 20036
Phone: 202-783-5550
Fax: 202-783-1583
E-mail: naccho@naccho.org
Web site: www.naccho.org

National Association of Local Boards of Health
1840 East Gypsy Lane Road
Bowling Green, OH 43402
Phone: 419-353-7714
Fax: 419-352-6278
E-mail: nalboh@nalboh.org
Web site: www.nalboh.org/

Public Health Foundation
1220 L Street, N.W., Suite 350
Washington, D.C. 20005
Phone: 202-898-5600
Fax: 202-898-5609
E-mail: info@phf.org
Web site: www.phf.org/

CHAPTER

7

Acquiring and Managing Data

The Effective Use of Health Information

Pamela Butler
David Pollick

Chapter Objectives

After reading this chapter, readers will:

- Understand the need for collecting health information.
- Identify several sources of secondary health information.
- Know how to collect primary health information.
- Recognize how to integrate and apply health information in a local health department setting.

Chapter Summary

To create a healthier community, it is essential to identify and characterize its current and past health status. A local health department has the responsibility to document the needs, resources, and capacity of the community to improve the health of its citizens. This responsibility was underscored by the Public Health Steering Committee of the United States Public Health Service as early as 1994. At this time, the committee identified 10 essential services for public health (Turnock, 2004).

1. Monitor health status to identify community health problems.
2. Diagnose and investigate health problems and health hazards in the community.

3. Inform, educate and empower people about health issues.
4. Mobilize community partnerships to identify and solve health problems.
5. Develop policies and plans that support individual and community health efforts.
6. Enforce laws and regulations that protect health and protect safety.
7. Link people with needed personal health services and assure provision of health care when otherwise unavailable.
8. Assure a competent public health and personal work force.
9. Evaluate effectiveness, accessibility, and quality of personal and population-based health services.
10. Research for new insights and innovative solutions to health problems.

A local health department should strive to become a knowledgeable authority on the health of its community. Health assessment is the first step in the continuous health improvement cycle, providing a process for data-driven planning, action, and evaluation. Participation provides a prime opportunity for the local health department to collaborate with a number of organizations at various levels (local, state, national) to significantly impact the health of local citizens.

This chapter is intended to be a practical guide for the local health department on how to acquire and use health information for community health assessment and other important activities such as evidence-based grant writing, health improvement programs and interventions, and public health information and education. A discussion of how to conduct a community health assessment is contained in Chapter 4.

Case Study

The members of the municipal committee were locked in a heated argument. Councilperson Smith was saying that the health status of many in the community was inadequate. In particular, many people could not receive adequate dental care. Councilperson Jones countered that the community was a healthy place to live, work, and raise a family. He had seen data that substantiated his position! Both turned to the mayor for support. How should the mayor reply to the two council members?

INTRODUCTION

This chapter is appropriately subtitled *The Effective Use of Health Information*. Readers are reminded to remember that data are important friends. The "laws" below provide a humorous overview that has an all-too-often familiar ring of truth:

Finagle's Laws of Health Information
The information you have is **not** the information you want.
The information you want is **not** the information you need.
The information you need is **not** available.

To monitor, diagnose, investigate, and mobilize communities to action, factual baseline information must be collected and analyzed for trends, areas of health concerns and needs, specific populations most at risk, and gaps in the local services and health improvement interventions and programming. Many kinds of information and data sets are available to meet these needs. Gathering data can be a very productive activity. However, without careful thought and preparation, it can become a monumental waste of time and resources as well as a great source of frustration. It is essential to learn which sources of health data and information will yield the best return with a small investment. The process of identifying, measuring, and reporting community health status and health needs provides information by which community priorities can be established.

To perform a basic assessment of a community's health status, the local health department should select a set of standardized health and social status indicators. Health status indicators provide the information base for larger planning, advocacy, and action strategies that utilize existing resources in a community. They are benchmarks by which change is measured over time.

Properly managed and presented data sets help to create a sense of shared responsibility for community health and well-being. They draw attention to problems and negative trends before they become damaging. Such health information can help to mobilize citizens to set priorities, establish goals, and participate in community planning. The use of community health indicators helps to articulate health needs and assists health care and social service providers when planning how to best meet a community's identified needs.

Health information can be found in both quantitative (numerical) and qualitative (descriptive) forms. It can also be divided into two major categories: primary and secondary. Primary data are obtained directly from surveying, talking, and interacting with residents in a community, whereas secondary data sources contain information freely available to any member of the public. Typically, secondary data has been collected by some entity for another purpose (Miller and Price, 2001). Every good health assessment begins with an eye toward data that have already been collected. Secondary data may be reported by rate, percent, or by total count. A rate compares events affecting populations over time. The numerator of this mathematical summary expresses the number of deaths, disease, disabilities, and so on, whereas the denominator defines the population at risk during a specific time interval. Rates may be crude (general), specific (reflecting age, gender, race, or ethnicity), or adjusted (specific ages) and are typically expressed in terms of events per 1,000 or 100,000 population or for a particular period of time, most commonly a year. Percentages express health, demographic, and socioeconomic data points as a proportion of a larger group or set, whereas a total count tracks actual numbers. Examining secondary data sets is the logical first step in the process of assessing the health needs of a community.

SECONDARY DATA

In 1988, the Institute of Medicine released a report entitled *The Future of Public Health*. This report identified the core functions of public health departments to be assessment, policy development, and assurance. Assessment includes the collection, analysis, and dissemination of information on the health of the community. This led to the Healthy People and Healthy Communities initiatives of the 1990s. As an outcome of these initiatives, the Centers for Disease Control and Prevention (CDC) developed a set of consensus indicators (CDC, 1991). These indicators were chosen because they were readily available and could be provided by state health departments. The State of Ohio was among the first to adopt the consensus indicators, doing so in 1996. Once adopted by states, the consensus indicators were employed in some early state health assessments.

This initial set of core data, first presented in July 1991, was chosen because it provided a reasonable assessment of health status that could yield useful trends over time. The initial data also provided a standard for states and local communities to begin monitoring and comparing progress toward the Healthy People 2000 objectives. Though minimal and now limited in scope, these indicators continue to be applicable to Healthy People 2010 objectives. More complete details, including definitions, of the CDC consensus indicators are contained in Appendix A at the conclusion of this chapter.

Input from six public hearings was incorporated to draft the target objectives for Healthy People 2010. These objectives are efforts to guide the nation during the first decade of the twenty-first century. The final set of Leading Health Indicators were selected on the basis of their ability to motivate action, the availability of data to measure progress, and their importance as public health issues (U.S. Department of Health and Human Services, 2000) The Leading Health Indicators provide several objectives and target goals and include the following areas of focus: physical activity, overweight and obesity, tobacco use, substance abuse, responsible sexual behavior, mental health, injury and violence, environmental quality, immunizations, and access to health care.

Each state has the option to modify this core set of health assessment indicators. In its *Leading Health Indicators for Healthy People 2010: Final Report* (1999), the Institute of Medicine provides leading health indicators for health determinants and health outcomes, life course determinants, and prevention-oriented measures. A set of environmental health measures was developed to augment the consensus set of health status indicators. Additional environmental health indicators have been suggested. However, few local health departments have completed environmental health assessments, and basic data sets for environmental factors vary from state to state. The suggested environmental health measures to augment the Consensus Status set of health indicators is summarized in Appendix B at the end of this chapter.

PRIMARY DATA

Although secondary data sources provide a baseline community profile that often initiates the health assessment process by stimulating dialogue and building consensus between key stakeholders of a community, information may still be missing. During the investigative process, data gaps may be identified. This leads to the search for additional information. Primary data collection methods typically are used to answer specific questions. Primary data are new and original information that are obtained by those conducting an assessment.

Primary data facilitates community health problem solving, planning, decision making, and prioritizing. Primary research can be subdivided into two categories: qualitative and quantitative. Qualitative research includes studies conducted on smaller groups of participants when seeking answers to concerns and questions. Key informant interviews, focus groups, group process, and the Delphi technique are examples of methods used to collect qualitative data. Surveys are an example of a quantitative study method. If conducted using appropriate methods, surveys yield data that are statistically valid. Such data can be used to make predictions. All of the following methods can be help to build consensus among the key stakeholders in a community:

- **Key informant interviews.** Every community has individuals who, by virtue of their position, may have useful insights regarding the health and well-being of the community. These individuals may include representatives of government, business, the clergy, and health or human service professionals. These people are usually recognized for some form of leadership. Interviews are conducted on an individual basis, using a prearranged and selected set of questions.
- **Focus groups.** Participants, often 5 to 10 persons who are willing to share information and insights, are brought together and asked organized questions for discussion to gain information and an appreciation of their belief systems about one or more well-defined issues.
- **The group process.** A larger group of individuals, usually 30 to 40, is divided into small groups to acquire information, make action lists,

brainstorm, and write fast. A slightly modified group technique—the nominal group process—helps to set goals, identify problems, and obtain suggestions for solving issues.

- **The Delphi technique.** This method of data collection evokes information, judgments, and perceptions from individuals without bringing the contributors together. Data collection can occur through the use of e-mail, fax, or traditional mail.
- **Surveys.** This method is a type of quantitative primary research tool that collects data from a sample audience. Widely used survey instruments currently associated with health assessments include the Behavior Risk Factor Surveillance System (BRFSS) for adults 19 to 65 years of age and the Youth Risk Behavior System (YRBS) for youths 12 to 18 years of age. Both are available from the CDC. A number of other survey instruments are suitable for different categories of investigation. Tools obtained from the CDC are especially effective for local health departments because they allow the users to compare their findings with regional, state, and national results. This allows for better benchmarking of the community's overall health status.

PRESENTING HEALTH DATA

Once data sets and responses to questions have been collected and compiled, the information must be presented in a form that is easily understood by all members of the community. Traditionally, tables, graphs, hand-drawn charts, and maps have been used to display data and information. Often, graphics and text are prepared with an orientation toward research and publication rather than to convey information in a direct and noncomplex way. Before the advent of computers, preparation of such data was very labor-intensive, requiring many hours to produce a finished product. With the advent of the computer, vast amounts of data and information can be captured, integrated, and selectively displayed with relative ease. Computer-based graphics programs can present data quickly and accurately and in versatile and often interactive formats.

Health departments and health planners must grapple with problems that can multiply in scale, intensity, variety, and complexity. The best possible means of analyzing and communicating this information must be determined. Computer graphics often provide an effective way to communicate information about complex issues and problems. Compared with tables and charts, computer-generated graphs and maps usually provide a clearer view of information. Maps are especially effective in conveying how data change over time as well as providing a sense of spatial orientation. Maps also allow individuals to quickly and easily visualize large volumes of data and information.

The downside to using computer graphics can be the time required to enter, code, and prepare data, which is often required for mapping. Time must be invested in learning how to manipulate computer software. Maps and graphics can also be used indiscriminately and inappropriately. Judgment must be used when deciding which graphic to present and determining what information will be conveyed.

A visual representation of the data set often enhances a reader's understanding and effectively communicates an idea with clarity and efficiency. The graphical illustration of quantitative data greatly enhances its appearance and effectiveness and offers the ability to present large amounts of information in a small space. Tables, charts, and graphs are convenient ways to clearly show data. When data are displayed in such a way, data patterns, trends, and variances become more obvious and recognizable (Soukup and Davidson, 2002).

An important consideration is how to best display the results in the appropriate graphic format. Charts and graphs must have an appropriate title that explains what the data measure. On line and bar graphs, the X- and Y-axes must be appropriately labeled with correct units of measure.

An easy way to create a graph is to enter data into a spreadsheet program such as Microsoft Excel or ClarisWorks. These programs will generate a graph using the entered data. Many types of graphics can be used to represent data sets. These include tables, graphs and pie charts, flow charts, drawings, diagrams, and photographs. Diagrams represent abstractions, operating principles, networks, and hierarchies within an organization while simultaneously displaying causality among the items. Flow charts depict steps in a process, whereas photographs show realistic views of objects in meaningful perspective. Bar graphs, line graphs, and pie charts are the three basic types of graphs.

It is often difficult to decide which type of chart is most appropriate to represent a particular data set. In most cases, the key to producing an effective chart is simplicity. Choose the graph that best expresses the results. A variety of charts and graphs are described in Appendix C at the end of this chapter.

Although a word-processing program usually provides many different styles for tables, for the purposes of report writing it is best to stick with simple formats. A clearly presented table is far more appealing to the eye. Typically, the font size used in tables is one to two points smaller than that used in the body of the text of a report. In most word processors, the quickest way to create a table is to paste data from a spreadsheet. After pasting the data, simply select (highlight) all of the rows and columns of the table and choose the Autoformat option from the Table menu. The word processor will automatically format the table. When inserting captions (titles), it is usually best to insert the caption above the table. It is often better to insert a figure caption below the figure.

The basic graphic-creation principles can be applied to specific health data. Two types of data are frequently required by health planning agencies: general demographic data related to health and specific data geared to particular objectives. Special studies may be required to obtain the latter data. Because it is important to learn as much as possible about the community prior to assessment, social indicators should be captured and considered whenever possible. The U.S. Census Bureau maintains a useful Web site (quickfacts.census.gov/) for creating multiple visual representations of information. National, state, and local general population data by age, gender, race or ethnicity, and population density by geographic location can be found. These varied data sets help to identify specific target populations who should be included in all phases of health assessment, planning, and evaluation. (See **Figure 7-1**)

Socioeconomic factors can reflect the ability of a community to provide the resources needed for community members to live productive, independent, and prosperous lives. These factors have been extensively studied and inversely correlated with overall health status. For example, leading socioeconomic indicators can be trended to show graphical representations that include: types of employment, unemployment rates (See **Figure 7-2**), median/mean income levels for individuals and families, education levels obtained (See **Figure 7-3**), high school graduation and dropout rates, poverty rates, numbers of individuals and families served by Medicare and Medicaid programs, uninsured rates, and the number of people who are homeless or in need of public assistance.

General health status information can be obtained through state health department vital statistics reports, including an analysis of mortality (leading causes of death), morbidity (leading causes of illness), and years of potential life lost. Mortality statistics identify leading causes of death, which are often reported by total numbers and by age-adjusted and crude rates per 1,000 or 100,000 population. Crude rates are calculated using the actual number of deaths reported for a given population during a given time interval and are not age sensitive. Age-adjusted rates express the expected number of deaths as if the population had the same age distribution as the standard population. **Figures 7-4** and **7-5** provide examples of mortality rates. Age-adjusted rates give health departments the ability

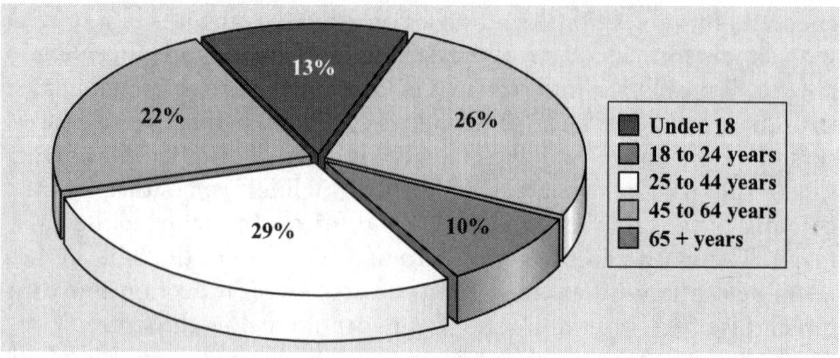

Figure 7-1 County Percent Population by Ages, 2000.
Source: U.S. Census, 2000

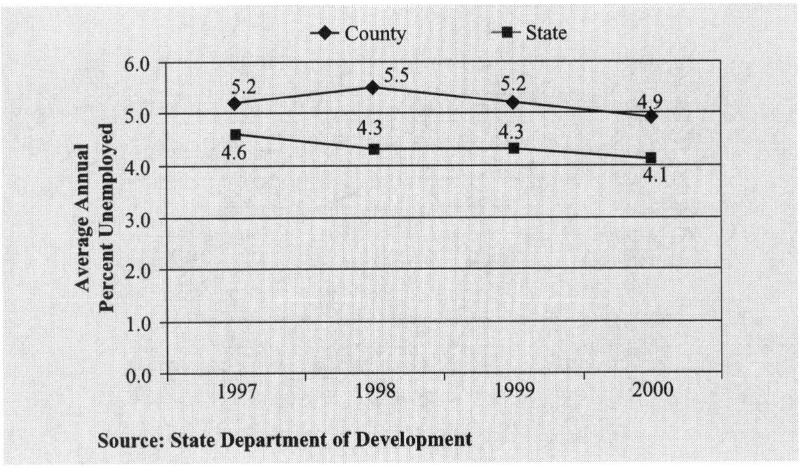

Figure 7-2 County Unemployment 1997–2000.

to compare local area statistics with adjacent or similar counties and regions. Both rates should be obtained and compared with counties that have comparable populations. Raw or unadjusted data may give the impression that a county or community has higher-than-average crude mortality rates. When age-adjusted figures are examined, they may compare favorably to the state and region (Turnock, 2004).

Another morbidity-based measure is years of potential life lost. This statistic factors out the number of deaths that occur after the age of 65 or 75, placing a larger emphasis on the causes of death affecting younger populations. Heart disease, cancer, and cardiovascular diseases are the leading causes of mortality for the total population of the United States.

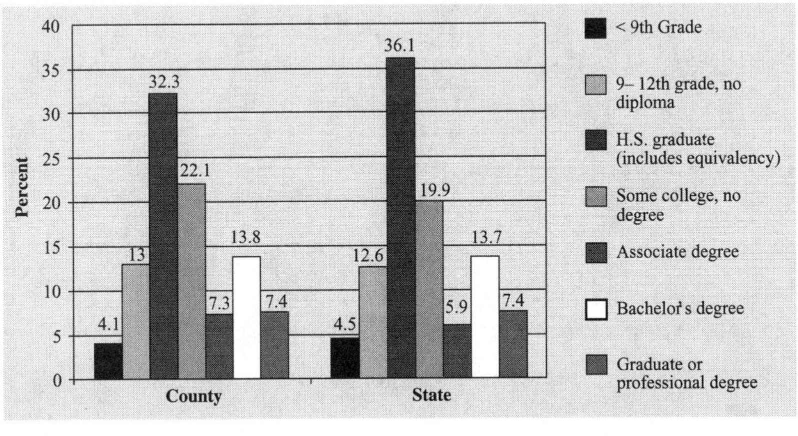

Figure 7-3 Education Attainment of Population 25 Years and Over, 2000 Census.

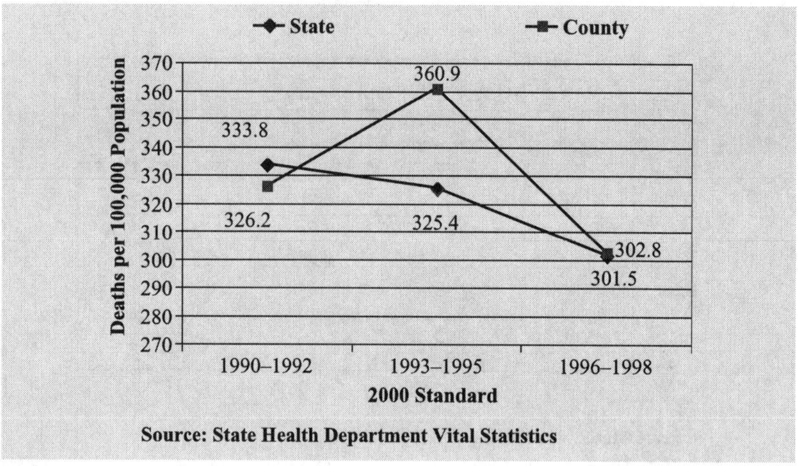

Figure 7-4 Heart Disease Age-Adjusted Mortality Rates 1990–1998.

However, these figures can be misleading, because the majority of deaths occur among members of an older population. When the causes of death for senior populations are factored out, the true causes of mortality for those who are younger can be identified (**Table 7-1**).

Whereas mortality rates describe the most extreme health outcomes, morbidity statistics provide insights into the illnesses that are currently impacting the health of a community. Morbidity rates measure the incidence or prevalence of disease in a specific population, geographic area, or other grouping of interest such as age or gender cohorts. **Figures 7-6** and **7-7** provide examples of graphs displaying morbidity data.

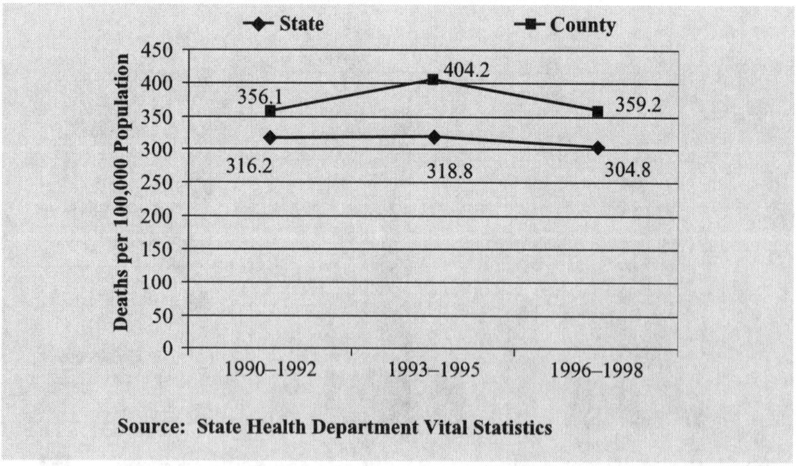

Figure 7-5 Heart Disease Crude Mortality Rates 1990–1998.

Table 7-1 Comparison of Years of Potential Life Lost and Leading Causes of Death for the United States, 1999–2000

Years of Potential Life Lost (Before Age 65)	Leading Causes of Death (Total Population)
1. Unintentional injuries	1. Heart disease
2. Cancer	2. Cancer
3. Heart disease	3. Cardiovascular disease
4. Perinatal period deaths	4. Chronic lower-respiratory disease
5. Suicide	5. Unintentional injuries

Source: 2002 National Center for Health Statistics (NCHS) Vital

Incidence is defined as the number of new cases of an illness or condition; prevalence measures the total number of cases reported within a defined population during a specified time period. Both the incidence and the duration of the illness or condition affect prevalence.

Health status data can be presented in a high-impact and powerful fashion through the use of mapping techniques. A number of very effective computer-mapping tools are available to apply the data contained in health status databases. Mapping can often provide a clearer view of health information than charts or tables. Changes in data over time can be tracked by series mapping. Multiple variables can often be displayed if they are spatially contiguous. Large volumes of data can be visualized quickly, providing at least a relative understanding of the magnitude and location of one or more variables. Conversely, creating clear maps usually requires a large amount of data to be coded. The raw data must of-

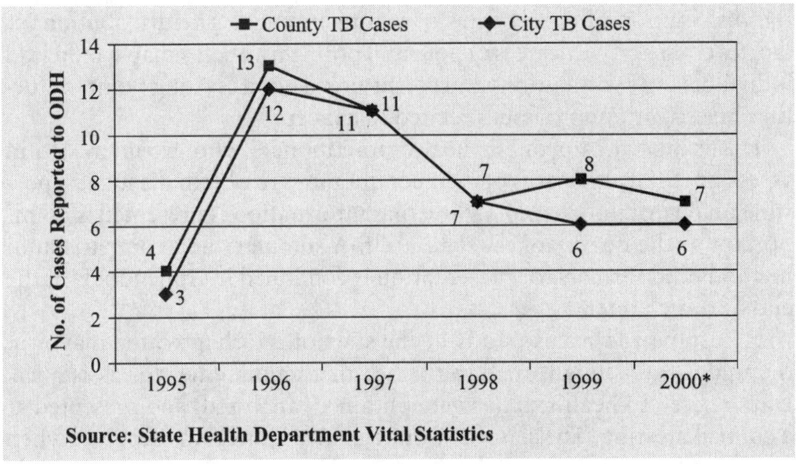

Figure 7-6 County TB Morbidity 1995–2000.

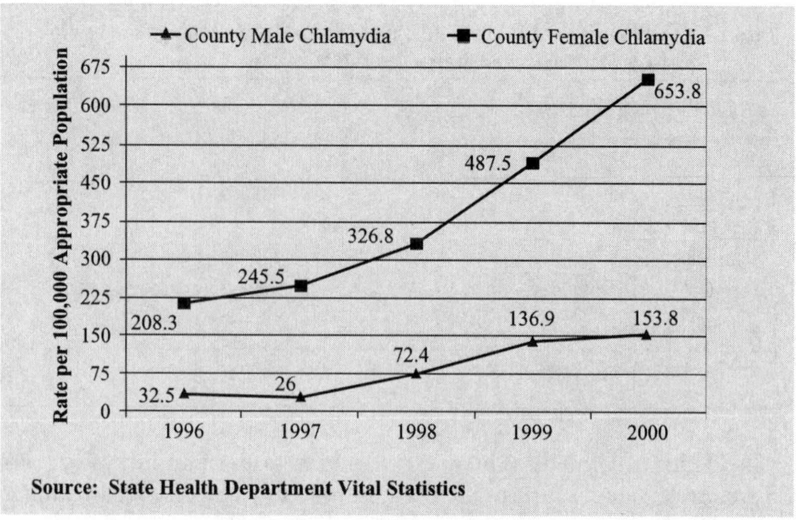

Figure 7-7 County STD Rates by Gender 1996–2000.

ten be tailored to meet the specific requirements of computer software programs. The temptation to map data indiscriminately must be resisted. The type of map must be carefully chosen to ensure an effective and accurate presentation of the data.

The following map (see **Figure 7-8**) represents a nine-year, age-adjusted average rate of total cancer deaths in Ohio. The mapping software uses a spreadsheet with a county identifier number and an associated rate in an adjacent column. The rates are then divided into mathematical intervals, which correspond to values on a gray scale. The county's cancer rate value is then displayed on the map. The result is an interesting spatial distribution of cancer rates over time in Ohio. The distribution indicates comparative degrees of potential problems. Such a map would lead individuals to ask questions and constitutes a good starting point for further investigation into issues related to cancer.

It is important for public health practitioners who are interested in assessing the health status of their communities to obtain the highest possible quality of information. How that information is presented is as important as the quality of the data itself. A summary and comparison of methods and formats for presentation is contained in Appendix D at the end of this chapter.

Returning to the case study at the start of the chapter, the mayor in the initial case study turned to the health commissioner for assistance. Data related to health status were obtained, analyzed, and presented at a council meeting. The claim of Councilperson Jones was accurate when all members of the community were considered as an aggregated, single entity. However, when subgroups were created using residence areas, two neighborhoods were found to have only one doctor each, and both were

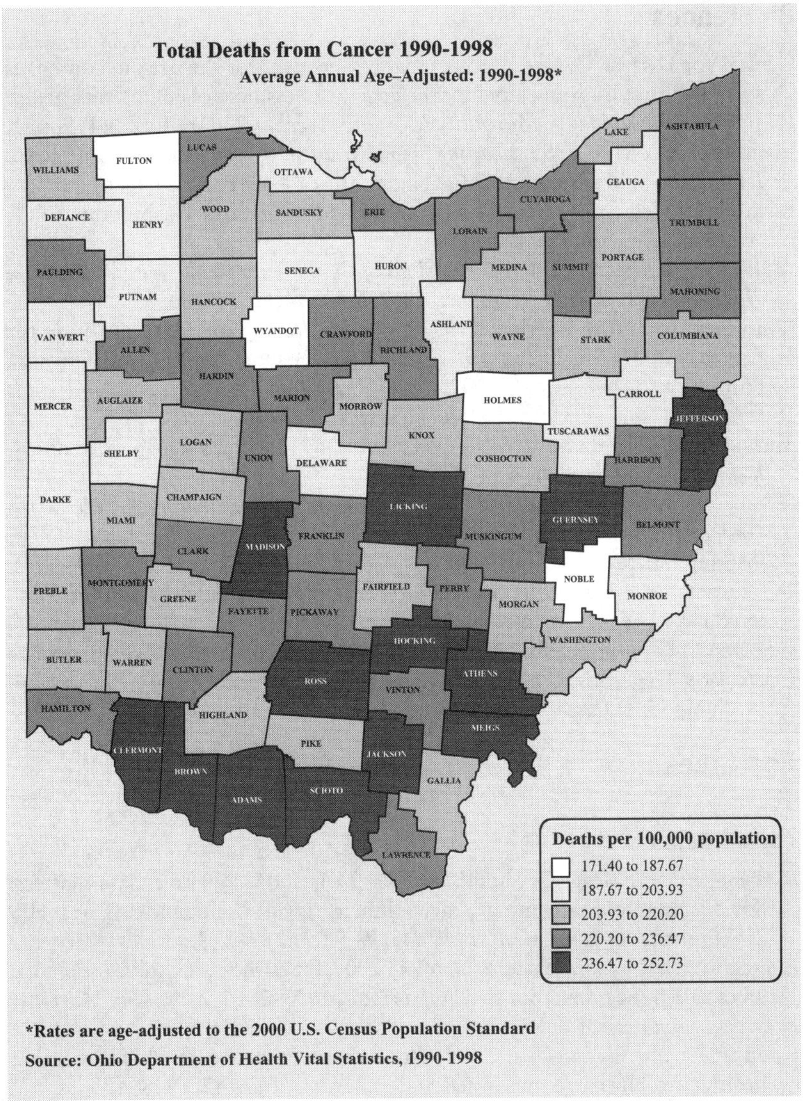

Figure 7-8 Total Deaths from Cancer 1990–1998.

without dentists. Adding to the problem, public transportation did not reach the new hospital that had been relocated to the outskirts of town where space was available. New routes were established for public transportation buses to serve the new hospital during the hours from 5:30 A.M. to 12:00 midnight. A contract to provide van service during the night was signed in the next month. The department of health opened a small clinic to provide health care services to people living in the underserved neighborhoods. A dental office has been included. The health department is currently recruiting a dentist.

References

Centers for Disease Control. 1991. Health objectives for the nation: consensus set of health status indicators for the general assessment of community health status—United States. *Morbidity Mortality Weekly Report* 40(27):449–451.

Institute of Medicine. 1999. *Leading Health Indicators for Healthy People 2010: Final Report.* Washington, D.C.: National Academy Press.

Institute of Medicine. 1988. *The Future of Public Health.* Washington, D.C.: National Academy Press.

Miller, D.F., and Price, J. 2001. *Dimensions of Community Health with PowerWeb: Health and Human Performance.* New York: McGraw-Hill.

Ohio Department of Health. 1997. *Ohio Public Health Plan: A Guide for Community Health Assessment.* Columbus, OH: Ohio Department of Health.

Soukup, T., and Davidson, I. 2002. *Visual Data Mining: Techniques and Tools for Data Visualization and Mining.* New York: Wiley.

Turnock, B.J. 2004. *Public Health: What It Is and How It Works*, 3d ed. Sudbury, MA: Jones and Bartlett.

U.S. Department of Health and Human Services. 2000. *Healthy People 2010: Understanding and Improving Health.* Washington, D.C.: U.S. Government Printing Office.

U.S. Department of Health and Human Services. 1992. *Healthy People 2000.* Sudbury, MA: Jones and Bartlett (reprint).

U.S. Department of Health, Education and Welfare. 1979. *Healthy People: The Surgeon General's Report on Health Promotion and Disease Prevention.* Washington, D.C.: U.S. Government Printing Office.

Resources

Periodicals

Barbeau, E.M., Krieger, N., and Soobader, M.J. 2004. Working-class matters: Socioeconomic disadvantage, race/ethnicity, gender, and smoking in NHIS 2000. *American Journal of Public Health* 94(2):269–278.

Centers for Disease Control and Prevention. 2004. Prevalence of cigarette use among 14 racial/ethnic populations—United States, 1999–2001. *Morbidity Mortality Weekly Report* 53(3):49–52.

Chen, A.Y., and Escarce, J.J. 2004. Quantifying income-related inequality in healthcare delivery in the United States. *Medical Care* 42(1):38–47.

Gilbert, G.H., Duncan, R.P., and Shelton, B.J. 2003. Social determinants of tooth loss. *Health Service Research* 38(6 Pt 2):1843–1862.

Hillemeier, M.M., Lynch, J., Harper, S., and Casper, M. 2003. Measuring contextual characteristics for community health. *Health Service Research* 38 (6 Pt 2):1645–1717.

Norris, J.C., van der Laan, M.J., Lane, S., Anderson, J.N., and Block, G. 2003. Nonlinearity in demographic and behavioral determinants of morbidity. *Health Service Research* 38(6 Pt 2):1791–1818.

Books

Best, S.J., and Kreuger, B.S. 2004. *Internet Data Collection.* San Francisco, CA: Sage Publications.

Chambers, R.L. 2003. *Analysis of Survey Data.* New York: Wiley.
Lawson, A.B., Browne, W.J., and Vidal-Rodeiro, C.L. 2003. *Disease Mapping with WINBUGS and MLwiN.* New York: Wiley.
Maxwell, N. 2003. *Data Matters.* New York: Springer-Verlag.
Tufte, E.R. 2003. *The Cognitive Style of PowerPoint.* Cheshire, CT: Graphics Press.
Tufte, E.R. 2001. *The Visual Display of Quantitative Information,* 2d ed. Cheshire, CT: Graphics Press.
Tufte, E.R. 1997. *Visual Explanations: Images and Quantities, Evidence and Narrative.* Cheshire, CT: Graphics Press.
Tufte, E.R. 1990. *Envisioning Information.* Cheshire, CT: Graphics Press.

Web Sites

- American Cancer Society:
  www.cancer.org
- Federal Statistics (FedStats):
  www.fedstats.gov/
- Health and Human Services Data Council:
  aspe.os.dhhs.gov/datacncl/index.shtml
- National Institutes of Health:
  health.nih.gov/
- Ohio Department of Health:
  www.odh.state.oh.us/resources/reports/oh_plan/phpcont.htm
- The National Committee on Vital and Health Statistics:
  www.ncvhs.hhs.gov/
- The National Health Information Infrastructure:
  aspe.hhs.gov/sp/nhii/
- U.S. Census Bureau:
  www.census.gov

Organizations

Centers for Disease Control and Prevention
1600 Clifton Road
Atlanta, GA 30333
Phone: 404-639-3311
Public inquiries: 404-639-3534 or 800-311-3435
E-mail: www.cdc.gov/netinfo.htm (Web form)
Web site: www.cdc.gov/

Health Resources and Services Administration
Parklawn Building
5600 Fishers Lane
Rockville, MD 20857
Phone: 301-443-3376
E-mail: ask@hrsa.gov or comments@hrsa.gov
Web site: www.hrsa.gov/

National Association for Public Health Statistics and Information Systems
801 Roeder Road, Suite 650
Silver Spring, MD 20910
Phone: 301-563-6001
Fax: 301-563-6012
E-mail: jay@kma.net
Web site: www.naphsis.org/

National Center for Health Statistics
Division of Data Services
3311 Toledo Road
Hyattsville, MD 20782
Phone: 301-458-4636
Web site: www.cdc.gov/nchs/nvss.htm

Public Health Foundation
1220 L Street, N.W., Suite 350
Washington, D.C. 20005
Phone: 202-898-5600
Fax: 202-898-5609
E-mail: info@phf.org
Web site: www.phf.org/

U.S. Department of Health & Human Services
200 Independence Avenue, SW
Washington, D.C. 20201
Phone: 202-619-0257 or 877-696-6775 (toll free)
Web site: www.hhs.gov/

U.S. Department of Labor Bureau of Labor Statistics
OCWC/OSH—Suite 3180
2 Massachusetts Avenue, NE
Washington, D.C. 20212-0001
Phone: 202-691-6179
Fax: 202-691-6196
E-mail: feedback@bls.gov
Web site: www.bls.gov/iif/home.htm/

APPENDIX

A

Healthy People 2010 Objectives and Targets

Table 7-2 Early Centers for Disease Control and Prevention Consensus Indicators and Healthy People 2010 Objectives and Targets

Outcome	Measure	Numerator	Denominator	HP 2010
Infant mortality	Infant mortality rate per 1,000 live births	Number of deaths under 1 year of age	Number of live births	Objective: 16-1c Target: 4.5 infant deaths per 1,000 live births
Total deaths	Total deaths per 100,000 population	Number of deaths (ICD-9 numbers 1-E999)	Total population	Objective: None Target: Not applicable
Motor vehicle crash deaths	Motor vehicle crash deaths per 100,000 population	Number of motor vehicle crash deaths (ICD-9 numbers E810-E825)	Total population	Objective: 15-15a Target: 9.0 deaths per 100,000 population
Work-related injury deaths	Work-related injury deaths per 100,000 full time workers	Number of work-related injury deaths	Workers 16 years and older	Objective: 20-1a Target: 3.2 deaths per 100,000 workers
Suicides	Suicides per 100,000 population	Number of suicides (ICD-9 numbers E950-E959)	Total population	Objective: 18-1 Target: 6.0 suicide deaths per 100,000 population
Homicides	Homicides per 100,000 population	Number of homicides (ICD-9 numbers E960-E978)	Total population	Objective: 15-32 Target: 3.2 homicides per 100,000 population

continues

Table 7-2 continued

Outcome	Measure	Numerator	Denominator	HP 2010
Lung cancer deaths	Lung cancer deaths per 100,000 female population	Number of lung cancer deaths (ICD-9 number 162)	Total population	Objective: 3-2 Target: 44.8 deaths per 100,000 female population
Female breast cancer deaths	Female breast cancer deaths per 100,000 population	Number of female breast cancer deaths (ICD-9 number 174)	Total female population	Objective: 3-3 Target: 22.2 deaths per 100,000 population
Cardiovascular disease deaths	Cardiovascular disease deaths per 100,000 population	Number of cardiovascular disease deaths (ICD-9 numbers 390-448)	Total population	Objective: None Target: Not applicable
AIDS incidence	AIDS incidence per 100,000 population	Number of incident AIDS cases	Total population	Objective: 13-1 Target: 1.0 new case per 100,000 population
Measles incidence	Measles incidence per 100,000 population	Number of incident indigenous measles cases	Total population	Objective: 14-1e Target: No cases of indigenous disease
Tuberculosis incidence	Tuberculosis incidence per 100,000 population	Number of incident tuberculosis cases	Total population	Objective: 14-11 Target: 1.0 new case per 100,000 population

Table 7-2 continued

Outcome	Measure	Numerator	Denominator	HP 2010
Primary and secondary syphilis incidence	Primary and secondary syphilis incidence per 100,000 population	Number of incident primary and second-ary stage syphilis cases	Total population	Objective: 25-3 Target: 0.2 cases per 100,000 population
Low birth-weight prevalence	Percentage of live-born infants weighing under 2,500 grams at birth	Number of live-born infants weighing under 2,500 grams at birth	Number of live births for whom birth-weight was recorded on the birth certificate	Objective: 16-10a Target: 5 percent of live births
Teen births	Number of live births to females 10–17 years of age as a percentage of total live births	Number of live births to females 10–17 years of age	Total number of live births	Objective: None Target: Not applicable
First trimester prenatal care	Percentage of women delivering live-born infants who received prenatal care during the first trimester (three months)	Number of women delivering live-born infants who received prenatal care during the first trimester	Number of women delivering live-born infants for whom entry into prenatal care was recorded on the birth certificate	Objective: 16-6a Target: 90 percent of live births

continues

Table 7-2 continued

Outcome	Measure	Numerator	Denominator	HP 2010
Childhood poverty	Proportion of children under 15 years of age living in families at or below the poverty level	Number of children under the age of 15 living in families at or below the poverty level	Number of families	Objective: None Target: Not applicable
Air quality	Proportion of persons living in counties exceeding U.S. EPA standards for air quality during the previous year	Number of persons living in counties exceeding U.S. EPA standards for air quality during the previous year	Total population	Objective: None Target: Not applicable

APPENDIX B

Environmental Health Measures

Table 7-3 Suggested Environmental Health Measures to Augment the Consensus Status Set of Health Indicators

Measure
Incidence of water-borne diseases from chemical infectious agents per year
Incidence of food-borne outbreaks/illnesses per year
Incidence of vector-borne diseases per year
Incidence rate of asthma morbidity as measured in asthma hospitalizations
Pounds of toxic releases to air per year
Percent of private wells with unsafe results due to bacteriological and chemical contamination

Source: Ohio Department of Health. 1997. ***Ohio Public Health Plan: A Guide for Community Health Assessment,*** Appendix D, Table 2, pages 39–40.

APPENDIX C

EXAMPLES AND DESCRIPTIONS OF CHARTS AND GRAPHS

Area Chart

An area chart displays the relative importance of values as they vary with a constant (e.g., time). Although similar to a line chart, an area chart emphasizes the amount of change (magnitude of values) rather than the constant and the rate of change. An example is shown in **Figure 7-9.**

Bar Chart

A bar chart shows individual figures at specified times or illustrates comparisons between items. The stacked subtype shows relationships to a whole. If the categories on a bar chart are organized vertically and the values arranged horizontally, this emphasizes comparisons and lessens the importance of a constant. An example is provided in **Figure 7-10.**

Bar Graph

A bar graph is used to show relationships between groups. The two items being compared can be independent. A bar graph provides an effective method for displaying relatively large differences. The column chart is a variety of bar graph that shows variations over a range of constants or illustrates comparisons among items. The stacked subtype depicts relationships to a whole. Although similar to a bar chart, the categories of a column charts are organized horizontally and the values are displayed vertically. An example is provided in **Figure 7-11.**

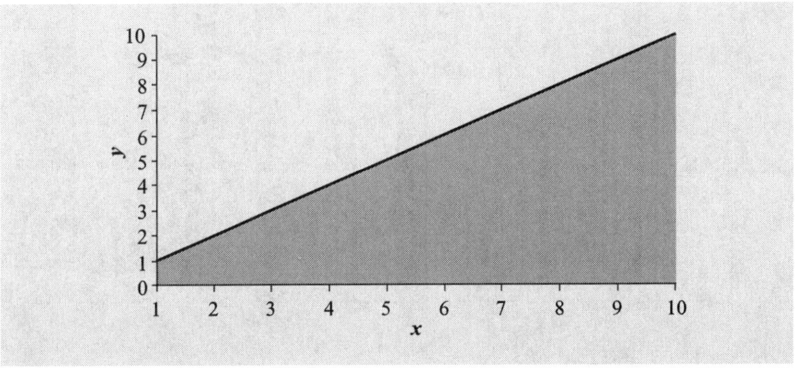

Figure 7-9 Area Chart.

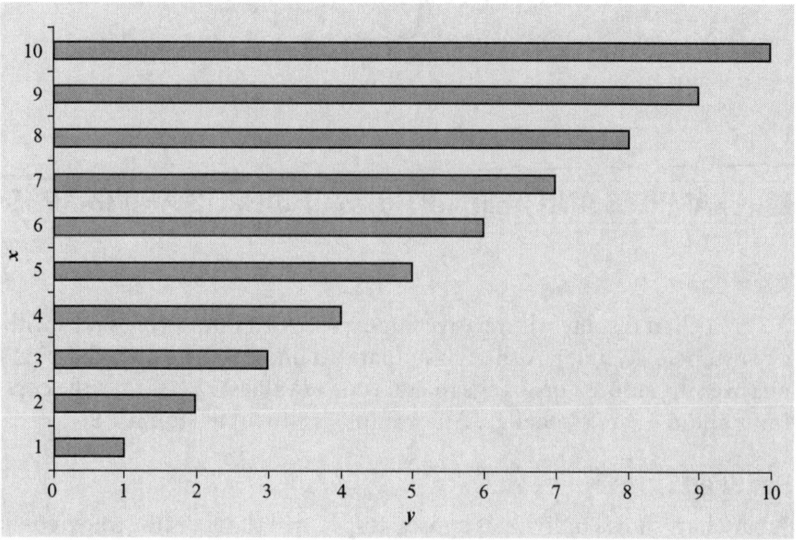

Figure 7-10 Bar Chart.

Line Chart

The line chart can show trends of continuous data over time using a common scale. Although similar to an area chart, a line chart emphasizes the flow of a constant and rate of change rather than the amount of change. A line graph is used to show continuous data (how one variable affects

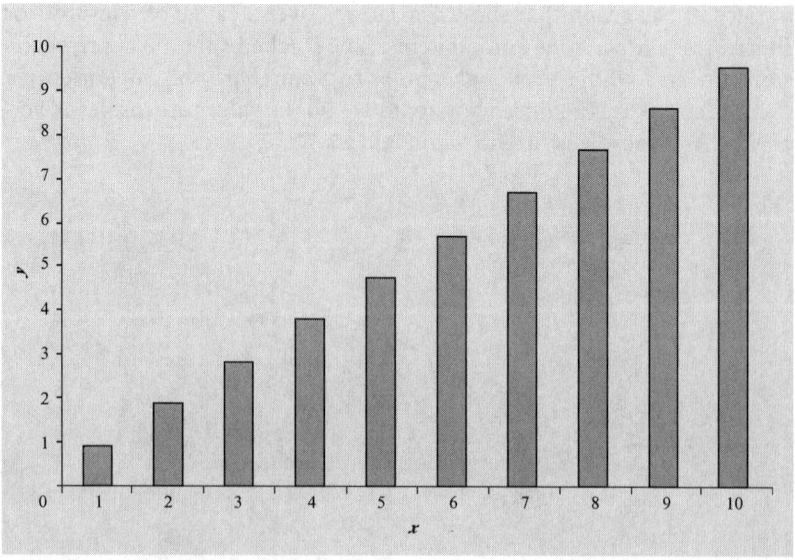

Figure 7-11 Bar Graph.

another). This variety of graph is needed to show the effect of an independent variable on a dependent variable. When there is a need to show trends or changes in data at uneven or clustered intervals, an XY, or scatter, chart is usually more appropriate than a line chart. **Figure 7-12** shows a line chart.

XY Chart

The *XY*, or scatter, chart shows the relationship or degree of relationship between numeric values in several chart data series or plots two groups of numbers as one series of *XY* coordinates. The *XY* chart can show uneven intervals, clusters of data, and similarities between large data sets. It is also appropriate for discontinuous data. This is one of the most commonly used graphs for representing scientific data. An *XY* chart is shown in **Figure 7-13.**

Pie Chart

A pie chart shows the relationship or properties of parts to a whole. This chart type is useful for emphasizing one or two significant elements. This kind of graph is needed to effectively display percentages. A pie chart is shown in **Figure 7-14.**

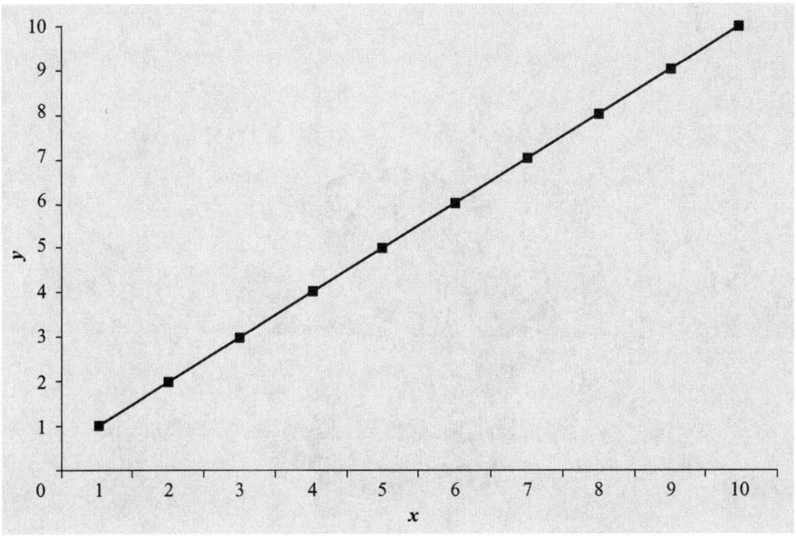

Figure 7-12 Line Chart.

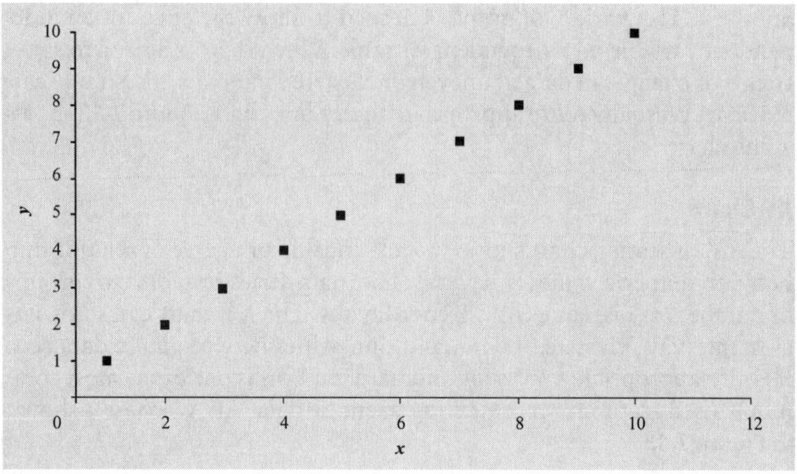

Figure 7-13 XY or Scatter Chart.

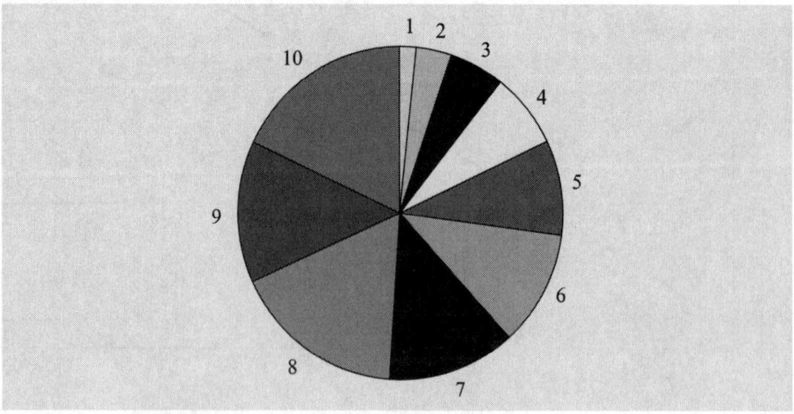

Figure 7-14 Pie Chart.

APPENDIX D

Categories of Charts

Major Categories of Charts		Graph (plot)	Map	Diagram	Table	Other Charts
Primary Function	Key features	Quantitative patterns & comparisons	Spatial & directional relationships	Nonquantitative interrelationships	Preciseness of information & ease of reference	Differs depending on specific chart
Quantitative	Shows patterns and/or relationships of quantative data at a point in time	Area graph Bar graph Circle graph Column graph Line graph Nomograph Polar graph Radar graph Scatter graph Trilinear graph	Contour map Demographic map Distorted map Elevation map Prism map Shaded map Smooth statistical map Weather map		Analytical table Bidirectional table General table Quantitative table Reference table Spreadsheet	Icon comparison chart Pie chart Proportional chart Ranking chart Unit chart Venn diagram
Quantitative	Shows patterns and/or relationships of quantitative data at a point in time	Area graph Candlestick chart Cash flow graph Column graph Control chart Index graph Line graph Run chart			Analytical table General table Quantitative table Reference table Spreadsheet	Comparative chart Icon comparison chart Point & Figure chart Proportional chart Stair chart Unit chart
Quantitative & Nonquantitative	Shows how/where things are distributed or located	100% graph Border plot Box plot Histogram Pareto graph Population pyramid Probability graph Quantille graph	Block map Blot or patch map Dot density map Geological map Pin map Profile map Topographical map Weather map	Block diagram Network diagram Voroni diagram	Analytical table Frequency table General table Percent table Quantitative table Reference table Spreadsheet	Business matrix Conceptual chart Floor plan
Nonquantitative	Relates time and activities			CPM chart PERT chart Time line	Calendar Time table	Explanatory chart Gantt chart Loading chart Milestone chart Scheduling chart
Nonquantitative	Shows how non quantitative things are organized, interconnected, or interrelated		Network map Ray map Road map Strip map Thematic map	Schematic: Block diagram Cause & effect diag. Conceptual diagram Flow chart Network diagram Organizational chart Relational diagram Venn diagram	General table Pictorial table Reference table	Conceptual chart Dendrogram Distributed channel chart Exploded diagram Gantt & milestone charts Minimum spanning Process chart Structure diagram
Nonquantitative	Shows how non quantitative things proceed		Flow map Weather map	Schematic: Conceptual diagram Decision chart Flow chart PERT & CPM charts Process chart Tree chart	Analytical table General Table Reference table Spreadsheet	Conceptual chart Gantt & milestone charts Illustration chart Process chart Vector chart
Nonquantitative	Shows how non quantitative things evolve or work			Schematic: Conceptual diagram Flow chart Process chart	Analytical table General Table Reference table Spreadsheet	Conceptual chart Cross-section Exploded diagram Illustration chart Pictorial Chart
Nonquantitative	Shows how to do things			Calculation chart How-to diagram Procedural diagram		Calculation chart How-to chart Illustration chart Pictorial instruction

Figure 7-15 Summary of Formats of Presentation.

CHAPTER

8

Public Health Constituencies

Eric Zgodzinski
L. Fleming Fallon, Jr.

Chapter Objectives

After reading this chapter, readers will:

- Be familiar with important constituency groups.
- Appreciate how rural, suburban, and urban health departments differ.
- Understand some political issues that impact public health departments.
- Recognize that there are limits to the activities of public health departments.

Chapter Summary

Most public health departments use the same list of 10 essential services to define their domains of service. Local differences in demographic and typographic configurations affect the programs that are offered. Programs in rural, suburban, and urban departments may be quite different in appearance and scope. They are designed to reach different constituency groups. Politics and political processes also affect the design and operation of health departments. Public health departments are limited in the programs and services they can offer. These are imposed by the nature of the discipline and by local fiscal resources.

Case Study

Jamie was a big city health commissioner who relocated to a small town prior to retirement. Jamie assumed the role of health officer using the same mind-set that had served her well in her previous position. After only a few weeks, Jamie was having problems with getting ideas across to the local board. Jamie became concerned that she would not succeed in a small town. What advice or words of wisdom would you offer to Jamie?

INTRODUCTION

Organizational behavior provides insights about how to motivate people. Management theories assist supervisors in guiding their subordinates. Core public health functions define the basic activities of an effective local health department. Publications discuss research and perspectives on management issues and many other topics related to implementing public health programs. However, few documents provide guidance for advancing programs or functioning within a specific system, such as a rural, suburban, or urban department. Departments in each of these settings have different concerns, needs, and issues related to funding, staffing, political milieus, as well as programs that are or should be offered. This chapter explores differences in these environments, focusing on concerns and issues unique to rural, suburban, and urban health departments.

RURAL DEPARTMENTS

The basic public health needs that are served by public health departments are essentially consistent. The resources available to address those needs vary with the density of the population being served. By definition, health departments serving rural populations have the least dense populations. The main industries in rural areas are often agriculture, timber, and mining. Delivering services to dispersed populations presents significant challenges. Agencies supported by state subsidy on a per capita basis obviously receive less money than agencies in more densely populated areas. This limits the number of staff and a department's ability to deliver services. A tax levy may have to be implemented to provide additional funding to adequately deliver services mandated by a state legislature or the federal government.

Transporting staff is a prominent issue in rural departments. More time is required to cover greater distances. The result is a proportionately larger allocation of work time to travel. Travel time is necessary but nonproductive.

Rural departments may also have a different mix of programs compared with larger departments. Smaller communities tend to be close-knit. Persons receiving services are likely to also be social companions. The same is true for politicians who control funding streams. This is a double-edged sword. Close relationships may facilitate delivery of services and advice but may impair its reception. Politicians may be more likely to provide financial support, but they also may be more likely to interfere with program administration.

Rural constituents typically have different lifestyles than their urban cousins. Mining and timber companies often offer some medical care services for their employees and dependents. Farming is different. Many farmers lack health insurance. Migrant workers often lack access to health care services. Many rural health departments are responsible for providing basic health care services. Rural dwellers tend to be politically conservative and resistant to offers of assistance by government agencies. Although such resistance is often minimal with regards to health care services, it is nonetheless a barrier that must be overcome.

Major programs for constituents in rural departments include household sewage and well water inspections. With a lack of infrastructure for these necessities, each household addresses these issues on an individual basis. Rural departments also have municipal centers that require scaled-down versions of programs found in suburban or urban areas.

SUBURBAN DEPARTMENTS

Suburban departments are unique in that they often face both rural and urban concerns. Funding sources within suburban departments tend to be adequate. They receive per capita apportionments, license fees, and grants. The tax base in suburban areas is usually sufficient to fully fund health departments. With increased population, there is usually an increase in services provided. The number of available staff is also usually adequate due to sufficient funding. Special tax levies are much less common in suburban areas than in rural regions.

Suburban health departments, unlike their rural counterparts, usually serve individuals who are comfortable with government agencies. People living in suburban areas tend to have more formal education than do their rural or urban neighbors. As a result of these two factors, less work is usually needed to convince constituents of the value of departmental programs and services.

Suburban departments, with their increased populations, serve a variety of income levels. For some, the health department may provide a supplement to medical care services provided elsewhere in the jurisdiction. Funding levels may permit the implementation of an increased number of screening programs. Vector control programs also are important. With older housing stock, there is more concern about mice and other transmitters of disease. Industry presents issues and challenges. Programs for constituents address air pollution and solid waste issues. Food-safety concerns in suburban departments grow as the number of restaurants increases. The number and mix of challenges faced by suburban departments differs from those of rural or urban health departments.

URBAN DEPARTMENTS

Due to the size of population that they serve, urban departments often are complex. Urban departments usually have the largest number of staff and the greatest financial resources available to conduct public health programs. However, stiff workloads and increased bureaucratic concerns accompany this luxury. Larger departments usually do not have the intimacy between staff and constituents that smaller departments do. Most often these departments have multiple levels of management and staffing, which adds levels of decision making and communication. All health departments encounter food-borne illnesses, but urban departments address them more frequently than rural departments. This is simply due to the greater number of restaurants and other food-serving establishments. Urban departments also must deal with increased numbers of industries as well as abandoned former industrial settings. The increased concerns associated with industrial settings include toxic chemicals, industrial accidents, and areas of environmental contamination.

With an increased population, increases in the incidence of infectious diseases can occur. For this reason, epidemiology and surveillance programs are usually larger and better organized in urban settings than in other departments. They are also better funded.

Vector programs are often major concerns within urban settings. With the population size and condition of the housing stock, rats can generate a large portion of a department's workload. Mosquito-control efforts can be extensive due to standing water concerns in containers and other man-made sites that support mosquito breeding. Rats, roaches, mosquitoes, and other vermin are concerns for constituents in all types of departments. However, in urban settings these problems are disproportionately large.

Larger populations are often quite diverse. Urban departments must recognize that their constituents range from people with low incomes to those who are very wealthy. Reaching diverse communities often requires a variety of approaches. Programs ranging from breast and cervical cancer screenings to lead remediation provide convenient examples. Individuals who lack insurance for such services often utilize breast and cervical cancer screening programs. Lead remediation programs are aimed at owners and residents of older housing stock.

POLITICS

Politics is a factor in all societies. Public health is not exempt from political concerns. Although local political processes may differ, political concerns must be addressed. The main concern shared by all public health departments is to enlist the support of politicians. If politicians do not become friends of the department, they must at least respect its goals and activities. Public health departments often underestimate the importance of political entities. Frequently, local politicians or political entities attempt to dictate how public health should do its job and the problems that it chooses to address. The public health department is often asked to undertake activities that are not within the department's purview. Public health leaders must find ways to tactfully decline such requests. This is a difficult but necessary task.

Maintaining both public and political health requires tact and frank discussions about the tasks public health can and cannot undertake. Public health departments exist to protect the community health. They cannot be used for purely political gain. Public health departments require financial support from politicians and should be held accountable for the prudent use of allotted funds. However, politicians must allow public health departments to focus on their goals and not be asked to assume tasks outside the parameters of the discipline. It is appropriate for public health departments to assume responsibility for health-related issues. It is inappropriate for public health to supervise a public works department. Public health departments should heed requests of political entities if they relate to health issues. Particular issues can differ depending on the size of a health department and the population it serves.

THE DOMAIN OF PUBLIC HEALTH

It is often difficult for public health leaders to decide which programs are relevant to public health. There is no simple concept that fully guides public health leaders in conducting their jobs. Chapter 4 describes an assessment process that can be used to identify areas of need within a community or health district.

Figure 8-1 addresses the issue of defining public health for particular locations. The three points of the triangle represent the main functions of public health. The first is epidemiology, the study of the distribution of disease in large groups of people. The second is concern for disease or injury. These concerns focus the efforts of public health practitioners. The third is education. This enables public health to try and change behavior, thus improving health throughout a community. The circle represents causes that may or may not be parts of public health. Programs or services that are within the triangle are sound. Those programs that fall outside the triangle but within the circle may be locally relevant. Programs outside the circle are not likely to be within the realm of public health.

Consider a request for a boat safety program. Elements of the proposed program may fall within the triangle. Analyzing the numbers, locations, and times of boating accidents is an epidemiological problem.

Figure 8-1 Relevance Diagram.

Teaching boat owners and operators how to tie knots, use flares, adjust personal flotation devices, or read charts does not fall within public health's typical area of educational expertise. If the program was public health concerns with water skiing in a contaminated lake, that would fall in the triangle and be a public health concern. The epidemiology portion would be the study of infectious diseases among the water skiers. The concern would be the infectious disease. Finally, the education would be why the water should not be used for recreation. Applying Figure 8-1 requires that users think critically about the issue at hand.

CONCLUSION

For the most part, the essential elements of public health do not change. The number and specific nature of most basic health services remain constant. Only the programs change. Public health is only as effective as its leaders allow their departments to be. Even the smallest of departments can excel and provide services appropriate for the size and location of the areas that they serve.

In the initial case study, Jamie was having difficulty in a new job. Some uncertainty accompanies the start of any new position. Moving to a health department with different demographic parameters compounds the dilemma. However, the essentials of public health do not change. Rural, suburban, and urban departments have differences in local issues that must be understood and appreciated.

Jamie had to meet the main stakeholders and understand their concerns and constituencies. Because local needs differ, Jamie had to become familiar with the relative importance of local issues in the new health department.

Jamie read the most recent community needs assessment. Meetings with local political leaders were scheduled and held. Jamie met with all

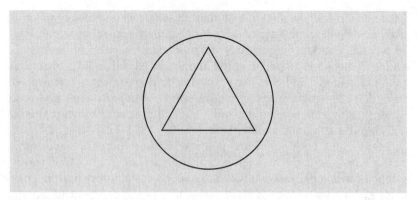

of the health department divisional heads. After three months, Jamie finally felt prepared to assume all of the duties of the new job.

Resources

Periodicals

Hajat, A., Stewart, K., and Hayes, K.L. 2003. The local public health workforce in rural communities. *Journal of Public Health Management and Practice* 9(6):481–488.

Parsons, R.J., Murray, B.P., and Dwore, R.B. 2003. Trends in rural healthcare delivery in the United States, 1990–1999. *Journal of Hospital Marketing and Public Relations* 14(2):23–36.

Rohrer, J.E., Kruse, G., and Zhang, Y. 2004. Hispanic ethnicity, rural residence, and regular source of care. *Journal of Community Health* 29(1):1–13.

Scala, M. 2003. Developing rural information and assistance programs. *Issue Brief-Center for Medicare Education* 4(7):1–4.

Books

Aguirre-Molina, M., and Molina, C. 2003. *Latina Health in the United States: A Public Health Reader.* New York: Wiley.

Baer, D.L. 2003. *Doctors in a Strange Land: The Place of International Medical Graduates in Rural America.* Lanham, MD: Rowman & Littlefield.

Loue, S., and Quill, B.E. 2001. *Handbook of Rural Health.* New York: Kluwer.

Stamm, B.H. 2003. *Rural Behavioral Health Care: An Interdisciplinary Guide.* Chicago: American Psychological Association.

Web Sites

- American Medical Student Association:
  www.amsa.org/programs/gpit/ruralurban.cfm
- Johns Hopkins Urban Health Institute:
  urbanhealthinstitute.jhu.edu/news-r.html
- National Association of Rural Health Clinics:
  www.narhc.org/about_us/about_us.php
- National Health Information Center:
  www.health.gov/NHIC/NHICScripts/Entry.cfm?HRCode=HR1229

Organizations

American Public Health Association
800 I Street, NW
Washington, D.C. 20001-3710
Phone: 202-777-2742
Fax: 202-777-2534
E-mail: comments@apha.org
Web site: www.apha.org/

Centers for Disease Control and Prevention
1600 Clifton Road
Atlanta, GA 30333
Phone: 404-639-3311
Public inquiries: 404-639-3534 or 800-311-3435
E-mail: www.cdc.gov/netinfo.htm (Web form)
Web site:www.cdc.gov/

National Association of County and City Health Officials
1100 17th Street, Second Floor
Washington, D.C. 20036
Phone: 202-783-5550
Fax: 202-783-1583
E-mail: naccho@naccho.org
Web site: www.naccho.org

National Association of Local Boards of Health
1840 East Gypsy Lane Road
Bowling Green, OH 43402
Phone: 419-353-7714
Fax: 419-352-6278
E-mail: nalboh@nalboh.org
Web site: www.nalboh.org/

National Rural Health Association
One West Armour Blvd, Suite 203
Kansas City, MO 64111-2087
Phone: 816-756-3140
E-mail: mail@NRHArural.org
Web site: www.nrharural.org/

CHAPTER

9

Interactions with Local Government

L. Fleming Fallon, Jr.
Peter Schade
Eric Zgodzinski

Chapter Objectives

After reading this chapter, readers will:

- Understand how politics and public health differ.
- Appreciate that politicians and public health officials must work together.
- Understand political isolation.
- Recognize that politics requires interactions that often are not agreed on by all parties.
- Know that political activities are cyclical.
- Understand the importance of clarity in missions and messages.

Chapter Summary

Politics involves compromise and adaptation. The political process is cyclic and usually linked to election periods. Because politicians often control economic resources, public health professionals and politicians must work in harmony. Having clear missions and goals are important to the success of each individual actor and to their collaborative interaction. Political isolation cannot be sustained without negative results.

Case Study

Bryan, the new Deputy Health Commissioner for Finance, was settling into his office. His recently awarded Master of Public Health degree hung on the wall. The interview process of last month now seemed only a blur. Bryan was quite comfortable with the first two duties of his new job, accounting and money management. However, the third item on his list of duties was new to him: Act as a liaison with the county commissioners with regards to fiscal matters. His supervisor had outlined the department's expectations for him earlier in the morning. Bryan was to establish relationships with the county commissioners. His longer range objective was to increase the health department's budgetary allocation. He knew that the budget for the next fiscal year had been finalized last month. He also knew that general elections would be held in six months. What steps should Bryan contemplate?

INTRODUCTION

Contemporary public health practitioners face a myriad of hurdles, barriers, and overall challenges when working with the people, programs, and projects needed to accomplish an objective. One of the more common approaches to overcoming these challenges is collaboration. Many traditional and nontraditional programs are being developed through collaboration. The core functions of public health are often successfully achieved due to collaborative efforts.

Public health agencies must develop proactive attitudes when interacting with local governments to achieve programmatic success. A key ingredient in obtaining such success is cooperation with city councils, county commissioners, township trustees, state general assembly members, mayors, county executives, public safety officials, citizen groups, and the media. Defining the relevant offices and individuals in local government is a process that involves all of the members of a public health agency. As might be expected, these interactions with local government officials and employees must have the full support of a board and become a part of the culture of an organization.

DEFINING LOCAL GOVERNMENT

Before interacting with local government officials, jurisdictional and political boundaries must be determined. Jurisdiction refers to the area within which a local public health agency has the legal power to act. Political boundaries refer to lines drawn on a map. These approximate the power boundaries of a jurisdiction. Political boundaries also refer to the acceptability of particular actions or philosophies within an area. In short, this refers to current concepts of political correctness. Most traditional legally mandated programs are limited to jurisdictional boundaries. Some newer nontraditional and emerging programs cross jurisdictional boundaries. Such crossing of jurisdictional boundaries will increase the need to clarify rules and responsibilities with local governments not only in the local jurisdiction, but also in areas contiguous to the health department as well.

As a first step in interacting with the local government, identify the local government structure of the immediate jurisdiction. This can be accomplished by inquiring at the county courthouse or local government office. It is essential that the board participate and approve of any programs or proposed procedural agreements that involve persons or units from other jurisdictions.

After identifying the political structures within the jurisdiction, plan how to make contact with individual politicians and how to get them involved. The ability to communicate with members and agencies of local government is an acquired skill. Identify the members of local government that should be included in the overall function of the health department. Brief these people on the issues affecting the community. Many of these individuals will embrace working with the public health department, viewing it as a win–win opportunity.

Some of these interactions must be planned. Begin with a simple telephone call or a hand shake and then request a meeting. Be sure to follow-up on any meetings or conversations. Such interactions often will lead politicians to call upon the public health agency when contentious issues arise or when they need advice on emerging issues facing those they represent.

Most agencies have some relationship with the local government. Public health staff members must be sensitive to government sponsorship and participation in public health programs. The goals of politics and public health programs may not be totally congruent. Initial relationships lead to more extensive ones. The process of building trust and programs is continuous.

The staff of public health agencies must be empowered to actively meet and inform members of the political hierarchy about activities being conducted by the local public health agency. Using strategic planning with local government support and endorsement is one of the key elements of successful programs. However, keep in mind that not all interactions are positive and that some stakeholders will decide not to participate. Interactions between the local government and the public health department require much energy, skill, and hard work.

Health commissioners, nurses, sanitarians, health educators, and other members of public health organizations must realize that political–public health interactions are cyclical. Politicians come and go, and the need to keep them continuously informed is sometimes difficult. Attending council meetings, hosting mayoral meetings, and discussing issues with trustees, commissioners and public safety officials will strengthen programs and increase involvement among stakeholders.

The media can be useful in strengthening the interaction process. For the sake of good governance and to be proactive, it is useful to establish interactive relationships with members of the media. Additional discussion of this topic is contained in Chapter 30.

CUSTOMER SERVICE

In some government agencies, customer service is lacking. In fact, many agencies have reputations that reflect their poor customer service. In some cases, health departments may fail to provide good customer service. Health departments may forget that they exist to serve the general public and that they must respond to the public's needs in a rapid and effective fashion. This may mean undertaking trivial tasks such as finding a telephone number for another department or performing non-public-health-related tasks such as helping with compliance with blood-borne pathogen regulations. Taking a cue from many organizations in private industry, customer service should be a prime concern. Having a policy of sound customer service means providing timely responses and adequate communications with members of the general public. Unfriendly and unhelpful interactions should be avoided. Ideally, they should not be tolerated within public health.

Public health has the responsibility to provide good customer service not only to the general public but to politicians as well. Many individuals in public health shun the political process. Erroneously, they dismiss it as being irrelevant. For many public health workers, politicians and the political process may evoke feelings of concern and apprehension. However, it is just as important to provide customer service to politicians as it is to serve the general public. In many instances, politicians who ask for a problem to be addressed or for information are likely to be doing so on behalf of a citizen. It is important to act on requests from politicians in a timely manner.

Responses to requests or complaints from politicians should be acted on as soon as is practical. However, a system of prioritization must be created and respected. If resources are being directed at a food-borne-illness investigation or an influenza immunization clinic, a complaint about blowing litter can be postponed for a few hours until resources can be freed to address the concern. It is also important to make a call to or follow-up visit with the politician who made the request to provide information and bring closure to the problem.

Timely responses and follow-up are important to members of the general public as well as politicians. Good customer service creates a favorable attitude toward public health. This becomes helpful when requesting support for tax levies or when signing new contracts. More importantly, it is the job of professionals in the field to serve and improve the public's health. Good customer service is a major element in achieving this goal.

POLITICAL INSULATION

Interacting with the local government and politicians is time-consuming. Some public health agencies feel political pressures to a greater degree because health department leaders are largely unacquainted with political leaders. Because of the lack of familiarity, these leaders do not connect on issues. Agencies experiencing the most pressure are typically those lacking interactive relationships with local politicians.

Several rough starts between regulatory and political officials may be required before positive ongoing relationships are finally established. The public health agency should be proactive and avoid unnecessary conflicts. By interacting, agency members are often able to create solutions before a crisis erupts. Quite often, when politicians require answers, public health officials are the resources to whom they turn. By creating proactive interactions with politicians, public health will be able to address those issues that it controls, not to sensationalized stories. A disease outbreak provides a convenient example. Governmental leaders that are given regular updates on disease prevalence are less apt to be surprised by an unexplained rise than those who are not briefed on a regular basis and learn about an outbreak through the media. Some public health agencies are not politically isolated. This is evident when local governments call for action and try to influence a health department without regard for the core functions of public health agencies. In reality, no agency is isolated from politics. True political insulation does not exist. It is simply less present in some circumstances. Political insulation tends to be issue specific. The more contentious an issue is, the harder one must work at the interaction process. Interaction with local government will lead to more success and better relationships than remaining aloof from the political process. The interactive process requires time to develop. It will be stronger between some entities than others. For this reason alone, public health practitioners must recognize the phenomenon of political insulation. In most cases, it can be minimized or eliminated.

LOCAL GOVERNMENT AND THE COMMUNITY

The interaction process usually begins with a specific need. The process of working with local government is much easier when the entire community is involved. Politicians embrace projects that create opportunities for themselves and for the communities they serve. Public health is in a unique position to assess, develop, and ensure that its programs result in a better life for those served. Community utilization is a key to forging new relationships with members of local government and in maintaining interaction on a continual basis. Local government will support public health efforts if they are linked to programs that promote community health, especially those that contribute to healthy lifestyles. Using a public health organization's resources is an excellent way to become a bridge builder between the local government and the community. It is important to remember that the public health organization's staff members and leaders are independent parts of the community being served by local government.

Strategic planning is a useful tool. For instance, a public health agency can plan a health fair for seniors, collaborate with local government for support, and then kick off the event. This produces the win–win situation that everyone desires. Community involvement is important for successful participation by local government officials. Public health agencies must respond to the needs of the communities that they serve, preferably in a proactive manner. However, reactive responses are common occurrences in public health due to the nature of disease prevention.

PREPARE TO BE NEEDED AND PREPARE TO BE BLAMED

Interaction is a neutral word. It does not define the positive benefits or reveal the negative aspects of working with others. However, when health department and government leaders interact, the majority of benefits are likely to be positive due to the rapport that has been established.

Public health must be prepared to be needed. It must be able to respond to situations and issues or to provide support for local government efforts to serve the community. Positive interactions will help politicians to see the importance of the public health agency.

Public health agencies must be ready to respond, and members of local governments must be prepared to rely on them. Although this may seem to be a natural process to many in the public health field, it often is quite foreign to local government officials who fail to recognize the importance of public health agencies. This is public health's dilemma. Public health organizations must ensure that local government understands public health's role in the community. When public health's role or purpose is not clearly understood by members of local government, then public health must be prepared to be blamed when negative issues arise. When members of local government and public health proactively work together to interact on issues, most negative outcomes can be prevented.

Failure to interact with the local government is often associated with a failure to interact with the media and the community at large. Negative situations become harder to overcome. The energy required to conduct damage control can easily outweigh the energy and resources required to build a positive interactive relationship with local government, the media, and the community in the first place.

CYCLES OF INTERACTION

Change is an element of both politics and public health. Responsibilities evolve as duties for individuals change over time. The interaction process is a cycle that is often laborious, but one that is necessary for the survival of public health.

Interaction with members of local government can be successful. The chances for success are increased when public health workers identify the cyclic processes that are inherent to each local government entity or office and to community demands. The process of interacting is more than merely discussing plans with someone new. Rather, it involves adopting an open-minded view of the issues. The interaction process, through the cycles of use, will become a venue for communicating on a broad variety of issues. To prevent lapses in communications due to natural cycles of interest, plan to communicate and remain active in the interaction process.

Local government members will accept assistance from public health during times of need, when attempting to enact a health-related ordinance or statute, when increasing efforts to bring a project to fruition, and during elections. The time immediately before an election and during the immediate post-election settling in period require the greatest amount of planning by public health if it is to remain connected with members of local government. One should interact with the local government as an entity, not as a collection of individuals. This concept of interacting with a group of people rather than with the same people on an individual basis is often muddled. When interacting, keep the issues on the table and focus on them. Avoid individual interests that may negatively affect the overall success of the process.

The natural cyclic nature of government is a positive trait. Cycles force the periodic examination of the programs administered by public health organizations. These cycles of change enable public health administrators to maintain a constant influence on interactions with local government officials.

CLEAR MESSAGES, VISIONS, AND MISSIONS

Successful interactions depend on valid information. The information relayed by members of a local health agency must be concise, clear, and represent the core values of public health. Mixed signals are often sent during interviews at the state and national levels. Local interactions rely on a smaller number of stakeholders from public health interacting with members of local government. The usual result is that a clear local message is sent and received. This is why public health organizations should work with representatives of state and federal governments who have offices in a local district. Conflicting issues will arise at the statewide level. Previous interactions with state legislators increase the chances that they will communicate with members of the community and with each other when decisions must be made for the issues at hand. Ideally, each local health department should develop an interactive relationship with members of local government and state legislators. This will facilitate the passage of public-health-driven issues and decrease the number of reactive responses.

A clear message, a clear vision, and a clear mission are vital for local government, the community, academia, industry, the media, and other stakeholders to embrace public health and ensure that its infrastructure is not only maintained but also rebuilt as needed. Interaction with local government is a process that involves an entire public health agency. Leaders must identify the political structure that is necessary to build this interaction. Leaders also must define the common denominators for success that will enable this interaction to grow and to become part of an organization's culture.

CONCLUSION

Experts define politics as the art of achieving results through a process of accommodation and compromise. In the United States, most government officials are elected. This defines the often-unstated priority for many politicians—reelection. Without reelection, there is no job continuity. Recognizing this fundamental aspect of government often helps to put some of the actions and activities of government officials into perspective.

The goals of elected political officials and public health agencies usually include improving the health and well-being of people living in the area served. Occasionally, an elected official will propose a public health program in an attempt to generate votes. If the proposed program is consistent with the goals of public health, it should be considered. If it is not consistent with an agency's goals or strategic plan, it should be carefully reviewed and discussed by a group of people representing diverse interests in the community.

Mutual support is a reasonable goal for agencies and elected officials. Nonsupport usually leads to future problems. Achieving a middle ground or compromise position requires tact. There are few absolute guidelines to offer on this subject. Each stakeholder (the public health administrator and the elected public official) has a short-term goal. These goals may differ. Over the long term, each stakeholder will require the support of the other to achieve good health for the population.

Returning to the case study, in the short term Bryan decided to meet with the county commissioners. He scheduled appointments with all five of them. Three of the meetings were pleasant and cordial. One seemed neutral at best; and one was difficult. The difficult meeting was with a commissioner who was not from Bryan's own political party. Bryan then looked up the terms for each commissioner. At that point, he decided that active participation in partisan politics might not be in the best interest of the health department.

Bryan cultivated relationships with all five commissioners. He spent extra time trying to find something in common with the commissioner from the opposite party. He purposely kept political discussions to a minimum. Bryan looked for venues in which the county commissioners could be seen as helping to improve community health. He sent regular updates to each commissioner.

At the end of his third year on the job, Bryan evaluated his position. The commissioners did not find him to be threatening. In fact, all accepted and respected him. Budgetary allocations for public health were increasing despite relatively austere economic conditions. The one fact that Bryan could not readily explain was his now-pleasant relationship with the difficult commissioner from the other party.

Resources

Periodicals

Barr, D., Fenton, L., and Edwards, D. 2004. Politics and health. *Quarterly Journal of Medicine* 97(2):61–62.

Fox, D.M., Kramer, M., and Standish, M. 2003. From public health to population health: How law can redefine the playing field. *Journal of Law and Medical Ethics* 34(4 Suppl):21–29.

Monson, A.Z., Hardy, G.E. Jr., and Thompson, E. 2003. Are we prepared for tomorrow's health challenges? *Journal of Law and Medical Ethics* 34(4 Suppl):33–38.

Ortolon, K. 2003. The carrot and the stick. *Texas Medicine* 99(10):43–46.

Books

Kraft, M.E.E., and Furlong, S.R. 2003. *Public Policy: Politics, Analysis, Alternatives.* Washington, D.C.: CQ Press.

Purdy, M., and Banks, D. 2003. *Sociology and Politics of Health.* New York: Taylor & Francis.

Web Sites

- State and Local Government on the Net: http://www.statelocalgov.net/index.cfm

Organizations

National Association of Counties
440 First Street NW
Washington, DC 20001
Phone: 202-393-6226
Web site: www.naco.org/

National Association of Towns and Townships
444 North Capitol Street, NW, Suite 397
Washington, DC 20001-1202
Phone: 202-624-3550
FAX: 202-624-3554
Web site: www.natat.org/

PART III

Managing Subordinates

CHAPTER 10

Fundamentals of Management: Theory and Applications

L. Fleming Fallon, Jr.

Chapter Objectives

After reading this chapter, readers will:

- Understand important management theories
- Appreciate basic organizational structures and concepts
- Apply span of control
- Construct planning aids

Chapter Summary

Skill in management is an absolute requirement for success as a health department executive. Management, in one form or another, is practiced by most people in their jobs almost every day. Even those in positions that are supervised and that require only the performance of repetitive tasks will find an understanding of management to be helpful. Knowledge of management improves relations between the people in an organization. Most professional employees are required to perform some managerial tasks. Because management is so pervasive, improved knowledge of managerial theory and practice will lead to enhanced job satisfaction and success.

The aim of this chapter is to delineate some basic concepts of management, both in theory and in actual practice. This chapter presents four theoretical models relating to management and motivation. In addition, some myths of motivation are considered. Developing supervisory skills and the importance of delegating responsibility are discussed. The chapter also considers the training and development of subordinates as well as the critical issue of fairness when interacting with others.

Case Study

The new health commissioner was adjusting her desk chair. It was her first day on the job. Her predecessor had been in the position for more than 20 years. The board told her that the department would not be difficult to run. During her interviews, she had heard rumors about how difficult the employees of the health department could be. She thought about running the department. No, she preferred to manage it. That might be difficult with almost 20 people reporting directly to the health commissioner. The public works division also might be a problem. The health department's budget seemed adequate, and the board said it would back her decisions. The problem of transforming the health department into a model organization occupied her thoughts. What advice would you offer to the new health commissioner?

FUNDAMENTAL GOALS AND ACTIVITIES OF MANAGEMENT

Citing a classic definition, management is one of the basic tools used to achieve the mission of an organization (March, 1958). One of the most fundamental aspects of any organization is its mission statement. The mission statement states why the organization exists. It delineates the activities that the organization will engage in. It provides a focus for all of the organization's activities.

Management provides the framework and basis for the system of controls needed to maintain any organization. The fundamental process of control is circular. Plans are made and elaborated. They are derived from the goals addressed in the organization's mission statement. Plans of action are devised to achieve these goals. The purpose of such plans is to translate goals into reality—to provide guidelines for the activities of an organization. Periodically, all plans should be subjected to review and audit. Were the objectives of the initial plan met? Were budgets and other resources sufficient? Did members of the organization work smartly and in concert to implement plans, or were efforts fragmented, overlapping, counterproductive, or ineffective? The results of this type of audit can be used to plan new strategies, programs, and activities or to modify existing ones. In this manner, the cycle of activities continues (**Figure 10-1**).

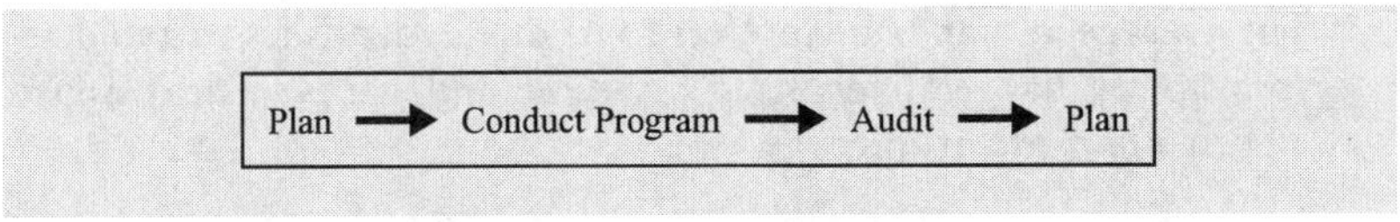

Figure 10-1 Cycles of Activities.

The process and techniques of forecasting are used to translate the abstract goals from the mission statement into realistic objectives for the organization. Forecasting methods vary in their sophistication. Frequently, an educated guess or hunch provides guidance for implementing the elements of an initial plan by giving actual values to forecast numbers. All too often, the same forecasting method is used in subsequent audits and reviews.

A slightly more sophisticated approach to forecasting involves either inflating present goals by a set percentage rate (often 10 percent, because this can be done mentally) or averaging the rate of recent growth to arrive at a future goal. Computing a moving average to account for recent trends is more accurate, but this approach is less frequently used. Other methods, such as regression equations, also exist. Such methods are infrequently employed by people who are not economists.

MANAGEMENT THEORIES

The most familiar form of organizational structure is the classic bureaucracy. This structure is widely used by governments, militaries, and churches and was first systematically described by Weber (Gerth, 1958). Bureaucratic theory states that regular duties are known to all; that there is a hierarchy of jobs, authority, and responsibility; and that written documents govern the conduct of the organization or institution. The advantage of a bureaucracy is that a rational code of conduct is substituted for rule by the whim of whoever is in charge. Bureaucracy also ensures that jobs are more likely to be distributed to individuals having specialized competence to handle them. The so-called "pecking order" found in most organizations is bureaucratic in nature.

Three major theories describe the attitudes and behavior of individuals toward subordinates within an organization. A widely discussed theory of human relations within an organization was suggested by Douglas McGregor (1967). It is commonly referred to as Theory X and is a traditional view of direction and control. Theory X has three major tenets:

1. The average human being has an inherent dislike of work and will avoid it if at all possible.
2. Because of this human characteristic of disliking work, most people must be coerced, controlled, directed, and threatened with punishment to get them to put forth adequate effort toward the achievement of organizational objectives.

3. The average human being prefers to be directed, wishes to avoid responsibility, has relatively little ambition, and wants security above all other considerations.

This theory is historically consistent with the attitudes of management and the rise of unions, vis-à-vis, the existence of an adversarial state between labor and management.

To some, Theory X seemed unduly harsh. Over the past four decades, alternative methods of management have evolved. More humanistic, they have been collected into theoretical form and labeled Theory Y. This theoretical position integrates individual and organizational goals. The assumptions of Theory Y can be summarized as follows:

1. The expenditure of physical and mental effort in work is as natural as play or rest.
2. External control and the threat of punishment are not the only means for bringing about effort toward achieving organizational objectives. Individuals will exercise self-direction and self-control in the service of objectives to which they are committed.
3. Commitment to objectives is a function of the rewards associated with their achievement.
4. Under appropriate conditions, an average human being learns not only to accept but also to seek responsibility.
5. The capacity to exercise a relatively high degree of imagination, ingenuity, and creativity in the solution of organizational problems is widely, not narrowly, distributed in the population.
6. Under the conditions of modern industrial life, the intellectual potentialities of an average individual are only partially utilized.

This theory reflects an attitude of trust on the part of employers. It implies that people are inherently ambitious and responsible rather than lazy and irresponsible. Theory Y has been implemented most frequently and successfully in managerial situations and in states having so-called sunshine laws that do not permit mandatory union membership as a condition of employment. Where older labor–management relationships continue, supervision using Theory Y tenets has been difficult to implement.

A recent theory of management has been imported primarily from Japan (Ouchi, 1981). Theory Z has not been as completely delineated as have the older theories. It extends many of the Theory Y notions relating to the inherent worth of people. With this theory, management makes longer-term commitments to its employees. It also expects a high degree of loyalty from them. Management sponsors activities and programs extending past working hours. There is a feeling of family among all parties. In Japan, it is uncommon for workers to change employers.

In some respects, Theory Z resembles the paternalism that was common in some U.S. companies in the mid 1800s. However, today the Theory

Z approach to management is not commonly used in the United States, although some firms have taken steps in that direction. A number of employers now provide employees with health clubs and physical fitness programs, daycare facilities, and other off-the-job activities. However, in the United States many employees frequently change jobs. One major firm that had a no-layoff policy was International Business Machines (IBM). Insiders and observers have both noted the strong corporate identification among workers at IBM was due, in part, to management's heightened attention to benefits for employees and their families, both on and off of the job. Competitive pressures and demands for productivity have reduced the implementation of Theory Z management in the United States.

The decline in the Japanese economy and the fall in the price of the yen have had strong impacts on Japan. Companies have started to lay off workers. The prevalence of Theory Z has been reduced as companies have reacted to competitive pressures.

John Stacey Adams (1965) proposed a theory of motivation that was based on the notion of equity. All individuals seek a fair balance between what they put into their jobs and what they get from them. Adams proposed that people form perceptions of fairness or balance by comparing their own situations with those of other colleagues. People are also influenced by partners, colleagues, or friends when they establish these benchmarks.

Inputs typically include attributes such as effort, skill, loyalty, hard work, commitment, ability, adaptability, flexibility, tolerance, determination, enthusiasm, trust in one's supervisor or superiors, support of colleagues and subordinates, and personal sacrifice. Outputs usually include tangible elements such as financial rewards, benefits, perquisites and pension arrangements, and intangibles such as recognition, praise, travel, promotion, training opportunities, a sense of achievement, and simple thanks. People need to feel that there is a reasonable balance between inputs and outputs. In short, people want to be treated in a fair and equal fashion.

If people feel that inputs are fairly and adequately rewarded by outputs, then they will feel happy in their work and motivated to continue inputting at the same level. Conversely, if people feel that their inputs outweigh the outputs, then they become unmotivated in relation to their jobs and employers. People respond to this feeling in different ways. In general, feelings of inequity are proportional to perceptions of the disparity between inputs and expected outputs. People will undertake actions to reestablish balance and equity. Some people reduce their levels of effort. They may become inwardly disgruntled or outwardly rebellious. Others try to improve their outputs by making demands for greater pay or seeking alternative employment. Equity theory can be summarized as follows:

1. Employees compare their inputs or personal value with the outcome received and mentally compute a personal input–outcome ratio that is compared with similar computations for other employees.
2. If employees perceive equity or feel that they are receiving a fair deal, they are content and may be further motivated to excel in their jobs.
3. When employees perceive inequity or injustice, they respond to the inequity by taking some action such as lowering productivity or output, reducing quality, increasing absenteeism, or seeking a different job.

Scientific management was systematically described by Frederick Taylor (1998). The concept of the most productive use of time is central to this theory. Time is managed by measuring the length of tasks with a stopwatch and then organizing a sequence of activities so as to minimize both extraneous motion and wasted time. The pace of an assembly line and its associated tasks are frequently organized by using scientific management principles. The theory's appeal is largely intellectual: minimizing wasted time and motion. Few executive or professional jobs lend themselves to this organizational principle.

Management and motivation are intertwined. Many important theories of motivation are discussed in Chapter 11.

MANAGERIAL STRUCTURE

The bureaucratic theory of organizational behavior also provides the most common model of managerial structure. Most organizations are hierarchical. Typically, several individuals report to a single supervisor. This is referred to as the *span of control.* Historically, the optimum span of control has been thought to be from three to seven individuals reporting to the same person. The advantage of this type of structure is that reporting relationships and supervisory responsibilities are clearly delineated. The disadvantages are that communications are frequently slowed and the organization is slow in responding to changing conditions. However, in the past few years, the span of control has increased in response to cost-cutting measures imposed by senior managers. It is not uncommon to find supervisors with 20 or more directly reporting subordinates in many U.S. businesses. In addition, the number of supervisory layers has also decreased.

APPLIED MANAGEMENT THEORY

The ability to delegate tasks is one of the most fundamental aspects of a successful manager. Some small organizations never grow significantly because the founder or head is unable to delegate work. Accepting this concept, it follows directly that subordinates and staff must be effectively employed. When possible, all should understand their departmental and organizational missions. Individual objectives should be linked to larger organizational goals.

It is important to distinguish between motivation and satisfaction. The former refers to the drive and effort required to attain a goal. The latter refers to the contentment derived when a goal has been met. The two can exist independently of each other. A more complete discussion of motivation theory is provided in Chapter 11. An effective manager understands what motivates each staff member. Then, to the extent possible within the organization, positions and tasks are structured to best utilize the skills and talents of individual employees.

Effective managers prepare their subordinates for promotion. Employee advancement is one indicator of managerial success. As part of the strategic planning process, many companies include succession planning for their employees. This process gathers results from individual testing and supervisor evaluations and then integrates them into the overall corporate goals.

Decision making is a key component of effective management. Although final decisions are frequently made by a single individual, input should be solicited from many sectors. It is useful to know the environment in which the decision will be made. Understanding the larger organizational milieu and culture is quite helpful. The implications of the decision must be weighed. Components to be considered may include the benefits that will be derived; economic, resource and opportunity costs; the mechanics of implementation and obstacles that may be encountered; political fallout; and future consequences at all levels. Alternatives should be subjected to the same scrutiny before being accepted or rejected. Each decision presents an opportunity for creativity. Within a complex organization, many decisions must be compromises. Compromise optimizes all the factors considered rather than maximizing a single aspect of the decision.

A health department is often, but not always, headed by a board of health. This body is responsible for and has final authority over the direction of the health department's affairs. It also has the responsibility to hire, evaluate, and discharge the health officer or health commissioner. The titles and eligibility requirements for health department leaders (health officer or commissioners) vary from state to state. Generally, a board will limit itself to establishing policy, reviewing progress and activities, and approving plans for the future.

PLANNING AIDS AND DEVICES

The timely completion of assignments is a prime ingredient in successful management. Managing and supervising progress are also important activities. To complete activities in a timely manner, individuals and organizations commonly use several planning aids. However, it is useful to understand planning and feedback cycles before any discussion of specific planning methods is undertaken. Detailed plans frequently are prepared on an annual basis. Many effective health departments have a five-year strategic plan that is annually reviewed and brought up-to-date.

The value of extensive strategic planning was questioned in the 1980s. However, the successful health departments that exist today are generally those that did not abandon strategic planning. Annual and strategic plans should be dynamic and well-used documents. Too often, they permanently reside on shelves after they are completed.

The clarity and specificity of plans increases as their time frame nears the present. As the time horizon in a plan approaches the present, the level of detail increases. Two common units of time are the quarter and year. Financial status is reported quarterly and summarized annually. Program success or failure is often measured quarterly so that programs can be modified before significant time elapses.

The simplest pictorial representation of the components required to complete a task is a time line (see **Figure 10-2**). With a time line, the different steps of a project are written down in chronological order. A slight refinement of this approach is to divide a line into equal time intervals and then note the events or activities on the line, with appropriately scaled space to represent the amount of time needed to complete the step. The time line is extremely simple to construct and is unambiguous. However, it only depicts order and does not show interrelationships and simultaneously occurring steps.

Henry L. Gantt developed an early pictorial system for use in planning and task allocation in the early part of the twentieth century (see **Figure 10-3**). Gantt recognized that overall program goals should be considered as a series of interrelated steps. He also appreciated the limitations of the time line. A Gantt chart depicts a series of events as bars that cross equal units of time on a chart. The advantage of a Gantt chart is that the manager gains a clear understanding of the timing and interrelationship of all of the component events of a project. One disadvantage is that the chart does not show dependent relationships between different project steps. However, the Gantt chart is both easy to construct and interpret.

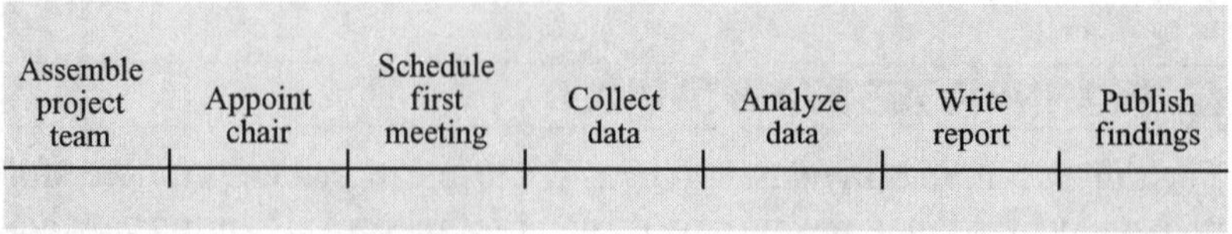

Figure 10-2 Time Line.

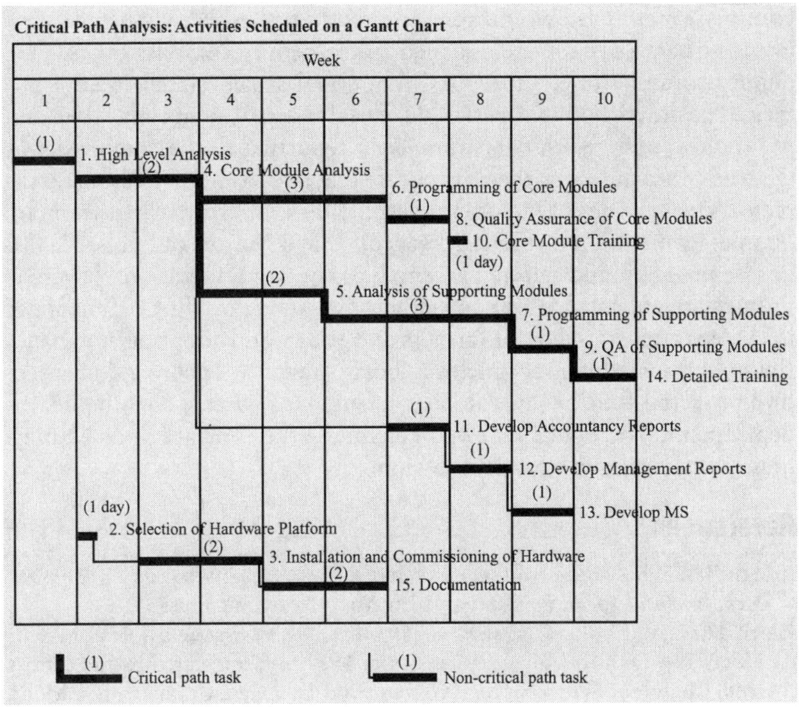

Figure 10-3 Gantt Chart with Critical Path

Source: MindTools http://www.mindtools.com/, 2003

CONCLUSION

Management is the art of utilizing all available resources to accomplish a given set of tasks in a timely and economical manner. A complete job description for a successful manager would include skill in diplomacy, coercion, politics, psychology, budgeting, evaluation, and a host of other attributes. Each individual manager evolves a personal style within an organizational culture. No two positions or individuals are exactly alike. A successful manager must be able to allocate resources and motivate subordinates to accomplish goals often imposed from external sources (i.e., upper management). A successful manager is one who understands the local organizational milieu as well as the larger environment in which it exists. The theories discussed in this chapter are only guidelines. Effective managers are a valuable asset to any organization in which they function.

Let's return to the opening case study. After reflecting for many minutes, the new health commissioner took out a pad and started to make notes. She would meet with the mayor and propose that public works be moved out of the health department. The mayor accepted her proposal. Next, she reconfigured the health department, appointing two deputy commissioners who would report directly to her. Newly established groups of employees were assigned to the deputy commissioners. One deputy commissioner supervised functional areas related to environmental health; the other supervised the health department clinic, the nursing service, and health educators. Also reporting to the commissioner were an office manager, the finance director, and the human resources director. Over the next year, she sent each of her subordinates to seminars on management. One voluntarily enrolled in a Master of Public Health degree program and selected an emphasis on administration. "There is the most logical candidate to replace me," she thought. The Commissioner led by example, striving for fairness and equity and adopting a managerial style that she later recognized as being similar to Theory Y. In her second year, the first of several large grants was awarded to the health department. The board renewed her three-year contract after 12 minutes of discussion in executive session.

References

Adams, J.S. 1965. Inequity in social exchange. In L. Berkowitz, ed., *Advances in Experimental Social Psychology.* New York: Academic Press.

Gerth, H.H., and Mills, C.W. (eds). 1958. *Max Weber: Essays in Sociology.* Fair Lawn, NJ: Oxford University Press, pp. 196–239, translated by the editors from Chapter 6, *Wirtschaft und Gesellschaft,* Tubingen, Germany: JCB Mohr, 1925. See Weber's essay "Bureaucracy."

March, J.G., and Simon, H.A. 1958. *Organizations.* New York: John Wiley and Sons.

McGregor, D. 1967. *The Professional Manager.* New York: McGraw-Hill.

Ouchi, W.G. 1981. *Theory Z: How American Business Can Meet the Japanese Challenge.* Reading, MA: Addison-Wesley.

Taylor, F.W. 1998. *Principles of Scientific Management.* New York: Engineering & Management Press (reprint of 1911 edition).

Resources

Periodicals

Bradley, E.H., Holmboe, E.S., Mattera, J.A., Roumanis, S.A., Radford, M.J., and Krumholz, H.M. 2003. The roles of senior management in quality improvement efforts: What are the key components? *Journal of Healthcare Management* 48(1):15–29.

Davis, J.A., Savage, G., and Stewart, R.T. 2003. Organizational downsizing: A review of literature for planning and research. *Journal of Healthcare Management* 48(3):181–201.

Gershon, H.J., and Jackson, W.C. 2003. The value of market research. *Journal of Healthcare Management* 48(3):152–155.

Gershon, H.J. 2003. Strategic positioning: Where does your organization stand? *Journal of Healthcare Management* 48(1):12–14.

Guo, K.L. 2003. An assessment tool for developing healthcare managerial skills and roles. *Journal of Healthcare Management* 48(6):367–376.
Mott, W.J. 2003. Developing a culturally competent workforce: A diversity program in progress. *Journal of Healthcare Management* 48(5):337–342.
Scott, G. 2003. The roles of the senior-level executive. *Journal of Healthcare Management* 47(1):9–12.

Books

Drucker, P.F. 2003. *Peter Drucker on the Profession of Management.* Cambridge, MA: Harvard Business School Publishing.
Drucker, P.F. 1999. *Management Challenges for the 21st Century.* New York: Harper.
Duncan, W.J., Swayne, L., and Ginter, P. 1997. *Handbook of Health Care Management.* Boston: Blackwell Publishing.
Dunn, R. 2002. *Haimann's Supervisory Management for Healthcare Organizations,* 7th ed. Chicago: Health Administration Press.
Hammon, J.L. 1998. *Fundamentals of Medical Management: A Guide for the New Physician Executive.* Tampa, FL: American College of Physician Executives.
Kovner, A.R., and Neuhauser, D. 2000. *Health Services Management: Readings and Commentary,* 7th ed. Chicago: Health Administration Press.
Rainey, H.G. 2003. *Understanding and Managing Public Organizations,* 3d ed. San Francisco: Jossey-Bass.
Shortell, S.M., and Kaluzny, A.D. 2000. *Essentials of Health Care Management.* Albany, NY: Delmar.

Web Sites

- Academy of Management:
  www.aomonline.org/
- American Health Information Management Association:
  www.ahima.org/
- Journal of Health Care Management:
  www.ache.org/PUBS/jhmsub.cfm
- Medical Group Management Association:
  www.mgma.com/
- Society for Human Resource Management:
  www.shrm.org/

Organizations

American College of Healthcare Executives
One North Franklin Street, Suite 1700
Chicago, IL 60606-4425
Phone: 312-424-2800
Fax: 312-424-0023
E-mail: ache@ache.org
Web site: www.ache.org/

American College of Physician Executives
4890 West Kennedy Blvd., Suite 200
Tampa, FL 33609
Phone: 800-562-8088 or 813-287-2000
Web site: www.acpe.org/

American Management Association
1601 Broadway
New York, NY 10019
Phone: 212-586-8100
Fax: 212-903-8168
Web site: www.amanet.org/index.htm

National Institute for Health Care Management Research and Educational Foundation
1225 19th Street, NW, Suite 710
Washington, D.C. 20036
Phone: 202-296-4426
Fax: 202-296-4319
E-mail: nihcm@nihcm.org
Web site: www.nihcm.org/

Public Health Foundation
1220 L Street, NW, Suite 350
Washington, D.C. 20005
Phone: 202-898-5600
Fax: 202-898-5609
E-mail: info@phf.org
Web site: www.phf.org/

CHAPTER

11

Organizational Behavior

L. Fleming Fallon, Jr.

Chapter Objectives

After reading this chapter, readers will:

- Understand the conceptual foundations of organizational behavior.
- Appreciate the history of organizational behavior.
- Describe structural factors related to organizational dynamics.
- Know how to work with informal groups in an occupational setting.
- Understand the strength of informal groups.
- Comprehend informal channels of communication.
- Apply organizational theory to resolve conflict.
- Recognize how politics can be understood using organizational theory.
- Know how to change the behaviors of organizational subordinates, peers, and supervisors.

Chapter Summary

This chapter presents the conceptual foundations of organizational behavior. Structural factors related to organizational dynamics are reviewed. The strength and mores of informal groups are discussed, as are informal channels of communication within an organization. Understanding organizational behavior provides useful methods for managing employees. Astute managers will study their employees as individuals and in groups, discern the idiosyncrasies and strengths of groups within their organizations, and use those insights to achieve agency goals.

Case Study

Pat was concerned. The health commissioner had asked Pat to form a task force to study the district's readiness with regards to bioterrorism. The names of several talented young staff members came to Pat's mind. However, they worked in different divisions of the health department. Pat's concern stemmed from observations of jealousy among employees. Budgetary restrictions had reduced the amount of raises that could be awarded. Staff in the epidemiology section had worked extensive amounts of overtime to complete a key report over the last few months. These staff members had forged strong ties during the project period. The commissioner had rewarded their efforts with salary increases that were larger than average for the department. Should all of the task force members be drawn from the epidemiology department? What would happen to the working relationship among the people who were not selected for the new task force? How would people in other departments feel about being passed over for inclusion on the task force team? This concern was especially acute among the group of rising stars. What advice would you give to Pat?

INTRODUCTION

Managers manage people. This is the norm for successful administrators. A successful manager understands people. However, simply knowing what makes people tick is only a portion of the information that must be mastered by a successful manager. Groups have their own dynamic patterns of behavior. Formal organizational structures exert an influence on the social aggregations of employees who work within them. Organizations are affected by interpersonal and intergroup factors. Positional or organizational authority is accompanied by the need to understand political factors. Unfortunately, understanding alone will not change people's behavior. A successful manager must be familiar with different theories and styles of leadership as well as methods of shaping the behavior of both individuals and groups.

From the perspective of a public health professional, organizational behavior can be defined as the study of how groups function and the psychological underpinnings contributing to that functioning. Many of the theories that have been developed to analyze and explain individual behavior have been applied to groups of people. Several of the following tenets concerning individual behavior are usually included as significant components of organizational behavior:

- **Causality.** Forces acting on people are responsible for human behavior. These forces can be internal or external to an individual. They can be due to the influence of genetics or the environment.

- **Directedness.** Human behavior is not only caused, it is also pointed toward something. This is referred to as being goal-directed (i.e., people want things).
- **Motivation.** As a result of analyzing underlying behavior, a push, want, need, drive, or motive can be found to explain most rational actions taken by individuals.

Each person has an individual constellation of behaviors. When individuals are combined into groups, the behaviors of the individual group members become summed. Even though they are the summation of personal behaviors, group behavior and group dynamics are not always similar to individual behaviors. It is important to review the determinants of individual behavior before attempting to explain the behavior of groups.

CONCEPTUAL FOUNDATIONS

Abraham Maslow (1943) made a major contribution to the understanding of individual behavior with his five-level hierarchy of needs. According to Maslow, the most basic needs of any individual are physiologic: air to breathe, water to drink, and food to eat. An organism must have all of the elements needed to exist. The next level of needs is concerned with safety. People require shelter and a feeling of protection from the physical elements of their environment. The third level of needs is concerned with love, affection, and belonging. Individuals want to be near and interact with other people. The importance of groups begins to emerge at this level.

The next higher level of needs is concerned with esteem, both from within an individual and within the external groups to which people belong. Individuals seek approval from others in their group. Self-esteem is based on personal capacity and achievement as well as respect received from others. Self-esteem arises from two needs. The first of these is an inner desire for strength, achievement, and independence. The second is a desire for recognition and appreciation by others. The highest level of need, the fifth level, is the need for self-actualization. Self-actualization refers to a desire for self-fulfillment and the reaching of one's full potential. Other researchers have formulated theories that attempt to define individual needs (Aldorfer, 1972; Rokeach, 1973). Although their individual components differ, most of the theories are hierarchical in nature.

An important contribution of Maslow's theory is the notion that needs must be satisfied in ascending order. Higher-level needs can only be addressed when all lesser or lower-level needs have been satisfied. The love and the approval of peers become less important as the time since one's last meal increases. Difficulties at home effectively displace feelings of self-fulfillment. These examples may seem trivial, but an astute manager tries to understand more about subordinates when problems develop than simply what has recently transpired on the job.

The sociologist Homans (1958) characterized social behavior as being an exchange. When in groups, people interact to receive a reward. Each person communicates with others in the group, and each tries to make a contribution to the group. In response, people in the group evaluate all contributions in light of the group's own norms of behavior. The members of the group, behaving in ways that are consistent with group norms, reward or punish the actions of individuals. Individuals react and either repeat the behavior (if it has been suitably rewarded) or adopt different behaviors in hopes of achieving a more satisfying reward. This behavior is similar to the operant conditioning paradigm postulated by Skinner (1953). Homans addresses the notions of conformity and the power of a group in shaping the behavior of its members. Applying these two theories, it becomes possible to direct the behavior of an individual by manipulating the group to which the individual belongs.

Whyte (1959) characterized organizational behavior with an interaction theory. Whyte's interaction theory has three main dimensions. First, interaction is synonymous with personal contact. Second, people interact when they engage in activities. Third, individuals have sentiments, the way they feel about the world around them. These three elements are fairly easy to quantify. Thus, change, which is a measurable deviation in any of the three elements, is quantifiable. Managers may find this theory useful in understanding the behavior of their subordinates and then initiating change. In an environment that increasingly relies on outcome measures, this theory has renewed appeal when applied to subordinates.

It is also helpful for managers to understand how to motivate individuals, because this information also contributes to predicting their behavior in groups. One major theoretical basis for understanding individual motivation has been elucidated by McGregor (1960, 1967). McGregor proposed two contrasting approaches to management: Theory X and Theory Y. The former assumes that people are inherently lazy and require both constant and close supervision to get them to produce. The latter asserts that people can and do assume responsibility for production and will reward management with increased production when they are allowed some measure of control over their own time and tasks. The implications for public health professionals applying McGregor's Theory Y are that individuals are able to accept responsibility over their jobs and will not abuse management's confidence when allowed a measure of autonomy and control. A Theory Z has been proposed by Ouchi (1981). This relates to the Japanese attitude of paternalism toward employees. Theory Z has been successful in Japan. However, it gained widespread but brief acceptance in the United States. Theory Z fell from favor when the Japanese economy faltered and American companies and organizations successfully increased productivity levels. These events occurred simultaneously in the 1990s. See Chapter 10 for a more complete discussion of Theories X, Y, and Z.

Another theoretical basis for motivation has been proposed by Herzberg (1966). In this paradigm, achievement, recognition, and the work itself bring satisfaction to individuals. These elements are called *motivators*. In contrast, some specific elements within the environment can bring dissatisfaction to individuals. These elements include interpersonal relations, company policy and administration, and working conditions. These elements are called *hygiene factors*. Two independent dimensions exist: (1) satisfaction and dissatisfaction and (2) motivation and hygiene. Because they are independent, less dissatisfaction does not result in more motivation. The fundamental implication for managers is that making jobs hygienic by improving working conditions, policies, or interpersonal relations only avoids dissatisfaction. When creating jobs that will motivate subordinates, supervisors will have to design jobs that satisfy intrinsically higher levels of needs.

STRUCTURAL FACTORS

An organizational structure and a hierarchy are necessary to effectively manage and coordinate the activities of large numbers of people. By their very nature, however, structure and hierarchy define and limit behavior.

The need for an organizational hierarchy has been both explained and justified by the concept of ownership. Ownership has a theoretical basis. All power and authority are vested in a company's owner. Because the Judeo–Christian tradition recognizes property as an extension of its owner, it is natural for an owner to unilaterally issue orders. Beginning with Adam Smith, classical economists have recognized that technology and the division of labor dictate the source and delegation of authority over the jobs of workers. Because the manager is the owner's appointee, authority still flows from the owner of the property.

Human differences due to cultural factors such as social class, caste, and prestige predate property. Such differences can also be used to explain the need for an organizational hierarchy. Using this approach, prudent people should be satisfied with their lot in life. This view was especially prevalent in nineteenth-century Europe. In the United States, the more popular explanation of class differences, leaders, and followers, was Social Darwinism (Hofstadter, 1992). Social Darwinism ascribed the evolution of control in an organization to a natural and random, rather than deliberate and non-random, process similar to the theory of evolution proposed by Charles Darwin in 1859. The theory of social Darwinism gradually fell from favor.

As corporations grew in number in America, the number of owners also increased. As ownership became increasingly disconnected and distant because of direct management through investment, the need for an organizational hierarchy became even more essential.

The evolution of a managerial structure is ultimately based on two fundamental needs. The first is the need to allocate people and jobs. Organizational effectiveness is not a result of all employees performing their tasks with equal ability. Employees have distinct differences in abilities and interests. Organizational effectiveness is due to people performing the jobs for which they are best suited. This requires that jobs are clearly defined and workers are assigned to the jobs for which they are most qualified.

The second need is that someone must be responsible for making unpopular decisions. The people who make these decisions must be differentiated from others in the organization on the basis of position and reward. The reward may be in terms of power, prestige, or psychological satisfaction other than money, but it must be present. The present-day system of rewards based on risk and responsibility has evolved from these fundamental needs of organizations.

The most common type of organization is the bureaucracy, or pyramidal hierarchy. In such a structure, authority flows downward from the top, and lines of communication are clearly delineated. Another form of organization is a matrix. The matrix structure brings together people with specific skills for specific short-term tasks or projects. When the task is completed, the people are reassigned to other groups who may need their particular skills or expertise. This is effective in some settings (primarily research and project-oriented operations), but it is difficult to administer and lines of communication can become blurred. Organizational structures are discussed in more detail in Chapters 5 and 10.

Once a hierarchical structure has been established, mechanisms are needed to support and maintain it. These mechanisms are management controls. They comprise a set of rules for operation and consist, in part, of objectives, plans, policies, and procedures. All organizations must have a purpose for existence or a mission. Goals and objectives should support the organization's mission. Strategic and detailed plans are formulated for different time periods in the future, becoming more detailed as their time frame approaches the present. Policies and procedures are a set of guidelines for day-to-day operations. Their purpose is to eliminate ambiguity and discrimination when interacting with employees. They provide guidance for managers in unfamiliar areas of organizational or agency operations. Frequently, these are collected and published and then made available to all employees (e.g., personnel policies, company handbooks outlining medical and insurance benefits). Individual departments may have internal procedure manuals that are used by department members. Examples of groups frequently having departmental policies include information systems, accounting and finance, medical, and legal. Job or position descriptions are control documents; they define the content and expected output from position incumbents.

Control does have a number of negative aspects. Once control has been established and accepted, standing plans and managerial protocols tend to limit organizational flexibility and individual initiative. It requires effort to keep policies, procedures, and controls up to date. The magnitude of this task is in direct proportion to the size of an organization. Existing policies may not apply to new conditions, and controls may relate to outdated or irrelevant factors. Rational plans that were developed to promote effectiveness may begin to interfere with the accomplishment of organizational objectives. A dynamic balance between spontaneity and control must be maintained. Effective managers frequently review control mechanisms to ensure that they continue to be timely, relevant, and effective.

Within every organization, tension exists between change and stability. To ensure effective interpersonal relations and efficient production, relative organizational stability is highly desirable. Without such stability, the advantages of the specialized division of labor are not realized, cooperative human relationships are hindered, and organizational control is handicapped. Within any organization, jobs are interdependent. The evolution of the process for replacing present job incumbents should be ongoing and is called succession planning. This planning may also be used to assist individuals in career advancement and preparation for future promotion. Department heads often maintain lists of potential candidates for key positions within their own functional areas. This minimizes organizational disruption when an individual vacates a position.

INFORMAL ORGANIZATIONS

Informal groups exist within the fabric of most formal organizations. These are usually peer groups. Each group has individual indicators of status and prestige. These have implications for a manager. A peer group serves three functions for an individual:

1. It satisfies complex needs.
2. It offers emotional support when identifying oneself and dealing with the world.
3. It assists in meeting personal goals.

Research has shown that employees who have minimal or no opportunity for social contact while on the job often find their work to be unsatisfying (Festinger, 1950; Mayo, 1946; Roy, 1960). The organizational cost of this lack of satisfaction can be measured in terms of low production, high turnover, and excess absenteeism. Personal self-image is derived, in large measure, from social image. A group provides its members with a guide to correct behavior. This is not correctness in terms of organizational written policies, but rather in terms of what is actually acceptable to the group.

Identification with the group is important. An individual has difficulty in holding out against the weight of an otherwise unanimous group judgment even when the group is clearly in error (Maslow, 1943). In an organizational setting, the group can assist individuals in solving specific problems and protect them from making mistakes. Individuals prefer to receive guidance, advice, and assistance from peers rather than supervisors or managers. As a bonus, the ability to render assistance often becomes a source of prestige for the giver. Hospital staff members provide a good example of this phenomenon. Attending physicians, medical residents, and nurses have their own informal rules of conduct, private jokes, and guidelines for seeking assistance. Nonconformity is punished by extra duty or withholding help during busy periods.

Groups usually refer to small numbers of individuals. A classic definition is provided by Berelson and Steiner (1964):

> A group is an aggregate of people, from two up to an unspecified but not too large a number. These individuals associate with each other in face-to-face relations over an extended period of time. They differentiate themselves in some regard from others around them. Finally, they are mutually aware of their membership in the group. (p. 47)

Membership in a group is related to both technology and the pace of work. Some type of physical closeness and an opportunity to communicate must exist before people can form mutually interacting groups. Sayles and Strauss (1966) described the progression of group development and how informal or group patterns of behavior evolve. Employees form friendship groups based on their contacts at work, the technological equipment that they use, and their common interests. These groups arise out of the fabric of an organization. However, once these groups have been established, they develop a life of their own that is almost completely separate from the working situations from which they emerged. This is a dynamic, self-generating process. After being brought together by the formal structure of an organization, employees begin to interact with one another. Increasing opportunities for interaction tend to create favorable sentiments toward fellow group members. In turn, these attitudes become the foundation for an increased variety of activities. Many of these are not specified by job descriptions. Some examples of these behaviors include special lunch arrangements, trading of job duties, fights with those outside of the group, and gambling on paycheck numbers. These increased opportunities for interaction build stronger bonds of identification. The group becomes something more than simply a collection of people. It develops customary ways of doing things. It evolves a set of stable characteristics that become very difficult to change or modify. In other words, the group becomes an organization in itself.

Members of many professional groups are able to differentiate themselves on the basis of clothing or other signs of elite status. Physicians frequently display stethoscopes prominently around their necks or wear surgical scrubs outside of a hospital. Nurses often wear their nursing school pins as decoration on clothing other than uniforms. Doctors use medical jargon as a means of establishing and maintaining group identity. The long hours worked by junior hospital staff often are a source of pride and an indicator of status within the group. Symbols of group membership and status do not end with the completion of residency training; they merely become more subtle. Board certification, professional recognition, academic rank, and the number of publications are all indicators of relative status.

Informal channels of communication also develop within the group (Fallon, 1974). These channels occur outside of normal, or formal, organizational channels. Informal channels are both effective and long-lived. Individuals use them to talk about ideas, share discoveries, and discuss common problems. Informal channels frequently cross established organizational or company boundaries and are relatively common among professionals. Researchers from different universities or medical centers often share ideas and data. Health commissioners in adjacent districts may share ideas or outcomes. Local health officers discuss common regional problems with each other at regional and national conferences. These contacts frequently provide professional support and reinforcement that might otherwise be unavailable due to the fact that professionals working on similar problems have offices that are situated in different locations.

Managers assign duties to individuals that are part of their job responsibilities. In theory, a manager should only be concerned that an assigned task is accomplished effectively and efficiently. However, other forces and factors can and do emerge. People usually like or dislike the people with whom they work; they are rarely neutral. These feelings encourage people to establish communications and perform activities with others in a variety of informal and usually unplanned patterns. An astute manager must understand and interact with these patterns to be optimally effective on the job.

The personal need for affiliation and group membership is well established. Yet once mutual relations and group standings have been established, many individuals become competitive and want to be perceived as having a higher status than their peers. Most people espouse equality, but as George Orwell (1946) stated, "Some want to be more equal than others." Prestige and status are frequently defined as sets of unwritten rules about the conduct that people are expected to show in the presence of others. Even within a small informal group, subtle differences in status begin to emerge.

There are two types of factors that are relevant to status: external and internal. External factors refer to influences that are brought to the workplace from the outside. These commonly include age, gender, race, education, and seniority. Internal factors are often consciously created when senior management creates and defines an organization. Titles, job descriptions, perquisites, offices, work schedules, mobility, and methods of evaluation all influence informal social structures. The title "Doctor" may sufficiently differentiate medical group members from other employees of a health department or health care organization. It does not perform this function in a university setting. It is interesting to note that within a strictly medical or health-related organization, the traditional signs of power and prestige are usually operative: office size, windows and their view, access to executive dining rooms, reserved parking, and the like. The same is true in university settings.

An effective manager must understand informal groups. If the group's basic attitude toward a company is positive, informal expectations can greatly assist management. A manager cannot treat people solely as individuals. It is particularly important to have an understanding of the relationship between formal and informal status systems and the impact of technology on informal social systems.

Difficulty is created for management when formal organizational goals or structures conflict with informal structures or status. This can happen when management's evaluation of positions or jobs does not correspond with the evaluation of the group. When this occurs, a manager must assume one of two extreme positions. The first is to rearrange the formal organization, policies, and procedures to accommodate the desires of the informal group. The second is to alter the norms or composition of the informal group. Compromise between these extremes is easier to accomplish. Conflict of this type is less common in professional settings than in blue-collar environments. Nevertheless, managers must be alert for it and seek methods of resolution that will have a minimal impact on the accomplishment of organizational goals and objectives and on the employees involved.

CONFLICT

When there is interdependence, the parties involved must establish relationships across boundaries—between individuals and among groups. This process is deliberate. It is an interaction of two or more social units that are attempting to define or redefine the terms of their interdependence. Stress and conflict frequently accompany such interactions. Three distinct types of conflict are of interest to the professional manager: interpersonal, intergroup, and specialist versus generalist.

Interpersonal conflict is probably the least important but most exaggerated type of friction. Managers often blame organizational problems on individual personalities or personnel incompetence. The traditional psychological explanation for interpersonal conflict is frustration. Thwarted individuals seek alternative methods to overcome their frustrations. In this process, they disrupt the normal activities of an organization. However, poorly structured organizational channels of communication frequently contribute to interpersonal conflict.

Organizational structure determines the flow of communications. A conscientious manager whose subordinates have interpersonal problems will benefit from a review of the organization's structure and workflow patterns. Individuals quickly grow tired of and resent communications that flow only in one direction. Similarly, subordinates are slow in adjusting to unexpected and uncontrollable changes in routine.

Unpredictability can also result from technological innovations as well as from modifications in organizational structure and policy. Stress is increased and subordinates become aggravated if change implies a status relationship that is different from one that was previously accepted. Stress is also amplified if change is unilaterally imposed without prior notice or consultation or if individuals perceive no functional or technological reason for change. When changes are necessary, a prudent manager informs subordinates early in the process and, if feasible, allows them to participate in decisions that affect their jobs or working conditions.

Intergroup conflict exists primarily between different interest groups within an organization, such as management, employees, and other work groups. Groups can be categorized as apathetic, erratic, strategic, or conservative. Apathetic groups are least likely to exert concentrated pressure on management. Their members are usually not very cohesive, and any group leadership is widely distributed. Erratic groups display inconsistent behavior towards management. Strategic groups are shrewd, carefully calculating how to apply pressure. They never tire of objecting to unfavorable management decisions or seeking loopholes in contract clauses and existing policies that will be beneficial to them. They continually compare their benefits to those of other departments within the company. Conservative groups are composed of elite members who are secure and powerful. They typically possess critical skills.

The success enjoyed by informal groups when bargaining with management is partially dependent on the internal strength or cohesion of the group. Cohesion assists the members in pursuing group goals. Members who engage in a common effort can strengthen cohesion. Cohesion has six dimensions: homogeneity, communication, isolation, size, outside pressure, and group status. Homogeneity reinforces a basic reason for the existence of many groups: Individuals seek out others who are similar to themselves. Groups having members with different backgrounds and interests are frequently ineffective in promoting their own particular interests. Competition between individuals can reduce group cohesion; stable group membership increases it.

Group members must be able to talk with each other. Lack of privacy and opportunity for discussion hinders group development. Both researchers and cartoonists have noted this when they discuss cubicles. The widely used partitions of contemporary offices are less expensive than permanent walls. They also tend to reduce group development and solidarity. Isolation of all group members from other employees promotes group solidarity, whereas isolation of individuals retards group solidarity. Small departments tend to be more closely knit than large ones, because larger groups tend to have fewer opportunities for informal communication and are more heterogeneous. This encourages fractionation into smaller cliques. This has the effect of creating small groups that offer more opportunities for group membership and interaction.

Under organizational pressure, communications among peers (lateral communication) tend to increase. Concurrently, communications between different levels of management (vertical communication) tend to decrease. Personal differences become minimized when presented with the threat of a common danger such as a tough supervisor. Strong management policies toward personnel may encourage the formation of strong informal groups to deal with the pressure. Finally, individuals prefer to identify with high-status groups.

The increasingly complex nature of modern health care organizations, the use of complex technological tools and concepts, and the need to increase productivity have contributed to the growth and importance of technological and clinical specialists. By definition and training, these individuals have advanced skills and specific knowledge. To the extent that supervisors lack these technical skills, they must carefully manage their subordinates. To be successful in their own supervisory positions, managers must rely heavily on specialists.

In contrast is the generalist. This is an individual who knows something about many positions but frequently not enough to displace a specialist. The generalist may not be a member of the specialists' group due to a lack of esoteric knowledge. The generalist is usually more expendable, thus having less job security. The generalist may have to use means other than technical knowledge to maintain a position, perhaps using the output of subordinates and politics. The traditional equation of authority with responsibility is less clear. This leads to problems in supervising and managing others. A subordinate is often unable to go to the supervisor for assistance with a technical problem. This can lead to resentment and feelings that the boss is incompetent. This notion was suggested almost a half century ago: The most symptomatic characteristic of modern bureaucracy is the growing imbalance between ability and authority (Thompson, 1963).

It is interesting to note the reversal of roles for specialists and generalists in contemporary health care. Generalists often have greater value to managed care systems than do specialists. They are the gatekeepers. Yet, they continue to be paid at lower rates than specialists.

Disputes over jurisdiction or turf have historically been common in public health organizations as different groups have tried to decide which one would assume the responsibility for leading a particular initiative or program. The historical result has been an informal arrangement known as a consultation. In addition to providing specialized expertise, a consultation serves an organizational need, allowing individuals to legitimately tread on the turf of others. The contemporary reality is that members of the same organization often provide consultations to each other, thus reducing turf infringements.

POLITICS

Political science is infrequently applied to group dynamics, yet it can make important contributions to understanding organizational behavior. In large organizations, human behavior responds to political variables, particularly authority. Analysis of motivation coupled with political explanations can be used to understand why systems of authority arise and why people continue to comply with their dictates. Before discussing applications, it is useful to understand what comprises authority. Most authority systems typically have five attributes:

1. It is deep seated, perhaps innate to the very being of either an individual or organization.
2. It is a system in which relatively few individuals make decisions for relatively many people.
3. Decisions are made on the basis of two different methods: standing and ad hoc. The former is carried out over a period of time and may affect many people. The latter is either an interpretation of existing or standing decision policies or is made because no explicit guidelines exist.
4. Decisions are communicated from managers to subordinates, who then implement them.
5. Subordinates will react to commands. Generally, they tend to obey. They may opt to disobey, but will incur sanctions or pay a price for this privilege.

Most small groups develop a system of customs and norms. Specific individuals emerge as leaders in the sense that group members accept their suggestions. Leadership may be accepted due to a leader's charisma. Another reason for acceptance of the leader is due to the leader's wisdom or judgment acquired from previous successful decisions or leadership experiences. Subordinates may obey because an individual has a particular position or office, and power is perceived as emanating from the position. Personal status and authority tend to reinforce each other. Finally, most cultures instill an ethic that individuals ought to obey both laws and persons of legitimate authority. In public health organizations, formal and informal hierarchies of power and status are frequently dissimilar.

Behavioral compliance can be analyzed in terms of rewards and penalties. Positive rewards make an individual feel good or provide desired actions or objects such as money, status, prestige, position, special treatment, or advancement. Negative rewards tend to be given in a hierarchy of increasing coercion with repeated applications. For example, if an individual does not react to a verbal suggestion, it is usually put into writing. A fine or suspension may follow the continued ignoring of suggestions or orders. Expulsion from the organization is the ultimate sanction.

It must be remembered that loss of a job means not only loss of income, but also the loss of group affiliation and personal self-esteem. People also obey commands to the degree that they have fear of or anxiety toward the organization issuing the orders. For most people, a job is more than simply a paycheck.

Peers cause another form of anxiety within an organization by exerting peer pressure. Individuals accept control by managers and executives because this also brings acceptance by the group. It is not unusual for peer pressure to be greater than organizational pressure. An adult with a family to support who quits a job but retains the respect of the informal group is not much different than a teenager who engages in deviant or rebellious behavior to keep the support of the peer group.

Peer pressure is especially powerful in public health care settings. Nonconformers may find themselves with unpleasant or difficult tasks to perform without the usual support or relief from other members of the group. Rival groups also can exert pressure. An individual who habitually abuses other colleagues usually gets neither resources nor assistance when help is needed with a project or program.

CHANGING ORGANIZATIONAL BEHAVIOR

Thus far, this chapter has been concerned with describing organizational behavior from both theoretical and experiential bases. However, knowledge must be applied for it to gain utility. This section addresses how a manager or supervisor can achieve changes in the behavior of peers and subordinates. Changes can be wrought by taking direct action, working through political channels, or by modifying the organization's structure.

One key form of direct intervention is leadership. Different names for this concept drift in and out of vogue. At different times in the past, all of the following have had periods of intense popularity: management by democracy (Tannenbaum and Schmidt, 1958); management by objectives (Drucker, 1974); Theory Y integration and self-control (McGregor, 1960); sensitivity training (Tannenbaum, Wechsler, and Massarik, 1961); and management by walking around (Peters and Waterman, 1982; Peters and Austin, 1987). The common denominator in all of these approaches is personal participation and interest in the affairs of one's subordinates.

Effective leaders are able to motivate their subordinates to think about problems they may encounter. As subordinates develop competence in their tasks, their self-esteem improves. Employees also learn to expect and receive respect from both supervisors and peers. Effective managers also promote good attitudes about the organizations in which they lead. Further, they continually review various aspects of their organization so that they can intercept and address problems before they grow and become insurmountable. An effective supervisor will discuss the details of a new program or project in advance rather than allowing an intern or inexperienced employee to look foolish at a meeting of senior managers.

Successful managers and supervisors also help to promote the careers of their subordinates. This includes both formal and informal ongoing training. Managers should project clear career paths for their subordinates. Within the limits of opportunity allowed by an organization, formal career paths should exist. Successful leaders understand that helping subordinates to succeed will reflect positively on themselves.

The essence of politics is achieving compromise and getting results. Organizations also seek positive results. Earlier in the chapter we delineated the behavioral dynamics of groups. A politically astute manager understands these rules of behavior and utilizes them for the benefit of an entire organization. This may involve establishing closer working relationships with informal leaders to improve the output of the entire group. Alternatively, it may mean promoting some goals of the group to rally support for a desired organizational goal. This must be done within the discretionary limits and guidelines allowed by the larger organization. This may also involve working behind the scenes to set the stage so that subordinates are allowed to shine. The possibilities are limited only by organizational guidelines, personal ethical standards, and individual imagination.

A final class of changes involves alterations to the existing formal structure of an organization. Such alterations may involve changes in authority, job duties, and responsibilities; modification of communication channels; and the alteration of the physical conditions of work.

Traditional management theory assumes an outward-looking posture and states that the job of a manager is to achieve common objectives using available resources within an allotted amount of time. However, this view of management is changing. Experts are urging that managers have more input into the development of organizational objectives and seek out and utilize any and all available resources within an organization (Rainey, 2003).

Consistent with this altered approach of shifting the responsibility for dealing with stress, contemporary managers must assume the task of absorbing and preventing stress. An important goal is to maintain organizational equilibrium. It is a manager's responsibility to design and adjust the work relationships of individuals so structural problems do not interfere with the effective performance of an organization. Frequently, simple changes of personnel can solve minor problems.

Finding an appropriate position and then placing a problem employee into it can be beneficial for both the sending and receiving group. Simply handing an unwanted employee to someone else will generate a group or organizational reputation that is likely to outlive the individual doing the dumping. Encouraging and maintaining open and appropriate communications between subordinates (laterally) and with supervisors (vertically) will improve managerial success. Years ago, observers noted that poor managers were characterized by either very high or very low levels of interaction relative to the usual level for a given position and organization (Richardson, 1961). Effective managers tend to spend more time responding to their subordinates and associates. They are more readily available and receive more contact from their subordinates (Rainey, 2003).

A key component of any manager's duties is to plan and modify the structure and flow of work to minimize any stressful patterns or factors that may hinder effective performance by individual workers. This may involve the use of organizational or physical buffers. If there are obvious external differences in the behavior or working conditions of two groups, it is sensible to limit interactions to the telephone, e-mail, and other electronic media. A manager must maintain a comfortable rhythm in the workflow of subordinates. This may involve scheduling, sheltering, or coaching subordinates. Workloads should be equitably designed and distributed. In the current climate of task specialization and electronic isolation, managers all too often react to the pressures of senior organizational leaders and simply demand increased output from their subordinates. Successful managers are careful not to routinely expect levels of production from their subordinates that they would be unwilling or unable to produce themselves.

SUMMARY

The pace and flow of work as well as the administrative processes by which they are controlled are fundamental for organizational success. Organizations have been characterized as being a system of relationships (Chapple and Sayles, 1962). Organization involves applying systems thinking and utilizing appropriate technology. Each organization is a collection of processes, procedures, policies, controls, formal authority structures, and leadership techniques. Among groups of organizations, it is unusual for changes in sentiment to precede changes in action or organizational rearrangement. Technology and organizational structures must be changed before group norms and values are likely to be successfully modified or altered.

This chapter has outlined various organizational theories and structures. The components of each have been examined and potential problems identified. Many lines have been devoted to understanding group dynamics and behavior. In addition to understanding one's subordinates and peers, an effective manager understands the organizational forces that exist in a local working environment. A willingness to listen to subordinates as well as superiors, to communicate using multiple methods, to be open to innovation, and to exhibit positive leadership traits should result in both effective and rewarding experiences as a manager.

Returning to the opening case study, Pat listened to the advice of two other experienced supervisors and then took the following actions. A description of the task force's duties and responsibilities was circulated among all health department personnel. All employees interested in working on the temporary task force were asked to write a single page letter indicating their interest, qualifications, and any special reasons why they should be selected. Members of the board of health were asked to rank the applicants for the task force. Information about this process had been given to employees. It accompanied the original letter that described the task force's activities. Pat made an effort to form two other temporary project task forces. Employees were allowed to participate on only one task force. Pat also included employees in a series of joint meetings with members of the health board to review and revise departmental goals. Over the course of a year, Pat included everyone who wanted to participate in some venue and succeeded in redirecting the focus of the employee groups to the mission and goals of the health department.

References

Aldorfer, C.P. 1972. *Existence, Relatedness, and Growth: Human Needs in Organizational Settings.* New York: Free Press.

Berelson, B., and Steiner, G. 1964. *Human Behavior—an Inventory of Scientific Findings.* New York: Harcourt, pages 325–334.

Chapple, E.D., and Sayles, L.R. 1962. *The Measure of Management.* New York: Macmillan.

Drucker, P.F. 1974. *Management: Tasks, Responsibilities, Practices.* New York: Harper and Row.

Fallon, L.F., Covitch, S.C., and Rothenberg, D.H. 1974. A study of informal information sources in an academic community. *Proceedings of the American Society for Information Science Annual Meeting* 11:260–263.

Festinger, L., Schacter, S., and Back, K. 1950. *Social Pressures in Informal Groups.* New York: Harper and Row.

Herzberg, F. 1966. *Work and the Nature of Man.* Chicago: World.

Hofstadter, R. 1992. *Social Darwinism in American Thought.* Boston: Beacon Press.

Homans, G.C. 1958. Social behavior as exchange. *American Journal of Sociology* 62(5):597–606.

Maslow, A.H. 1943. A theory of human motivation. *Psychological Review* 50(4):370–396.

Mayo, E. 1946. *The Human Problems of an Industrial Civilization.* Cambridge, MA: Graduate School of Business Administration, Harvard University.

McGregor, D. 1960. *The Human Side of Enterprise.* New York: McGraw-Hill.

McGregor, D. 1967. *The Professional Manager.* New York: McGraw-Hill.

Orwell, G. 1946. *Animal Farm.* New York: New American Library.

Ouchi, W.G. 1981. *Theory Z: How American Business Can Meet the Japanese Challenge.* Reading, MA: Addison-Wesley.

Peters, T., and Auston, J. 1987. *A Passion for Excellence: The Leadership Difference.* New York: Harper and Row.

Peters, T., and Waterman, R.H. 1982. *In Search of Excellence: Lessons from America's Best-run Companies.* New York: Harper and Row.

Rainey, H.G. 2003. *Understanding and Managing Public Organizations,* 3d ed. San Francisco: Jossey-Bass.

Richardson, F. L.W. 1961. Talk, work and action. *Society of Applied Anthropology* monograph 3.

Rokeach, M. 1973. *The Nature of Human Values.* New York: Free Press.

Roy, D.F. 1960. Banana time—job satisfaction and informal interaction. *Human Organizations* 18(3):158–168.

Sayles, L.R., and Strauss, G. 1966. *Human Behavior in Organizations.* Englewood Cliffs, NJ: Prentice-Hall, pages 89–104.

Skinner, B.F. 1953. *Science and Human Behavior.* New York: Macmillan.

Tannenbaum, R., and Schmidt, W. H. 1958. How to choose a leadership pattern. *Harvard Business Review* 2(2):95–101.

Tannenbaum, R., Wechsler, I., and Massarik, F. 1961. *Leadership and Organization.* New York: McGraw-Hill.

Thompson, V. 1963. *Modern Organizations.* New York: Knopf.

Whyte, W. F. 1959. An interaction approach to the theory of organizations. In Haire, M. (ed), *Modern Organization Theory,* pages 155–183. Boston: Wiley.

Resources

Periodicals

Barrere, C., and Ellis, P. 2002. Changing attitudes among nurses and physicians: A step toward collaboration. *Journal for Healthcare Quality* 24(3):9–15.

Crow, S.M., and Hartman, S. J. 2003. Responding to threats of workplace violence: The effects of culture and moral panic. *Health Care Management* (Philadelphia, PA) 22(4):340–348.

Dowd, S.B., and Root, A. 2003. The hospital manager and game theory: Chess master, poker player, or cooperative game player? *Health Care Management* (Philadelphia, PA) 22(4):305–310.

Jameson, C. 2003. Helping people change: The magic of motivation. *Journal of the Oklahoma Dental Association* 94(2):16–29.

Levin, R.P. 2003. Leadership skills and team development. Part III of the dental management pyramid series. *American Journal of Dentistry* 16(5):359–360.

Lipcamon, J.D. 2003. Managing change within the healthcare environment. *Radiology Management* 25(6):20–25.

McConnell, C.R. 2003. Accepting leadership responsibility: preparing yourself to lead honestly, humanely, and effectively. *Health Care Management* (Philadelphia, PA) 22(4):361–374.

Terry, P.E. 2003. Leadership and achieving a vision—How does a profession lead a nation? *American Journal of Healthcare Promotion* 18(2):162–167.

Books

Brimson, J.A., and Antos, J. 1998. *Activity-Based Management for Service Industries, Government Entities, and Nonprofit Organizations*. Boston: Wiley.

Greenberg, J., and Baron, R.A. 2002. *Behavior in Organizations: Understanding and Managing the Human Side of Work*, 8th ed. Upper Saddle River, NJ: Prentice-Hall.

Greenberg, J. 2004. *Managing Behavior in Organizations,* 4th ed. Upper Saddle River, NJ: Prentice-Hall.

Locke, E.A. 2003. *Blackwell Handbook of Principles of Organizational Behavior.* Boston: Blackwell.

Potterfield, T.A. 1999. *The Business of Employee Empowerment: Democracy and Ideology in the Workplace.* Westport, CT: Greenwood Publishing Group.

Schermerhorn, J.R., Hunt, J.G., and Osborn, R.N. 2002. *Organizational Behavior*, 8th ed. Boston: Wiley.

Web Sites

- Donald R. Clark:
  www.nwlink.com/~donclark/leader/leadob.html
- Human Resources Internet Guide:
  www.hr-guide.com/
- Journal of Organizational Behavior:
  www.jstor.org/journals/08943796.html
- Organization Development Network:
  www.odnetwork.org/
- Organizational Development Institute:
  members.aol.com/odinst/index.htm
- Society for Industrial and Organizational Psychology:
  www.siop.org/

Organizations

American College of Healthcare Executives
One North Franklin Street, Suite 1700
Chicago, IL 60606-4425
Phone: 312-424-2800
Fax: 312-424-0023
E-mail: ache@ache.org
Web site: www.ache.org/

American Management Association
1601 Broadway
New York, NY 10019
Phone: 212-586-8100
Fax: 212-903-8168
Web site: www.amanet.org/index.htm

American Psychological Association
750 First Street, NE
Washington, D.C. 20002-4242
Phone: 800-374-2721 or 202-336-5510
Web site: www.apa.org/

American Psychological Society
1010 Vermont Avenue, NW, Suite 1100
Washington, D.C. 20005-4907
Phone: 202-783-2077
Fax: 202-783-2083
E-mail: aps@psychologicalscience.org
Web site: www.psychologicalscience.org/

The Society for Organizational Learning
955 Massachusetts Ave., Suite 201
Cambridge, MA 02139
Phone: 617-300-9500
Fax: 617-354-2093
E-mail: info@solonline.org
Web site: www.solonline.org/

CHAPTER

12

Position Descriptions

L. Fleming Fallon, Jr.
Joseph A. Diorio, Jr.

Chapter Objectives

After reading this chapter, readers will:

- Understand the importance of a properly prepared position or job description.
- Know how to conduct a position analysis.
- Appreciate the contribution made by a position's incumbent.
- Know the components of a position description.
- Know how to create a position description.

Chapter Summary

Position descriptions are the documents upon which the operations and activities of any organization are based. They should support the mission, goals, and objectives of the organization that creates them. All job descriptions in an organization should use the same format and language. Well-written position descriptions include clearly delineated duties and responsibilities and describe compensable factors such as the level of responsibility, the number of persons supervised, the resources controlled, and the experience and minimum level of education needed to successfully complete the job.

Case Study

The health officer of a large suburban health department was planning for the future. The board had discussed creating a new position for someone to conduct training. One of the sanitarians had just completed a Master of Public Health degree. According to departmental rules, a search would have to be conducted to find the best candidate for the position. If the job description were written carefully, the sanitarian clearly would be the best candidate. Then there was the task of actually writing the position description. That task could be accomplished in a half an hour. The health officer set to work. What comments would you offer to the health officer?

INTRODUCTION

Managers must conduct a job analysis when preparing position descriptions. The format of a position description varies among and within organizations. Health departments may use separate formats for clerical, nonexempt positions and managerial, exempt positions. A position description generally has three main parts: identification information, a job summary, and a list of the principal duties performed. The process of generating a position description begins with an analysis of the job or position.

Positions, not individuals, are classified. Occasionally, the temptation exists to write a position description for a specific individual, tailoring the requirements and experiences so that a preselected person becomes the best candidate in a job search. This should be avoided. If the person leaves the position, the specifications will not change. Finding a replacement may then become very difficult. It is better for all concerned that the position description be written for the job and not for a particular person.

POSITION ANALYSIS

A job description is the most obvious and visible output of a job analysis. Comprehensive and accurate job descriptions, developed as a result of job analysis, are used when selecting, training, evaluating, and compensating employees.

The basis of any employment decision is job analysis, the most fundamental activity in human resource management. Accurate information about all positions is required to efficiently direct and control the activities and operations of any health department. Federal regulations and competition have increased the importance of job analysis. Because human resources are usually the largest cost element for most health departments, supervisors and managers must have current and accurate information about all positions in order to operate programs and deliver services in an efficient manner. Health departments have often omitted position descriptions, relying on the professional nature of many employees' duties. Position descriptions provide more than just guidance for an employee's day. They are integral to an agency's efforts to be fair and equitable to all employees. Health departments that do not have current position descriptions become vulnerable with regards to accusations of discrimination in employment practices. One way to defend against charges of unfair employment practices is to conduct job analyses and prepare job descriptions.

A job analysis includes the extensive study of a specific position and yields information for a position description. The person conducting a job analysis gathers information about positions from several sources. These include interviews with people currently in the position (also referred to as job or position incumbents), observation of the performance of the job's duties or tasks, worksheets or questionnaires completed by employees, and information from sources such as the *Dictionary of Occupational Titles*.

The position analyst will compile his or her findings and review the job analysis with the job incumbent. Once agreement is reached with regards to the job description's accuracy, the preliminary document is given to the incumbent's supervisor for review. Supervisors may add, delete, or modify descriptions of duties, knowledge, skills, abilities, or other characteristics. After supervisors approve individual position descriptions, they are forwarded to upper management for final approval. A final position description is prepared, signed, and dated. Copies are given to both the incumbent and the supervisor. A copy is also filed for future reference.

■ ROLE OF THE POSITION INCUMBENT

Job incumbents have an important role in the process of generating an accurate position description. Position incumbents can assist in the process of analysis by taking time to think about their job. They should keep a diary of work-related activities or make notes about their job duties. These should include all activities that occur during one complete cycle of duties. Typically, a year may be required to complete all job duties. Unless job analysis occurs when budgets are being prepared, budget-related tasks may be overlooked.

At the beginning of an analysis interview, incumbents should explain their concept of the job to the analyst. The analyst should try to make the job incumbent focus on the facts. Job incumbents should avoid overstating or understating characteristics of a position, such as duties, required knowledge, skills, or abilities. Both the analyst and the job incumbent should remain focused and minimize discussion of extraneous issues. Analysts are only concerned with the position. Personal performance, fairness of wages, complaints, and relationships with supervisors or coworkers are not relevant.

Upper managers determine the extent of a position's impact and the boundaries of a job. Position analysts do not determine consequences as part of their work. Such decisions are made by senior managers. For example, salaries will not be reduced or a position eliminated because of the analysis process. An analyst may recommend title changes or other position realignments, but the final decision is made by senior management.

■ ELEMENTS OF A POSITION DESCRIPTION

A position description usually includes the following elements: job identification information, a job summary, a principal duties performed section, and a job specification section.

The **job identification information** must include, at a minimum, the position title, the department location, and the last date on which the content of the position description was verified. Other data, such as the title of the supervisor, help to show how the position fits within the larger organization.

The **job summary** provides an overall concept of the purpose, nature, and extent of the tasks performed by the person in the position. In a well-constructed system, the job summary should relate to the mission statement of the department in which the position is located and to the global mission of the organization.

The section on **principal duties performed** presents job facts in an organized and orderly fashion. When preparing the principal duties performed section, a job is normally broken down into approximately five to eight functions for the purpose of describing the position. The job functions should be listed in order of decreasing frequency or occurrence; that is, the task that requires the most time to complete or is the most critical for a given position should be listed first. For each function listed in this section, a description of the job's activities (i.e., what is done on the job), how the task is accomplished, and why it is necessary should be provided. This is a convenient method of organizing a position description. It quickly and effectively communicates a great deal of information about a position to a reader unfamiliar with the job.

Position descriptions should be written using sentences that are clear and brief. Experts suggest using action verbs and the present tense. In preparing a job summary, the purpose of the position must be clearly stated. This statement should be as brief as possible while still accomplishing its purpose. Words should be carefully selected to convey the maximum amount of specific meaning. General or vague terms should be avoided unless they are absolutely essential as a substitute for a long and detailed explanation.

The principal duties performed section follows the job summary and includes major job functions, as previously outlined. Many organizations include a fourth section in their descriptions that covers job specifications. The **job specification** section outlines the minimum specific skills, effort, and responsibilities required of an incumbent on the job. Job specifications provide the basis and justification for values that will be assigned to factors used in evaluating a position. Factors are elements created by a job analyst and subsequently used when comparing different positions within a single organization. Job specification statements must describe the extent to which a given factor is present and the degree of difficulty encountered in the position for that factor.

When writing job specifications, individual statements should be definite, direct, and to the point. Any unnecessary embellishments or complicated sentences should be avoided except where they materially add to an understanding of the details contained in the statement. Any specifications that apply only to occasional duties should be indicated accordingly so that the percent of time or frequency with which the specification applies will not be overestimated.

Education requirements for a position description must be supported by the analysis of actual duties. Higher educational requirements are legal but must be such that the skills or training can only be acquired through formal education. Minimum levels of schooling must be used. Artificially high educational requirements are a form of discrimination. They are not only illegal, but also unethical. Skills must be supported by position analysis. These are factors that are linked to compensation. Other factors that must be compensated include the level of responsibility, the number of people supervised, the amount of funds managed, and the resources controlled.

Job specifications are then translated into position descriptions. These descriptions are for specific job categories, for example, Secretary 2, Nurse Aide 1, Sanitarian-In-Training, or Environmental Supervisor 1. The title indicates the major function of a position. The number after it may indicate the level of the position in the organizational hierarchy. Whereas job specifications may be recorded for individual incumbents, position descriptions are developed for general categories of jobs. Well-written position descriptions should contain the items listed in **Table 12-1**. An example of a completed job description in the described format appears in Appendix A, which can be found at the end of this chapter.

A position description becomes a very important human resource management document for managers and supervisors in that it sets out the major duties and responsibilities for persons in specific positions. In many cases, the position description may be detailed to the level where it can be used for performance appraisals and employee evaluations.

The preparation and verification of a position description and its specifications comprise the first step in developing a base salary compensation program. The next step in the process involves rating positions, or job evaluation. Job evaluation is essentially a comparison between available information for each position and rating scales that have been established to assist in determining order among many different positions. Job evaluation establishes the relative position of each individual position with respect to all jobs in an organization. Typically, the human resources

Table 12-1 Position Description Components

Component	Explanation
Title	Specific title for the job
FLSA[1] status	Exempt or nonexempt
Summary of duties	Major tasks to be performed
Salary range	The minimum, midpoint, and maximum for the job
Knowledge required	Specific training needed to perform the job; specific experience, both type and amount needed, to perform the job
Skills required	Specific skills expected
Effort required	Both mental and physical; any heavy lifting
Responsibility	Consequences of an error
Working conditions	Hazards or other poor working conditions
General statement	"Other duties as required"

[1]Fair Labor Standards Act

department performs the job evaluation. If it is a new or highly controversial position, an interdisciplinary job evaluation committee, composed of members from various sectors of an organization, may evaluate a job.

■ CONCLUSION

Many think that position descriptions are dry and uninteresting. However, they are important documents for any organization. Position descriptions should be closely linked to organizational goals and objectives. They are used when determining compensation levels. Job descriptions have a regular format, style, and language. They should be prepared with care and periodically reviewed for accuracy and currency.

Returning to the health officer who began to write a job description for the new training position, a pause would be in order. Job descriptions are not essays. They are based on an analysis of the new position. A thorough position analysis usually requires more than 30 minutes to complete.

The health officer apparently intended to specify a Master of Public Health degree as the minimum level of education for the job incumbent. While such a decision might appear to create a good opportunity for the sanitarian, formal schooling is not the only place where expertise in training can be obtained. An employee with several years of work experience who has had some leadership responsibilities should be able to become a successful trainer. Artificially high educational requirements are a form of discrimination. The health officer should be reminded that job descriptions are written for positions, not people. To ignore this advice is to court problems when seeking a replacement for the proposed new employee.

Resources

Periodicals

Hayes, H. 2002. Employee training and job descriptions. *Maryland Medicine* 3(1):39–41.

Loomis, C. 2003. You're the boss: Understanding your responsibilities as an employer. *Journal of the Oklahoma State Medical Association* 96(11):535–537.

Sachs Hills, L. 2004. Special considerations for hiring an office manager. *Journal of Medical Practice Management* 19(4):189–192.

Books

Byars, L.L., and Rue, L.W. 2003. *Human Resource Management*, 7th ed. New York: McGraw-Hill.

Farr, J.M., Ludden, L.L., and Shatkin, L. 2001. *Dictionary of Occupational Titles*, 2d ed. Indianapolis, IN: JIST Works, Inc.

Plachy, R.J., and Plachy, S.J. 1997. *More Results-oriented Job Descriptions: 226 Models to Use or Adapt—with Guidelines for Creating Your Own*, 2d ed. Chicago: AMACOM.

Wilson, M. 2004. *Volunteer Job Descriptions and Action Plans*. Loveland, CO: Group Publishing.

Web Sites

- America's Career Info Net:
  www.acinet.org/acinet/jobwrite_search.asp
- Delaware Association of Nonprofit Agencies:
  www.delawarenonprofit.org/JobDesc.htm
- Johns Hopkins University:
  hrnt.jhu.edu/compensation/gjd/
- Management Assistance Program for Nonprofits:
  www.mapnp.org/library/staffing/specify/job_desc/job_desc.htm
- O*Net Online:
  online.onetcenter.org/
- Office of Personnel Management, Overview of the Fair Labor Standards Act:
  www.opm.gov/flsa/overview.asp
- Rice University:
  www.ruf.rice.edu/~humres/Training/HowToHire/Pages/4.shtml

Organizations

American College of Healthcare Executives
One North Franklin Street, Suite 1700
Chicago, IL 60606-4425
Phone: 312-424-2800
Fax: 312-424-0023
E-mail: ache@ache.org
Web site: www.ache.org/

American Management Association
1601 Broadway
New York, NY 10019
Phone: 212-586-8100
Fax: 212-903-8168
Web site: www.amanet.org/index.htm

Management Assistance Program for Nonprofits
2233 University Avenue West, Suite 360
St. Paul, MN 55114
Phone: 651-647-1216
Web site: www.mapnp.org/library/guiding/motivate/basics.htm

Society for Human Resource Management
1800 Duke Street
Alexandria, VA 22314
Phone: 800-283-7476
Fax: 703-535-6490
Web site: www.shrm.org

The National Human Resources Association
P.O. Box 7326
Nashua, NH 03060-7326
Phone: 866-523-4417
Fax: 603-891-5760
E-mail: nhraadmin@humanresources.org
Web site: www.humanresources.org/

APPENDIX A

SAMPLE POSITION DESCRIPTION

JOB TITLE:	Department Controller
UNIT OR SECTION:	Administration
FLSA STATUS:	Exempt
DEPARTMENT:	Finance
SALARY RANGE:	(intentionally left blank)
BASIC FUNCTION:	Plans, directs, and coordinates on an efficient and economical basis all departmental accounting operational functions, including cost accounting, financial accounting, general accounting, information systems, and general office services.
SCOPE:	Work encompasses involvement in a broad range of accounting activities that are essential to the maintenance of departmental operations and the dissemination of financial information to the board and senior health department management.

SUMMARY OF DUTIES:

1. Directs all essential accounting operational functions in a timely and accurate manner, developing methods geared to providing management with information vital to decision-making processes.
2. Directs the development of methods and procedures necessary to ensure adequate financial controls within each of the accounting operational areas.
3. Performs analysis and appraisal of the department's financial status; prepares recommendations with respect to future financial plans, forecasts and policies.
4. Works closely with the Health Officer on confidential financial matters and expedites such matters to conclusion.
5. Directs this function within the accounting parameters established by departmental, state and GAAP rules and regulations.
6. Manages functional span in manner that fully complements and interfaces with all other agency components.

SUPERVISION EXERCISED:	NUMBER OF EMPLOYEES:
A. DIRECT: General supervisors; functional areas	2–3
B. INDIRECT: Supervisors and administrative and clerical personnel	15–20

TRAINING AND EDUCATION:
Certified Public Accountant (CPA) required; graduation from an accredited school.

EXPERIENCE:
Must have at least five years of experience in accounting with some supervisory responsibility.

RESPONSIBILITY:
Budget of $3,500,000 per year.

Responsible for all required board, state, and federal filings for tax and other financial purposes.

EFFORT:
Minimal physical effort required; no lifting.
Mental effort requires ability to concentrate on numbers for long periods of time and to work under sometimes severe deadlines.

WORKING CONDITIONS:
Works in well-lighted office; no exposure to hazards in the normal course of work.

The above constitutes a general summary of duties. Additional duties may be required.

APPROVALS:
By the supervisor, the health officer, and the human resources department.

DATE:

CHAPTER

13

Employee Recruitment and Selection

Diane Borst

Chapter Objectives

After reading this chapter, readers will:

- Know the major laws and regulations affecting the recruitment and selection process.
- Appreciate basic recruitment methods.
- Understand alternative methods for interviewing and selecting applicants.
- Assemble the components of a good orientation program to integrate the new employee into the workforce.

Chapter Summary

Recruitment and selection are key elements of contemporary public health care. Workers typically change jobs and careers three or more times in their lives. Labor turnover is costly and time-consuming. Choosing the right employee takes time, thought, and effort. By using the methods in this chapter, administrators can save their organizations time, money, and aggravation when recruiting, selecting, and orienting new employees within the concepts of applicable laws.

Case Study

Marysville is about 50 miles southwest of a major city. Its population has almost doubled in the past decade to approximately 60,000 people.

The main reason for this influx is the movement of several large industries into the Marysville area. The new industries include a national food distributor, a major tire manufacturer, and an automaker.

The long-time residents of Marysville have noted that the new people moving into town seem to have customs and preferences that are somewhat different from theirs. For example, the supermarket now carries a variety of fresh peppers and large sacks of white rice. Items such as okra, collard greens, and yams are readily available, as are plantains. Kosher products are also on the grocery shelves along with many Middle Eastern foods such as pita bread and hummus.

Until the new industries arrived, the local hospital was the largest employer in the area. It had a fairly stable workforce, with most employees having a minimum of 6 to 10 years of service. However, as opportunities became available in the new companies, hospital employees have been recruited away to fill the industry jobs.

The county health department, also located in Marysville, has had a cordial relationship with the hospital and has hired some employees from the hospital. The agency is geographically close to the hospital, and employees frequently eat lunch at the hospital cafeteria. The pay rates and benefits of the health department are comparable to those of the hospital. The secretary to the health commissioner has just resigned. The reason for leaving was due to spousal relocation. As the person responsible for human resources, how should you begin the process of hiring a new secretary?

Rather than wait until the end of the chapter to conclude this case study, commentary will be provided after each section. This change in format reflects the importance of employee selection for any organization.

INTRODUCTION

Employee recruitment and selection is usually coordinated by human resources. This responsibility may be shared among two or more people. More typically, it is a portion of the job duties of a single person. The importance of the human resources function is not proportional to the number of people handling the duties. Human resources is critical to all organizations and is not related to the size of the human resources department.

KEY ELEMENTS OF RECRUITMENT AND SELECTION

The Position Description

Chapter 12 provides information on the content and value of position descriptions. The first step in the recruitment process is to review the existing position description. This may be an opportunity to change or upgrade the job or to add or delete some of the position's duties. The position description will become the factual basis for recruitment, selection, and, later on, employee performance review. This is an important initial step.

Major Applicable Laws and Regulations

Most employers are covered by federal legislation that affects how employees are recruited. Although many laws and regulations impact employees and employers, those presented here refer only to the recruitment and selection of employees.

In 1964, the United States Congress enacted **Title VII of the Civil Rights Act.** This law prevents employers from discriminating in terms of recruitment, selection, compensation, privileges of employment, benefits, or terms of employment on the basis of race, color, religion, sex, or national origin. Most employers are covered under this act (Dessler, 2000). Specifically, public and private employers of 15 persons or more fall under the jurisdiction of this act. This includes all private and public educational institutions, the federal government, and state and local governments. Additionally, employment agencies are prohibited from discriminating in terms of the applicants they may refer to an employer.

The **Age Discrimination in Employment Act (ADEA)** of 1967 prohibits discrimination against persons who are between the ages of 40 and 70. The **Vocational Rehabilitation Act of 1974** prohibits employers with federal contracts of $2,500 or more from discriminating against handicapped persons and requires employers to take affirmative actions to hire handicapped persons.

The **Pregnancy Discrimination Act (PDA)** of 1978 requires employers to treat women affected by pregnancy, childbirth, or related medical conditions as they would all other employees for purposes of employment. This includes benefits coverage, if offered to employees in similar job classifications.

In 1990, the U.S. Congress passed the **Americans with Disabilities Act (ADA).** In 1992, this wide-reaching act was extended to cover employers with 15 or more employees. Not only are employers required to take affirmative actions to hire those with physical disabilities, they are also required to make reasonable accommodation to hire and employ such persons unless doing so would cause undue hardship to an employer.

Reasonable accommodation might mean, for example, installing a ramp for an employee who requires a wheelchair, changing a person's job duties to allow more sitting by someone who has a bad back, or installing a phone headset for a person with a hearing impairment. Individuals are defined as being disabled when they have a physical or mental impairment that substantially limits one or more of life's major activities (Dessler, 2000). Many court cases have attempted to arrive at a precise definition of disability as used in the act.

How does this apply to the case in Marysville?
An interviewer cannot ask a female applicant or employee if she is pregnant or planning to become pregnant. An interviewer cannot ask if a person is a U.S. citizen. However, it is legal to ask if the applicant has permission to work in the United States. Proof of permission to work (a green card) might be very important in the Marysville situation. It is also unlawful to ask applicants in what country they hold citizenship. A person cannot be asked for a date of birth during an employment interview. It is legal to ask if a person is old enough to work. After hiring, it is permissible to ask for proof. Finally, it is illegal to ask a job candidate if he or she has been arrested. A person does not have a criminal record until convicted in a court of law.

METHODS OF RECRUITMENT

New employees come from two major sources: (1) within the organization and (2) outside the organization.

Within the Organization

News of new openings tends to travel quickly in an organization. **Word of mouth** is generally quite informal and a very unscientific approach to recruitment, but it may be efficient in a smaller organization. Many employers advertise positions through **job postings**. When a position becomes vacant, the position is listed on one or more centrally located job-posting boards. The amount of information in the posting varies, depending on the size of the organization and the number of job titles. A posting can include a simple listing of the position's title, department, shift, and pay grade or a more complex listing of abilities and skills required or desired. Employers generally post internally for five to seven working days before moving to outside recruitment techniques. This gives employees a chance for promotion or change and encourages retention. An organization's **skills bank**, normally maintained by a human resources person or department, is another source for potential candidates.

Current employees may be a good source of referrals for new employees. Because a current employee is a known entity, there is a good probability that the referral will be of the same quality. This is more likely to occur than with a walk-in applicant. Some employers offer bonuses for successful employee referrals. Bonuses are paid after a new employee remains on the job for a minimum period of time, usually from three months to one year. The bonus amount depends on the organization, its needs and policies, and the practices of other organizations in the same area competing for the same employees.

How does this apply to the case in Marysville?
If the health department is small, fewer than 15 employees, word of the secretarial vacancy will travel rapidly throughout the organization. It will

be necessary to have a screening or internal application process in effect to ensure fairness in interviewing and selecting. If the health department has more than 15 employees, a job posting should be prepared and disseminated. This ensures compliance with federal laws and regulations.

Outside an Organization

There are two types of **employment agencies:** those that are free and those that are not. In general, state employment agencies and union referral halls are available without cost. State employment agencies are listed under each state's department of labor. Union referral (sometimes called hiring) halls will be known through an organization's collective bargaining agreement.

Private employment agencies, including search firms, will screen and interview qualified candidates prior to referring them to an organization. This can save time, especially if there is a small pool of applicants or if the position must be quickly filled. The cost of the employment agency fee is generally paid by the new employer. It is important to carefully review contract terms and fees before making a commitment to an agency to conduct a search. The usual fee is approximately 10 percent of a year's salary or one month's salary (Renckly, 2004).

Outside organizations, such as professional societies or special interest groups, provide another source for referrals. Typically, these referrals are free. Other potentially useful organizations include colleges, universities, programs and schools of public health, chambers of commerce, and specialized trade schools.

Printed **want ads** may appear in newspapers, journals, magazines, or at a particular point of service, such as a grocery store or a place where likely candidates may congregate. One employer has posted job openings in local places of worship (Hammer, 2003).

However, print advertising results in lead times. For example, an advertisement in a Sunday newspaper may not yield applicants until several days later. An ad placed in a professional journal or magazine may not be run for a month or more after it has been submitted. The cost of print advertising also can be high. A recent study by the Employment Management Association and reported in *The Fordyce Letter* estimated the cost per hire using print advertising to be $3,295 (Bolles, 2003).

The same study reported that the cost per hire using the **Internet** was $377, almost 10 times lower than the cost of print advertising (Bolles, 2003). Jobs can be posted on a number of different Web sites. Some of these sites are listed among the resources found at the conclusion of this chapter. Both employers and prospective employees use the Internet sites. If the hiring organization is very large, it may have its own Web site that can be used for recruitment.

Posting on the Internet can have several advantages. First, it is open to a wide range of applicants. Second, it is available around the clock, every day, whereas print media is only available for a limited amount of time. Third, it is less expensive than print advertising. However, listing jobs on the Internet also has its disadvantages. The pool of applicants may be so large that an organization may become overwhelmed. Resumes may arrive from areas so geographically distant that interviews are not feasible.

Many smaller communities have **public access TV or radio** and will air information about jobs available in the area. It is worth checking to see if this service is available.

Walk-ins and **write-ins** are people who send in a resume or apply for a job without knowing of a specific employment opportunity. These people should complete a standard application for employment that should then be kept on file. Some employers give walk-ins a brief interview as a courtesy and to assess applicants' potential for future employment. This is especially critical in a tight labor market.

Organizations should consider contacting local colleges or universities to arrange a structured internship program. This is especially true of Master of Public Health degree programs that are offered by programs and schools in public health. Academic credits can frequently be arranged. Organizations benefit by having a chance to assess the performance of students in preparation for possible future employment.

How does this apply to the case in Marysville?

When determining the optimal recruitment approach, an organization should consider the following: What is the likelihood of identifying qualified in-house candidates? Is it necessary to fill the secretarial vacancy immediately or can a temporary agency supply the service until a permanent replacement is hired? Does the health department have a file of prior applicants for this type position? How much time and money is the organization willing to spend to recruit for this vacancy? Given the advantages and disadvantages of different modes of advertising, which will work best in this situation? Are there colleges or universities in the vicinity of Marysville that offer degrees in public administration? Would they consider internships? Does the department have the managerial time necessary to devote to supervising an intern?

A want ad, print or electronic (Internet), may be necessary. The want ad should contain information about the position, such as a brief description of duties, the supervisor, and the location of the agency. Additional information may be added that describes why the job or organization might be attractive to an applicant. In the Marysville case, opportunities for growth, expansion of the organization, and flexible hours may be of interest. Comments about the local environment might include the attractiveness of the surroundings, opportunities for leisure activities, the quality of local schools, availability of parking, the competitive salary, the availability of the hospital, and childcare programs.

What qualifications does the candidate need? How many words per minute should the candidate be able to type? What software programs should the candidate know? What kinds of people and telephone skills are required? The nature and extent of additional information varies with the nature of the labor market in which the health department is competing.

All advertisements should indicate that the employer is in compliance with federal laws. Usually the phrase "An Equal Opportunity Employer" will appear at the bottom of each advertisement. This may be particularly important in the Marysville case, because so many persons of diverse origins have recently moved to the area.

Finally, how will the health department process contacts? Modes and preferences for contact such as telephone, fax, e-mail and in person should be indicated. Be sure to include the correct information for communicating with the department: organization name, mailing address, telephone and fax numbers, and any deadline for submission.

SCREENING, INTERVIEWING, AND SELECTING

Screening

Because there may be a number of applicants for a position, it is important to determine the important qualifications for the position and interview only those applicants meeting the minimum threshold. Selection criteria for an initial screening typically include education, skills, and relevant experience. A position description must be used as a guide. Prudent organizations keep detailed records of the process, noting data about people who are retained in the pool as well as those who are rejected during the initial screening. Reasons for inclusion or exclusion from an initial pool should be noted. These data may be needed for later reports that document compliance with relevant legislation. This step may be performed by the human resources department or by the hiring manager, depending on the size and policy of the organization.

How does this apply to the Marysville case?
Based on the position description, the organization will be able to determine the level of each of the areas mentioned in the preceding paragraph. For example:

- **Education:** Must be a high school graduate, preferably a graduate with a secretarial curriculum.
- **Skills:** Must be fluent in Word, Word Perfect, Excel, Access, and Outlook Express and know how to work on a PC platform; must have strong oral and written communications skills.
- **Experience:** Must have three to five years of secretarial experience in a public agency.

Interviews

An interview is a face-to-face conversation with an applicant. It may also be the first exposure of an organization and applicant to one another. The primary purpose of an interview is to determine the suitability and fit of an applicant to the open position. The result of a good interview should be a mutual understanding of the interests and abilities of both the employer and the applicant.

Preparing for the Interview

To prepare for a successful interview, interviewers should take a number of steps before an actual conversation begins:

- Read the position description. Job duties should be clear. An interviewer should be able to articulate these duties in a meaningful way to the applicant.
- Provide a list of basic questions that will be asked of all interviewees. This will ensure that all applicants are treated in a fair manner.
- Take the time to thoroughly read each applicant's resume. In busy times, it is easy to skip this step and conduct an interview without adequate preparation. Reading a resume and application prior to an interview gives confidence to the interviewer and saves the interviewer time by eliminating the need to ask questions that are already answered on the resume or application.

Conducting the Interview

One of the most stressful parts of a manager's job is interviewing candidates for employment. A number of techniques can make this task easier.

Establish Rapport

First, set the interviewee at ease. This can be accomplished by sitting across a table facing the interviewee rather than sitting behind a desk. A cup of coffee or tea or a soft drink may be offered. Second, begin by asking innocent questions: "How did you hear about this opening?" or "How was your travel time to arrive here?" Note that these are open-ended questions that cannot be answered with a yes or no response. This encourages interviewees to talk.

Describe the Job and the Organization

It is the potential employer's obligation to describe the position and the organization in a very honest fashion. The position can best be described by using the position description (see Chapter 12). At the interview, newsletters or brochures from the organization can be given to candidates to review. A rule of thumb is to ask if an interviewee has any questions about the potential job or organization.

Ask Questions

The next task is for the interviewer to begin asking questions. Behaviorally based interviews ask questions about how the applicant would respond under particular circumstances. For example, in the Marysville case, the interviewer could ask, "How would you respond if a person insisted on seeing me immediately?" Other behaviorally oriented questions include: "What did you like best about your last job?" and "What did you like least?" and "How do you handle a difficult or demanding person?"

This type of interview is sometimes referred to as being behaviorally-based. There have been notable successes with this type of interview. Women & Infants Hospital, a 2,600-employee facility that is part of the Care New England Health System provides an example. With a combined emphasis on quality improvement and the use of behaviorally based interview techniques, the organization improved its patient satisfaction, and its employee turnover rate declined to 8.5 percent per year, compared with the national average of 20 to 25 percent (Greengard, 2003).

It is important to remember the guidelines provided by federal laws and regulations regarding what can and cannot be asked during a pre-employment interview. Although sometimes difficult for an interviewer to maintain, **silence** is important. This is sometimes referred to as the 80/20 rule (Larson, 2000). Interviewers should talk about 20 percent of the time and listen about 80 percent of the time. Silence after a question will tend to force an interviewee to respond.

Post-Interview Evaluation

Allow time to reflect on the interview. What were the strengths and weaknesses of the applicant? How would such an applicant fit into the organization? A formal post-interview evaluation sheet is helpful to ensure that all interviewees are treated in a similar manner.

Types of Interviews

Interviews can be conducted in a number of different ways. Interviewers may use unstructured interviews, semi-structured interviews, or group interviews.

Unstructured Interview

This type of interview is free flowing and unplanned. It is usually a one-on-one conversation between an applicant and a prospective employer. The steps in the interview process outlined earlier can be valuable in this type of interview.

Semi-Structured Interview

Prior to the interview sessions, the persons conducting the interviews agree on the general topics or areas about which questions will be asked. For example, in the Marysville case, the interviewers might ask some standard open-ended questions, such as the following: What work experience did you enjoy the most? Why? What did you like least about your last job? Why are you changing jobs? Given your knowledge of this position, what do you think would be your major contribution to the job?

Group Interview

If the new person will be working in a small department or if frequent communication with other employees is required, an employment interview may be extended to include several people. The obvious advantages are that everyone hears the same responses and members of the group can evaluate the candidate from various perspectives. Interviewees sometimes feel that a group interview is intimidating. Such a structured interaction can demonstrate a candidate's ability to handle stressful situations and interact with a group of people.

Selection

Once a candidate has been selected, the rate of pay must be agreed upon, the necessary paperwork must be completed, and a date for the new employee to start work must be scheduled. Employment is contingent upon the following points, as applicable. Is the applicant of legal age to work? Does the person have permission to work in the United States? Can the applicant pass minimum physical requirements for the job?

How does this apply to the Marysville case?
Because there has been an influx of new people in the area, their permission to work in the United States should be carefully checked.

■ THE FIRST DAY ON THE JOB

A new employee will need to learn about the organization, its policies, its procedures, and its social structure. Orientation programs typically provide this information. Several important pieces of information are usually included in an orientation program. The person conducting the orientation should provide general information about the agency. For example, what programs and services are offered by the public health agency? What is the organization's main mission? What role does the agency play in the local health care system? Provide specifics about the organization. A copy of the employee handbook, if one is available, should be distributed. What are the goals and objectives of the group or program that has hired the new employee? What is its mission or focus? How many employees does it have? What are the structures of the agency and subgroup? How frequently and on what criteria are performance appraisals based? How long is the probationary period, if any?

Job-specific information should be provided. A copy of the position description should be provided and used to orient the new employee with the position's specific duties. Both the supervisor and the newly hired employee should review the job's basic tasks. Social aspects of the job should also be considered—no one wants to eat lunch alone on the first day at the job. Some organizations appoint a buddy or mentor for each new employee. The mentor introduces the new employee to others and fills in the social gaps not covered in a job description. Questions concerning storage of personal belongings while at work and the locations of restrooms and coffee or water stations may seem trivial. However, information about these basic needs will help the new employee adjust to the new position in a sensible and thoughtful manner.

Other approaches to socialization include meeting with the chief executive officer, holding roundtable discussions with managers and new employees, and training supervisors to orient new employees in a systematic manner (Hammer, 2003).

How does this apply to the Marysville case?
Any or all of the options mentioned could be used to orient the new secretary. The investment in time and effort will depend on the culture of the organization and its past history.

CONCLUSION

By using the techniques in this and other related chapters, an organization will be able to recruit, interview, select, and orient new employees in a timely and efficient manner. The newly hired members of the team will be knowledgeable of the rules and regulations regarding recruitment, selection, and their individual positions.

The new secretary from Marysville was hired after a seemingly complex search. The guidelines of the Equal Opportunity, Affirmative Action, and Americans with Disabilities laws were followed. The new secretary spent his first morning being oriented to his new job and coworkers. A mentor introduced him to other employees throughout the company. The new employee was familiar with both the professional and the social aspects of the job within three weeks.

References

Bolles, R.N. 2003. *What Color Is Your Parachute? 2004: A Practical Guide for Job-hunters and Career Changers*. Berkeley, CA: Ten Speed Press.

Dessler, G. 2000. *Human Resource Management,* 8th ed. Upper Saddle River, NJ: Prentice-Hall.

Greengard, S. 2003. Gimme attitude. *Workforce Magazine*, July, pp. 56–60.

Hammer, M. 2003. Optimas award managing change: Almost curtains. *Workforce Magazine*, August, pp. 54–55.

Larson, W.W. 2000. *Ten-Minute Guide to Conducting a Job Interview.* New York: Penguin.

Renckly, R.B. 2004. *Human resources,* 2d ed. Hauppauge NY: Barron's Educational Series.

Resources

Periodicals

Becker, C. 2003. Killer credentials: In wake of nurse accused of killing patient, the health system wrestles with balancing shortage, ineffectual reference process. *Modern Healthcare* 33(51):6–7.

Hekman, K.M. 2004. Hidden expenses: The true cost of adding a physician to your medical group practice. *Medical Group Management Association* 4(1):44–47.

Hills, L.S. 2003. Preliminary screening of job applicants in five steps. *Journal of Medical Practice Management* 19(3):143–145.

O'Rourke, G. 2003. The new face of healthcare. *Healthcare Management Forum* 16(4):35–36.

Priester, R., and Reinardy, J.R. 2003. Recruiting immigrants for long-term care nursing positions. *Journal of Aging and Social Policy* 15(4):1–19.

Books

Arthur, D. 2001. *The Employee Recruitment and Retention Handbook*. New York: AMACOM.

Byars, L.L., and Rue, L.W. 2000. *Human Resource Management*, 6th ed. New York: McGraw-Hill.

DeNisi, A.S., and Griffin, R.W. 2001. *Human Resource Management*. New York: Houghton Mifflin.

Foster, M. 2002. *Recruiting on the Web*. New York: McGraw-Hill.

Noe, R., Hollenbeck, J.R., Gerhart, B., Wright, P.M. 2000. *Human Resource Management: Gaining a Competitive Advantage*. New York: McGraw-Hill.

Wood, R., and Payne, T. 1998. *Competency-Based Recruitment and Selection*. New York: Wiley.

Web Sites

- America's Job Bank:
  www.ajb.dni.us
- Careerbuilder.com:
  www.careerbuilder.com/JobSeeker
- Monster.com Job Center:
  www.monster.com
- TopUSAJobs.com:
  www.topusajobs.com
- Workforce Management:
  www.workforce.com
- Yahoo.com Classifieds:
  classifieds.yahoo.com/?qsc=hotjobs

Organizations

American College of Healthcare Executives
One North Franklin Street, Suite 1700
Chicago, IL 60606-4425
Phone: 312-424-2800
Fax: 312-424-0023
E-mail: ache@ache.org
Web site: www.ache.org/

American Management Association
1601 Broadway
New York, NY 10019
Phone: 212-586-8100
Fax: 212-903-8168
Web site: www.amanet.org/index.htm

Management Assistance Program for Nonprofits
2233 University Avenue West, Suite 360
St. Paul, MN 55114
Phone: 651-647-1216
Web site: www.mapnp.org/library/guiding/motivate/basics.htm

The National Human Resources Association
P.O. Box 7326
Nashua, NH 03060-7326
Phone: 866-523-4417
Fax: 603-891-5760
E-mail: nhraadmin@humanresources.org
Web site: www.humanresources.org

U.S. Chamber of Commerce
1615 H Street, NW
Washington, D.C. 20062-2000
Phone: 202-659-6000
Web site: www.uschamber.com/default

CHAPTER

14

Wage and Salary Considerations

Joseph A. Diorio, Jr.
L. Fleming Fallon, Jr.

Chapter Objectives

After reading this chapter, readers will:

- Understand that people do not work solely for money.
- Appreciate the objectives of compensation programs.
- Know the differences between cash and noncash compensation.
- Understand the relationship between motivation and compensation.

Chapter Summary

This chapter is about money. Many people believe that money is the only reason that people accept and keep their jobs. Money is an important factor, but it is not the only reason that people remain in their jobs. Some forms of compensation are given in cash. Forms of noncash compensation include vacation, health and other types of insurance, sick time, paid time off, and retirement funding.

Case Study

Marlowe was in a quandary. At its monthly meeting last night, the health board approved the new epidemiologist position. The health officer was told to go ahead and make hire. "Don't delay because the work is piling up," the board president said. The health officer relayed the good news to Marlowe, giving permission to begin the search. What guidance would you offer to Marlowe?

INTRODUCTION

People work for the pay. This is a common myth. Money is a powerful motivation, but other factors provide more motivation than money. Elements of a total compensation program include both direct and indirect compensation. Direct compensation refers to salaries, bonuses, and other forms of incentive payment. Indirect compensation refers to employee benefits and perquisites, items that an employee typically receives in forms other than cash payments.

An optimum balance of direct and indirect compensation results from the interaction of organizational objectives, legal considerations, and employee motivation. Each of these factors is discussed in this chapter as it relates to the development of a total compensation program.

OBJECTIVES OF COMPENSATION PROGRAMS

Virtually all organizations have the stated objective of developing and maintaining a compensation program that attracts, retains, and motivates competent employees. Further, the compensation program should be designed and administered in a manner that provides adequate, equitable, and balanced treatment for all employees.

Despite having common purposes, the organizational objectives that shape individual compensation programs are sufficiently diverse that the result is a wide range of design variations. To help define their compensation programs, organizations must address several key questions. These are found in **Table 14-1.**

The literal bottom line for compensation is what the organization can afford to pay. This is determined by several factors, including available and ongoing financial resources and prevailing rates for a region and for specific skill sets of desired employees. The goal of compensation is to

Table 14-1 Key Questions When Planning Compensation

- How much can the organization afford to pay its employees?
- What are the prevailing wages within the profession and the industry?
- What are the prevailing wages within the local geographic area?
- How will the organization respond to cost-of-living changes?
- What are the impacts of unions upon wages within an organization, area, and industry?
- Does the organization want to be a wage leader or a wage follower?
- What form of compensation will result in the most efficient use of the organization's resources and maximize productivity?
- How will individual compensation rates be established?

most efficiently use organizational resources to maximize employee productivity.

The list of questions in **Table 14-1** is not all encompassing. When an organization faces unique competitive and economic circumstances, it must address additional compensation questions. Having developed a strategy or organizational philosophy for the direct (cash) portion of the compensation plan, a fair and equitable method for relating jobs to payment must be in place.

DIRECT (CASH) COMPENSATION

A main requirement of any direct compensation plan is to develop a base-salary compensation program. The development of a base-salary compensation program employs a number of techniques. Each technique or component has a purpose that must be communicated to managers at all levels. The components and purposes of direct compensation are listed in **Table 14-2.**

Each job or position must be described using a common set of parameters. Many organizations have their own guidelines or systems for classification. Consultants also are available to administer job analysis

Table 14-2 Components and Purposes of Direct Compensation Programs

Component	Purpose
Job analysis	Defines and describes a job. Provides crucial information for job evaluation, salary administration, recruitment, training, supervision, and organizational development.
Job evaluation	Establishes an organizational hierarchy among all jobs.
Job grading	Groups similarly evaluated positions to facilitate salary administration.
Incentive plans	Pays for output rather than merely for time worked; may be applied to individuals or groups.
Merit pay plans	Provides superior increases for superior performance.
Benefits	Provided on the basis of membership in an organization or membership in a specific class of employee within an organization.
General increases	Provided to all members of an organization. Generally used to reflect changes in the cost-of-living, general economic changes, or changing conditions within a defined labor market.
Maturity curves	Most commonly applied to professional employees. Pay reflects years of experience in a profession. Most versions include some provision for differentiating and rewarding individual performance.

Source: Farland (1991).

programs for organizations. Once all the positions in the organization have been analyzed, they must be evaluated. This, too, is a component of salary administration systems. It provides a relative ranking of and internal equity for all of the positions of an organization. Jobs that require similar skills, preparation, or experience are graded at similar levels.

Incentive plans are then prepared. These reflect an organization's compensation philosophy. Similarly, merit pay plans are drafted. These are intended to reward outstanding performance. Not all employees should receive merit pay at the same time or at the same rate. General increases are given to all employees. These reflect satisfactory completion of work responsibilities and are independent of quality or job performance. Some positions require employees with professional training. They often receive additional compensation to reflect their additional training requirements. Simply increasing their pay grade would skew the pay structure for the entire organization. Instead, these people are given professional bonuses. Such bonuses are based on maturity curves.

All positions in an organization must be evaluated. The process of developing position descriptions was discussed in Chapter 13. Once all positions in an agency have been evaluated and placed in a system that enables comparison of one position with others, salaries (direct compensation) must be established. Two major factors are considered when establishing salaries: external equity and internal equity.

External equity means that rates of pay in an organization are reasonable compared with other similar positions in a given area for people performing the same or similar job duties. Some regions of the country pay less for the same position than do others, so it is important to compare particular tasks (the duties within similar position titles that have the same tasks) from one agency to another. It is also important to compare similar-sized organizations to avoid unfair comparisons. For example, large or urban health departments may pay more than rural health departments for employees performing the same job. An outside human resources consultant commonly conducts salary or benchmark surveys to ensure fairness or external equity.

Internal equity means that all employees think that their pay is fair when compared to others with the same job title in the same organization. Motivation, performance, and incentive may be influenced by an employee's perceptions of equity or inequity. Periodic surveys, both internal and external, conducted by a human resources consultant, focus on ensuring both of these equities.

■ INDIRECT (NONCASH) COMPENSATION

In addition to the cash compensation (paychecks) that employees receive, many organizations also provide indirect compensation in the form of fringe benefits. A widely quoted estimate is that for every dollar spent on direct compensation, another 35 to 40 cents is spent on benefits. Examples of benefits that employers provide include those required by statute, such as Social Security, unemployment compensation insurance, and workers' compensation insurance. Employees may be required to contribute to these types of benefits.

Social Security has expanded from a form of basic pension coverage for about 50 percent of the workforce to a full-scale social insurance program available to over 90 percent of the total population. Although employees tend to equate Social Security with old age retirement entitlements, it also covers survivor, disability, and health insurance benefits. Social Security is a contributory benefit, with both employees and employers sharing the cost. Currently, employees contribute 7.65 percent of their first $87,900 of income. Employers also contribute 7.65 percent, up to the same dollar limit. The amount of income that is subject to Social Security taxes periodically changes.

Unemployment compensation insurance is administered by individual states. These programs are experience-rated as a means of encouraging employers to avoid terminations. Employers are taxed according to their record of terminations. Currently, the average standard tax rate for unemployment compensation insurance in the United States is approximately 2.75 percent of payroll (U.S. Chamber of Commerce, 2002).

Workers' compensation insurance is intended to provide health care, income maintenance, and survivor protection for workers disabled or killed due to occupational injury or illness. Like unemployment compensation insurance, organizations are experienced rated. Rates vary widely and are a function of job type, industry stability, and the state.

Additionally, organizations may provide benefits that are not mandated. These are generally categorized as health protection, retirement, and time off with pay. Some of these include health insurance, payment for child care, tuition assistance, pensions, discounts, recreation programs, recognition awards, and other nonmonetary incentives to enhance the productivity of employees.

Among these benefits may be an employer-sponsored **Employee Assistance Program (EAP)**. In the 1970s, employers began to recognize that there was a mutual benefit to providing assistance to employees who had non-work-related types of problems, also called "outside-of-work" problems. These outside-of-work problems, in the eyes of employers, were thought to lessen employees' attention and productivity on the job. Thus, employers began to set up services that could help employees and to refer them to programs that could assist them with their personal situations. Areas of assistance include problems with excessive use of alcohol, drug use, legal problems, difficulties with children or spouses, responsibilities for caring for elder relatives, as well as others.

An employee assistance program may be in-house (i.e., staffed by organizational employees) or it may be a contracted service, whereby employees are referred to outside service providers. In either case, two principles are paramount. First, staff members must voluntarily use an employee assistance program. A supervisor can suggest and recommend that employees use EAP services, but it cannot be mandated. Second, an employee assistance program must maintain confidentiality. A referring supervisor will not receive any information back from an EAP as to an employee's progress or status.

Health protection plans have changed dramatically over the last decade. Since 1991, the percentage of employees covered under a traditional indemnity or fee-for-service plan has dropped from 70 percent to less than 10 percent. Managed care plans such as health maintenance organizations, preferred provider organizations, and point-of-service plans have become the predominant forms of medical coverage. The need to control costs in this area has resulted in a greater degree of employee cost sharing. The percentage of employees covered by plans that require some form of cost sharing has grown from 19 percent in 1983 to approximately 60 percent in 2003 (U.S. Chamber of Commerce, 2002).

The Consolidated Omnibus Budget Reconciliation Act (COBRA) mandates that insurance benefits be extended to terminated employees at some cost to the former workers. This increases an employer's administrative costs for providing a competitive total compensation package.

In addition to health insurance coverage, organizations attempt to protect employees during times of illness or accident with a variety of other programs, including sick leave and disability insurance. Organizations providing **sick leave** generally allocate a set number of days per employee per year. The national average is slightly more than five days per year. Organizations vary widely in the practice of allowing employees to bank, or accumulate, their sick leave time. Under a banking provision, employees are permitted to carry unused sick leave forward to the next year. For financial reasons, this option has been significantly curtailed in recent years. In organizations where the accumulation of sick leave is permitted, it is common for many employees to have in excess of 60 sick days, representing a significant accrual expense for their employers. Many organizations annually buy unused sick days back from their employees. Other agencies provide financial incentives to employees who don't use their sick days, although the extent of this practice has not been accurately surveyed.

Employers are increasingly adopting **paid time off (PTO)** plans where employees accumulate an allotted number of days and then may use them in a more discretionary manner. For example, employees may bank their sick days into a PTO and then use them in the event of an illness of a child. This concept is becoming more popular because it provides flexibility to employees in today's workforce and recognizes the variety of outside demands on each employee.

Long-term disability insurance is a common benefit to protect employees from the financial devastation of a serious illness or accident.

Plans usually provide covered employees with a percentage of their wages during a period of disability. Typically, the benefits approximate 60 to 66 percent of an employee's base compensation. Payment of this benefit begins between three and six months after the onset of the disability, depending on the terms of the coverage.

Life insurance provides employees with a level of coverage equal to some multiple, usually one to two times, of their annual compensation. Although this basic coverage is usually provided at no cost to an employee, tax regulations require employees to pay taxes on the amount of premium provided to purchase coverage in excess of $50,000. In addition to basic life insurance coverage, many organizations provide employees with the opportunity to purchase a limited amount of additional life insurance coverage through a payroll deduction plan. This additional coverage tends to be restricted to one to two times the base salary.

Employee retirement plans include defined benefit and contribution plans. **Defined benefit** plans are those that use a formula to determine what actual benefits will be prior to retirement. Employees know well in advance of retirement what their periodic payout will be. **Defined contribution** plans set forth the amounts that employers and employees will each contribute. The actual amount of the periodic payout is not determined until the employee retires, because it will depend on investment income. Most contemporary plans are vested. This means that after a certain period of employment, usually 5 to 10 years, but possibly more, an employee has a right to the contributions made by the employer and to the final pension. This right is not forfeited if an employee seeks other employment.

■ EMPLOYEE MOTIVATION

The motivational aspects of compensation have generated numerous theories and much research. Within this section, only the highlights of some of the predominant theories will be discussed.

How important is compensation to employees? Several researchers have conducted studies in which employees were asked to rank up to 12 factors in terms of importance in providing job satisfaction (Vreeland, 1998). Pay has consistently been ranked in the middle in terms of providing job satisfaction, usually falling somewhere between the fourth and eighth positions. The rankings contained in **Table 14-3** are typical of the results of such a study.

Self-fulfillment, opportunity for advancement, and security were ranked ahead of compensation in this study (Vreeland, 1998). This does not mean that the motivational aspect of compensation can be ignored. Herzberg (1966), in defining his motivator–hygiene theory of job satisfaction, classified pay as a hygiene factor. In his theoretical structure, compensation is not capable of enhancing job satisfaction. However, the lack of compensation or inadequate compensation is a significant source of job dissatisfaction.

Table 14-3 Importance Ranking of Reward Categories

Category	Rank
Self-fulfillment	1
Opportunity for advancement	2 (tie)
Security	2 (tie)
Direct compensation	4
Working conditions	5
Social	6
Benefits/indirect compensation	7
Esteem	8

Source: Vreeland (1998).

A number of causal models relating compensation with job satisfaction have been developed (Vreeland, 1998). Basically, these models state that any employee behavior that appears to lead to a reward tends to be repeated, whereas behavior that does not appear to be rewarded tends not to be repeated. By establishing compensation as a reward for performance, organizations should, theoretically, be able to direct the efforts and behavior of the workforce into the most profitable activities for an agency. Additional discussions of employee motivation are contained in Chapters, 12, and 17.

CONCLUSION

This chapter has considered fundamentals of compensation and benefits. Well-managed and successful compensation programs must have goals that support the organization's mission, goals, and objectives. Money alone does not motivate employees. Compensation is conventionally divided into direct, or cash, items and indirect, or noncash, forms. Much time and creative effort has been expended on indirect compensation programs in recent years. Employee motivation is an important aspect of a compensation program.

Returning to the initial case study, Marlowe reached into a file and extracted a position description that had been prepared the previous month. The problem of establishing a competitive salary was next. Marlowe called several neighboring health districts and requested data on the salaries of their epidemiologists. She then requested salary information from the state association of local health boards. With these data, Marlowe established a pay range for the epidemiologist position. All health department employees receive the same package of benefits.

Marlowe conducted a successful search and hired an epidemiologist. After two weeks on the job, the new employee was heard to mutter

"Where did all of this work come from? Did the department pile it up when they were trying to hire?"

References

Farland, D. An investigation of the relative effectiveness of three models of job satisfaction (Doctoral Dissertation). Cleveland, OH: Case Western Reserve University, 1991.

Herzberg, F. 1966. *Work and the Nature of Man.* Chicago: World Publishing.

U.S. Chamber of Commerce. 2002. Employee benefits in medium and large firms. U.S. Bureau of Labor Statistics, Division of Financial Planning and Management, Washington, DC.

Vreeland, B. 1998. Rewards of work. *Working World*, July, pp. 6–14.

Resources

Periodicals

Bolster, C.J., and Hawthorne, G. 2003. Looking for answers. Boards struggle to find the proper way to compensate executives. *Trustee* 56(10):8–13.

Harknett K., and Gennetian, L.A. 2003. How an earnings supplement can affect union formation among low-income single mothers. *Demography* 40(3):451–478.

Holve, E., Brodie, M., and Levitt, L. 2003. Small business executives and health insurance: Findings from a national survey of very small firms. *Managed Care Interface* 16(9):19–24.

Mulvey, J. 2003. Retirement behavior and retirement plan designs: Strategies to retain an aging workforce. *Benefits Quarterly* 19(4):25–35.

O'Campo, P., Eaton, W.W., and Muntaner, C. 2004. Labor market experience, work organization, gender inequalities and health status: results from a prospective analysis of U.S. employed women. *Social Science and Medicine* 58(3):585–594.

Books

Beam, B.T., and McFadden, J.J. 2000. *Employee Benefits.* Dearborn, MI: Dearborn Trade.

Bereman, M.L., and Bereman, N.A. 2001. *Compensation Decision Making: A Computer-Based Approach.* Fort Worth, TX: Harcourt Brace.

Berger, L.A., and Berger, D.R. 1999. *The Compensation Handbook.* New York: McGraw Hill.

Fay, C.H., Knight, D., and Thompson, M.A. 2001. *The Executive Handbook on Compensation: Linking Strategic Rewards to Business Performance.* New York: Simon and Schuster.

Gerhart, B., and Rynes, S.L. 2000. *Compensation in Organizations.* San Francisco: Jossey-Bass.

Lawler, E.E. 2000. *Rewarding Excellence: Pay Strategies for the New Economy.* San Francisco: Jossey-Bass.

Martocchio, J.J. 2000. *Strategic Compensation: A Human Resource Management Approach.* Upper Saddle River, NJ: Prentice-Hall.

Rakich, J.S., Darr, K., and Longest, B.B. 2000. *Managing Health Services Organizations,* 4th ed. Baltimore, MD: Health Professions Press.

Risher, H. 1999. *Aligning Pay and Results. Compensation Strategies that Work from the Boardroom to the Shop Floor.* Chicago: AMACOM.

White, G., and Druker, J. 2000. *Reward Management: A Critical Text.* New York: Routledge.

Ziingheim, P.K., and Schuster, J.R. 2000. *Pay People Right: Breakthrough Reward Strategies to Create Great Companies.* San Francisco: Jossey-Bass.

Web Sites

- Manufacturer's Association of Central New York: www.macny.org/Consulting/wsa.html
- Monthly Labor Review Online: www.bls.gov/opub/mlr/1992/06/art3exc.htm
- Society of Human Resources Online: www.shrm.org/hrlinks/Links.asp?Category=9
- Wages: www.wage.org/doc/text/18salary.html

Organizations

American College of Healthcare Executives
One North Franklin, Suite 1700
Chicago, IL 60606-4425
Phone: 312-424-2800
Fax: 312-424-0023
E-mail: geninfo@ache.org
Web site: www.ache.org

American Management Association
1601 Broadway
New York, NY 10019
Phone: 212-586-8100
Fax: 212-903-8168
Web site: www.amanet.org/index.htm

American Psychological Association
750 First Street, NE
Washington, D.C. 20002-4242
Phone: 800-374-2721 or 202-336-5510
Web site: www.apa.org

Society for Human Resource Management
1800 Duke Street
Alexandria, Virginia 22314
Phone: 800-283-7476 or 703-548-3440
Fax: 703-535-6490
Web site: www.shrm.org/

U.S. Chamber of Commerce
1615 H Street, NW
Washington, D.C. 20062-2000
Phone: 202-659-6000
Web site: www.uschamber.com/default

CHAPTER

15

Employee Training

Charles R. McConnell

Chapter Objectives

After reading this chapter, readers will:

- Appreciate the importance of training and development as continuing activities.
- Be able to outline the essential role of department managers as teachers.
- Appreciate the importance of new employee orientation.
- Understand applicable principles in addressing staff training and development needs.
- View cross-training as a means for improving employee capability and departmental effectiveness.
- Know how to approach on-the-job training.
- Understand employee mentoring.
- Appreciate the importance of developing potential managers.
- Recognize how human resources can help managers meet departmental training needs.

Chapter Summary

Training assures the future of any organization. It helps to ease the transition into an organization and facilitates movement within it. Training takes many forms. New employee orientation, mentoring, and on-the-job and off-site training are common examples. Managers often provide training in formal or informal settings. Cross-training of employees with similar types of jobs provides organizational flexibility. Giving potential leaders developmental opportunities facilitates succession planning.

Case Study

"Monday mornings should not be so complicated." At least that's what Sam, the health commissioner, thought. The new epidemiologist was scheduled to report for work at 10:00 A.M. A second new employee was scheduled to begin on Friday. "Two new people on two different days in the same week," thought Sam with an air of defeat.

Sam had been reading about the importance of developing potential new managers. However, the usual departmental duties would not diminish. Because the previous Friday was a state holiday, the morning volume of e-mail was extra heavy. This was especially a problem because a prankster had spread Sam's e-mail address to Web sites that specialized in body-reshaping surgery or drugs to enhance performance. "Why couldn't both new employees start tomorrow?" mused Sam. What advice would you give to Sam?

INTRODUCTION

Senior managers in most health departments can be counted on to support and praise the value of continuing education. Unfortunately, many managers drop training and development when budgets become tight and expenses must be reduced. This is due, in part, to the difficulty of pinpointing cost savings that can be attributed to continuing education. Most individuals in management believe or know intuitively that education ultimately saves money. The problem is that there are no reliable ways to measure the results of education in terms of cost-benefit analysis. As a result, money spent on education is often viewed as resources that are expended with few tangible results.

As important as training and development are to every health department, in many instances they receive minimal attention from upper managers. Simply reminding department managers that they have a responsibility for employee development is insufficient. Managers should be encouraged to view training and development as an important method for keeping valuable employees interested and challenged.

Factors that motivate employees are found primarily in the nature of the work. Among the strongest motivating factors are the opportunity to do interesting and challenging work and the opportunity to learn and grow. Better-performing employees usually are so motivated. They are also the individuals who are most likely to leave in search of more interesting and challenging work and greater overall opportunity. One way for department managers to increase the chances of retaining their better employees is through visible support for training and development.

A department that places no emphasis on training and development may seem to be standing still. In reality, it is actually going backward. With technological, economic, legislative, financial, and social change constantly occurring, no department of health can afford to stand still. A certain amount of forward progress is necessary simply to remain abreast of change. Therefore, maintaining or improving the abilities of staff must be an ongoing effort. Continuing education is essential.

THE MANAGER'S ROLE IN EMPLOYEE TRAINING

Under the blanket heading of *training* is an entire range of employee development activities, from providing new employee orientation to assisting employees in moving up into management. Employee development should be one of the most important aspects of a manager's job.

Managers are likely to have greater depth and breadth of technical knowledge and expertise in the area or program they manage than is found anywhere else in the organization. Managers tend to be educated in the field in which they work. In addition, they have the advantage of practical education acquired through experience. Therefore, managers are primary resources for information about their departments and the work they perform. Department managers are uniquely positioned to pass on their knowledge and expertise to others. Department managers have the responsibility for maintaining and improving the capability and competence of their staff.

The importance of continuing education and training is underscored by the extent to which various accreditation and regulatory agencies assess training activities during their periodic surveys. Another indicator of the importance is the fact that many health care practitioners are required to provide evidence of a certain number of continuing education units each year to maintain their professional licensure.

From a manager's perspective, teaching should be an integral part of management's role. Teaching is an essential part of managerial delegation. Unfortunately, employee instruction is often overlooked.

NEW EMPLOYEE ORIENTATION

Each health department manager should have a new employee orientation plan for the agency. Orientation plans are required by accreditation and regulatory agencies.

An organization usually provides a general new employee orientation that addresses common matters. Ordinarily provided by human resources, the general orientation addresses such matters as the organization's structure and leadership, employee benefits, the performance appraisal process, the organization's dress code, employee parking, facility security, infection control, and universal precautions. Employee health and other benefits and the employee assistance program, employee work rules, and generally applicable policies are also typically included.

A department orientation should provide an introduction to the people in the agency and program area and to the physical space, equipment, processes, and special department policies. On-the-job guidance in getting started doing the work for which the new person was hired should also be provided. One of the most inappropriate ways of treating new employees is to simply allow them to begin working. Even experienced and well-educated new employees require some guidance concerning variations specific to a particular department and program area as well as time to ask questions about the new job.

As part of a new employee's orientation, it may help to appoint a mentor. This is an experienced person who can provide guidance through the new person's first few days or weeks on the job. Mentoring offers valuable benefits. It provides a personally guided orientation for the newcomer, and it affords an opportunity for further development to an experienced employee.

■ TRAINING TO CORRECT PERFORMANCE PROBLEMS

Training ought to be a manager's priority. However, it is not the manager's top priority, which is running a program area and getting out the expected work. Nevertheless, training is important, especially regarding new or revised work procedures and correcting performance problems.

In assessing employee performance, managers continually compare observed performance with expectations. Managers may have to be teachers when helping employees correct performance problems. When an employee displays performance problems that command a manager's attention, it is always appropriate to consider if reasonable efforts are being made to help the employee succeed. Many employees fail at their jobs because they were inappropriately trained, insufficiently oriented, or inadequately supported.

It may be necessary to impose a particular kind of education or training as a condition for continued employment. For example, an individual whose telephone manners have elicited many complaints may be required to complete a program in telephone etiquette. One whose job requires writing but who has experienced problems with written grammar may be required to take a remedial English language program.

■ DETERMINING DEPARTMENTAL LEARNING NEEDS

If a variety of learning needs seem to be present throughout a department, it may be helpful to conduct a needs analysis for basic learning. One approach consists of making a simple chart for each job description in the department, with columns indicating the required skills and rows listing the employees whose work indicates those activities. It then becomes a matter of assessing all employees in terms of whether their skills are adequate to meet normal job expectations. Each assessment that falls short of normal expectations indicates a learning need. This approach helps managers focus training activities on the areas of greatest need. In addition to managers' assessments, noticeable performance problems also indicate areas of need, as do tendencies toward repetitive errors or actions that generate chronic complaints by customers, coworkers, and others.

A manager's initial assessment of training needs is translated into training objectives. Learners must initially know where they are headed. Once this is determined, learners and managers can consider how to get there.

A learner's motivation is key to the eventual success of training. Managers must be prepared to help employees answer one particular question about what they are being asked to learn: "What's in it for me?" When correcting a severe performance problem, the answer may be as basic as "You get to remain employed." Numerous other responses are possible, such as "You get to learn something that may eventually help get you promoted" or "You get more variety in your work" or "You get to do something more challenging than what you've been doing."

EMPLOYEE TRAINING WITHIN THE DEPARTMENT

The following principles may assist a manager when addressing staff training and development needs. All employees who are expected to learn something deserve to know why they are learning, and all should be advised of specific goals and objectives. Employees learn better when they actually become involved in the process. The more hands-on or learn-while-doing components that can be incorporated, the more likely a training program will be successful. Employees will more quickly and accurately absorb material that applies to their daily work than material they view as irrelevant. Thus, in-department employee training should be practical and immediately applicable rather than theoretical.

Most employees will accept new ideas more readily if these ideas support their previous beliefs. New material, techniques, and processes are best presented within the context of a department's mission. For example, "We're still here to serve members of the community, but now it can be done more quickly and at lower cost." Some employees learn best when allowed to pursue their own areas of interest or needs at their own rate. For these employees, managers must provide clear expectations, necessary information and materials, and general guidance. Many employees must be encouraged to find learning pleasant. For some employees, the possibility of education of any kind essentially means going back to school, which renders them resistant to training. These people must be shown what's in it for them.

CROSS-TRAINING FOR EFFICIENCY

Department managers who supervise employees working in comparable positions in terms of job grade or pay scale have the opportunity to implement cross-training. For example, an office manager may have three clerical-level employees who are assigned in different capacities: a file clerk, a program secretary, and a data entry specialist. These three jobs reside in the same pay grade. As long as the three people simply do their own jobs, the department has limited flexibility. If one person is on vacation or is ill, no one is trained to assume the missing person's duties. If all three people are capable of doing all three jobs, the employees can be moved around as needed. Resources can be shifted as workloads or backlogs demand, and any of the three people can cover for any of the others as necessary.

This type of flexibility can be obtained by training the three employees in each other's jobs. This requires time and effort. Each person can train the other two people in the particulars of his or her job. The manager provides general guidance. This training will ultimately repay the time and effort involved. The department gains considerable flexibility in addressing backlogs and covering for vacations and illnesses. The individuals gain greater interests and challenges associated with their work through increased task variety.

ON-THE-JOB TRAINING

On-the-job training is appropriate under many circumstances. For some learning needs, it may be the best available approach. On-the-job training is best accomplished under the direct supervision of a manager or under the direct guidance of an experienced employee. Employees being trained on the job receive step-by-step instructions on how to accomplish a task while actually performing it. After employees perform the task a sufficient number of times under this direct guidance, the instructor may then reduce or eliminate the verbal guidance and simply watch the employee until assured that the activity is being performed in a satisfactory manner. Thus assured, the instructor may further withdraw to a position of being readily available to answer questions.

On-the-job training is not simply allowing employees to learn by trial and error with only a rough idea about any expected results. However, this is precisely what it becomes when managers decide that they are too busy to properly address training.

Improper or inadequate on-the-job training can be dangerous or destructive. Employees may learn to perform their tasks in a highly inefficient manner, creating inappropriate work habits that will become deeply ingrained and difficult to correct. It is far better for managers to ensure that sufficient time and attention are devoted at the start of the learning process so that on-the-job training can succeed as intended.

Another common but inadequate approach to training, or at least satisfying annual in-service education requirements, is to give staff members files or folders to review. Often, accreditation agencies or state regulations require these documents to be read. A reading package is circulated among the staff with instructions for each recipient to review the documents as required, check off to indicate that they have done so, and pass the material to the next person. This is the loosest and probably the weakest approach to training. Short of questioning each recipient in detail, there is no way to ensure that the material has been read and absorbed.

Most people recall a certain portion of information they hear (10 percent), a somewhat greater portion of what they both see and hear (20 percent), and almost all of what they see, hear, and do (90 percent). This suggests that the most effective job-related training should include a combination of lecture, demonstration, and hands-on practice.

Using multiple channels of sensory input increases the likelihood of learning. This is why personal reading alone may be the least effective way of learning, and why lecture alone is not a great deal better. When multiple senses are used simultaneously, the chances of learning increase. Repeating the same material after a lapse of time and presenting it in varying forms can be highly effective in ensuring that the material will be retained.

EFFECTIVE MENTORING

Mentoring can be most effective if it is officially sanctioned. It need not take place within the context of a formal program, but it should be acknowledged as an actively used employee development technique rather than simply an ad hoc practice whereby people might happen to link up with each other. The extent of the formality required may be minimal. The new employee and experienced employee or mentor are intentionally brought together by a department manager. All three parties agree on the objectives of the relationship, specifying what the new employee is expected to learn. The manager remains close enough to the process to be able to evaluate both the new employee and the mentor during and after the relationship period.

By officially addressing mentoring as a means of employee development, an organization sends a strong message to all employees concerning its commitment to their development. Although mentoring is one of the least costly development tools available, it can be extremely effective. Its visible use proclaims that the organization cares about the development of its people.

For a new employee, a mentor can be a valuable facilitator, sounding board, and source of advice and guidance. The mentor benefits as well. Mentoring can provide a sense of fulfillment and satisfaction, especially for a senior employee who is in need of additional challenge and who can benefit from more interesting work experiences. The process helps mentors further refine their skills and keep them sharp.

Employees most likely to realize significant benefits from a mentoring relationship are those who demonstrate a willingness to learn, are proactive in expressing this willingness, and are ambitious and enthusiastic. Effective mentors are able to assume full responsibility for their own growth and development. They are receptive to coaching and constructive feedback and have the ability to change behaviors based on positive experiences.

Experienced employees who are considered for mentoring responsibilities should be persons that are willing to serve voluntarily and give the undertaking the time and energy it requires. No mentor should ever be unilaterally assigned or forced to serve. Potential mentors should possess sufficient knowledge and expertise in the new employee's areas of responsibility. They should have good interpersonal skills such as patience, be supportive and friendly, and be effective listeners. Above all else, potential mentors should demonstrate an interest in the development of others.

■ DEVELOPING POTENTIAL MANAGERS

An essential part of every manager's responsibility is to help identify and develop new managers. This includes identifying and developing one or more potential successors. Many managers fall short of the latter need.

The development of potential successors is closely associated with the practice of proper delegation. This is the primary means by which succession planning evolves. It is an area of concern or threat for some managers. Such managers are insecure in their positions and fear the competition provided by intelligent, up-and-coming subordinates. Many managers simply do not think beyond the present. They are ill-prepared to imagine being moved up or out or becoming incapacitated and no longer able to function in their positions.

Development of a potential new manager may not occur within a department because it requires serious and progressively more delegation of responsibilities. This takes time and planning on the part of management. Such development requires delegation of tasks that are increasingly more responsible. Suitable tasks are often sufficiently appealing or important that managers retain them personally rather than give them up to subordinates.

At the very least, having a potential successor in the process of development means that managers usually have readily available coverage for vacations and illnesses as needed. No person is or should be absolutely indispensable. The loss or absence of a group's leader when there is no ready back-up person can create significant inefficiency and inconvenience to an organization.

A manager who entertains ambitions about advancing higher in an organization should take seriously the need to develop a potential successor. Higher management will often look closely at a manager's track record in delegating tasks and especially at whether that manager has one or more capable successors in the wings. Enlightened higher management may well conclude that a supervisor who has paid no attention to developing a potential successor shows little strength in delegation, a skill that becomes increasingly important as one moves up in an organization. Executives in an organizational hierarchy may be unwilling to promote a manager if doing so means having to conduct an external search for a successor or promoting an untried insider.

No manager wants to lose good employees. However, some of them are going to be lost regardless of what management does. Managers who put time and effort into developing potential successors may see many of them eventually lost to other departments or other organizations as they take advantage of opportunities to advance their careers. But these employees are likely to be lost to an organization if they are not given opportunities to develop. Some of them will be lost even sooner if they remain unchallenged in their jobs. Therefore, prudent managers should take full advantage of the talents that are available in their groups by delegating tasks to the better and more willing employees and helping them to develop.

Only rarely does a manager have anything to fear from a subordinate who is encouraged to develop and grow and learn some aspects of the manager's job. In fact, having one or two sharp, up-and-coming employees is often just what a manager needs to remain effective and continue to grow.

■ HOW HUMAN RESOURCES CAN HELP

It is customary for an organization's general new employee orientation to be presented or at least coordinated by human resources. As far as this orientation is concerned, ordinarily all a manager has to do is ensure that each new employee attends. However, some managers have to be reminded of the necessity for all new employees to attend the orientation. Some of these new employees may be filling positions that have been empty for some time, and the department may be behind in its work. Occasionally, managers may decide that new employees cannot be spared for the few hours required for orientation. There may be a tendency to regard orientation as just another human resources thing that intrudes on a manager's ability to run a program.

In most instances, a general orientation to the organization includes topics that are required by accreditation or regulations. Orientation then becomes partly a response to external requirements and partly a service performed to get new employees pointed in the proper direction.

Beyond ensuring that new employees attend the orientation, it is the responsibility of managers to be aware of training needs and to either attend to them or refer them as necessary. In addressing issues of employee training and development, the department manager should expect human resources to work with managers in diagnosing particular problems and determining the kinds of training or education that might be helpful, to provide certain kinds of needed training, to secure the involvement of other in-house training expertise, to identify external sources for specifically required training and determine how these sources are accessed, and to guide employees in using an organization's tuition-assistance program when appropriate.

Training needs should be addressed on a continuing basis, both to assess present circumstances to determine the skills and attitudes that must be adopted or improved to meet current needs and to attempt to determine future needs based on trends that appear to be coming during the next one or two years. Information for evaluating training needs can be gathered in a variety of ways, including questionnaires completed by managers and employees, focus group discussions, individual interviews with managers and employees, and exit interviews at which departing employees are asked for their opinions concerning developmental needs. Topics that are frequently mentioned merit consideration as potential program topics.

Human resources can contribute information relevant to determining training and development needs from direct contact with people on the job, both managers and rank-and-file employees; reviewing performance appraisals, performance improvement records, and disciplinary actions; and monitoring trends in public health.

In guiding any training and development activities, human resources may recommend involving both managers and employees in preparing training agendas and determining program content. It often starts with needs that employees appear to be the most strongly motivated to address. Human resources focuses on present jobs and needs first, then looks to the future, focusing primarily on behavior in the belief that if skills are appropriately implanted or modified then proper attitudes will follow. It will use on-the-job experiential learning to the maximum practical extent, supplemented with training from other sources.

In evaluating training efforts, human resources will attempt to determine whether the needs assessments that were conducted were accurate, whether targeted skills have been learned and incorporated into new behaviors, and whether employee attitudes appear to have been modified. Human resources must assess what has been learned and how this audit of results can support the next cycle of training.

CONCLUSION

Training and development should be ongoing and nearly continuous activities. Managers are central to training efforts, identifying needs and often serving as trainers. New employees must be properly and completely oriented to a health department as well as their own program areas. Cross-training provides flexibility, especially in times of crisis. On-the-job training is important and often conducted by a mentor. Potential new managers rarely emerge without assistance. They must be nurtured and developed by providing opportunities for them to actually supervise others or guide programs. Human resources personnel may provide assistance in training and development.

Returning to the harried health commissioner in the opening case study, Sam should seek volunteers to serve as mentors for the new employees. This would provide support for the new people and give Sam a chance to evaluate the leadership potential of two subordinates. Sam also should take the new employees to lunch on their third day of employment.

Although it would be efficient to provide one initial orientation session for both new employees, Sam should avoid the temptation. This would require the new epidemiologist to either start without any training or to waste four working days. Either alternative would send a negative message to the new employee.

One year later, both new employees were fully integrated into the health department. One of the mentors seized the opportunity to shine and was promoted seven months later. Both mentors reported increased job satisfaction. Sam had noticed the improvement in their job productivity. The epidemiologist volunteered to serve as a mentor in the future. Sam was still struggling with the daily volume of unwanted e-mail offers.

Resources

Periodicals

Longman, S., and Gabriel, M. 2004. Staff perceptions of e-learning. *Canadian Nurse* 100(1):23–27.

Price, J.H., Akpanudo, S., Dake, J.A., and Telljohann, S.K. 2004. Continuing-education needs of public health educators: their perspectives. *Journal of Public Health Management and Practice* 10(2):156–163.

Stengel, J.R., Dixon, A.L., and Allen, C.T. 2003. Listening begins at home. *Harvard Business Review* 81(11):106–117.

Sumrow, A. 2003. Motivation: A new look at an age-old topic. *Radiology Management* 25(5):44–47.

Books

Baume, S., Pink, D., and Baume, D. 2004. *Enhancing Staff and Educational Development.* New York: Taylor & Francis.

Bubb, S. 2004. *The Insider's Guide to Early Professional Development.* New York: Taylor & Francis.

Buckley, R., and Caple, J. 2004. *Theory and Practice of Training*, 5th ed. London: Kogan Page.

Stimson, N. 2002. *How to Write and Prepare Training Materials*, 2d ed. London: Kogan Page.

Wilcox, M., and Rush, S. 2004. *The CCL Guide to Leadership in Action: How Managers and Organizations Can Improve the Practice of Leadership.* San Francisco: Jossey-Bass.

Web Sites

- International Journal of Training and Development: www.blackwellpublishing.com/journal.asp?ref=1360-3736
- National Institute of Health: learningsource.od.nih.gov
- Training and Development Community Center: www.tcm.com/trdev
- Workforce Management: www.workforce.com/section/11

Organizations

American College of Healthcare Executives
One North Franklin, Suite 1700
Chicago, IL 60606-4425
Phone: 312-424-2800
Fax: 312-424-0023
E-mail: geninfo@ache.org
Web site: www.ache.org

American Management Association
1601 Broadway
New York, NY 10019
Phone: 212-586-8100
Fax: 212-903-8168
Web site: www.amanet.org/index.htm

American Society for Training & Development
1640 King Street, Box 1443
Alexandria, VA, 22313-2043
Phone: 703-683-8100
Fax: 703-683-8103
Web site: www.astd.org/astd

National Association of County and City Health Officials
1100 17th Street, Second Floor
Washington, D.C. 20036
Phone: 202-783-5550

Fax: 202-783-1583
E-mail: naccho@naccho.org
Web site: www.naccho.org

Public Health Foundation
1220 L Street, NW, Suite 350
Washington, D.C. 20005
Phone: 202-898-5600
Fax: 202-898-5609
E-mail: info@phf.org
Web site: www.phf.org

CHAPTER

16

Rewarding Employees

Kip E. Miller

Chapter Objectives

After reading this chapter, readers will:

- Understand the theories of motivation and their contributions to understanding what motivates individuals and groups, particularly in the workplace.
- Identify early reward research and understand its historical importance.
- Discuss practical ways to recognize and reward employees, especially in today's working environments and marketplace.

Chapter Summary

From the most selfless act of kindness to the most hideous, terrible deed, mankind has sought to study and understand why people do what they do. This chapter will review significant theories of motivation. Maslow, McGregor, Herzberg, Vroom, and others will be reviewed and explained in light of historical context. Theory is important because it explains past observations and predicts future ones.

Taking these theories and applying them to everyday life and work situations is important to the managers, directors, and supervisors who are in charge of groups of employees. This is especially important as society faces the challenges of a dwindling labor force and one that requires more job-specific education. Recruiting and retaining quality employees does not just happen. It takes a concerted effort on the part of management. This chapter will identify ideas that can enrich the work experience and the quality of an employee's contribution to an employer.

Case Study

The most junior member of a particular unit within a local health organization has been employed for 10 years. The average tenure in the unit is 15 years. The members of this unit, though by no means perfect, provide consistent service and require far less micromanagement compared with other units in the organization.

As often happens, once employees reach the top of the salary scale, providing meaningful incentives is difficult at best. Vacation time, sick time accrual, and wage caps have all been reached by every individual in the unit, so they cannot be paid more or have their benefit structure increased. Their supervisor wants to do something for them because they consistently receive positive feedback from customers, work cooperatively with the other units, and often complete projects ahead of schedule and with consistently good results. What motivates this unit to perform as it does?

INTRODUCTION

Theories are developed to explain past observations and predict future ones (Beck, 2000). The following is an overview of historical and contemporary theories of motivation. They have been chosen based on their contribution to understanding motivation and their utility for supervisors and managers.

MASLOW'S HIERARCHY OF NEEDS

Maslow observed that a person will start at the bottom of a pyramid, or hierarchy, and seek to satisfy basic physiologic needs such as obtaining food and shelter. Once these needs are met, an individual is then no longer satisfied. The individual then moves to the next level of the pyramid. Above the basic need to obtain food and shelter are four other levels: safety and security; love and belongingness; self-esteem; and, finally, self-actualization (Maslow, 1943). Safety needs on the job include physical safety as well as protection from layoff. Social needs bring to light that most people want to be part of a group. Esteem needs emphasize that individuals wish to garner the respect or esteem of other people. A promotion is an example of this. Finally, self-actualization is the art of reaching one's potential.

Maslow's model has some weaknesses. First, an individual's behavior may be in response to several needs at one time. Second, different individuals do not respond in the same manner at similar levels. For instance, not every person has the same level of need to belong to a group. Lastly, the model ignores the frequently observed behavior of individuals who tolerate a difficult job for the promise of future benefits. However, Maslow's observations offer a basic understanding of how individuals' responses to perceived needs motivates their attempts to meet those needs in a work setting.

MCGREGOR'S THEORY X AND THEORY Y

Douglas McGregor distinguished two approaches to management and workers: Theory X and Theory Y. McGregor did not imply that all workers could be described by one theory or the other. Rather, Theory X and Theory Y were seen as two extremes, with a complete spectrum of behaviors in between. Theory X assumes that people dislike work and must be coerced, controlled, and directed toward organizational goals. The theory also assumes that most people prefer to be treated in this way so that they can avoid responsibility. Theory Y emphasizes people's intrinsic interest in their work, their desire to be self-directed and seek responsibility and their capacity to be creative in solving business problems (McGregor, 1960).

An example may provide clarification. A sales manager of a company who gives credence to Theory X would establish sales quotas for the sales force. The sales force might be given a goal for the year that, if reached, would result in an all-expense-paid weeklong trip for the successful salesperson and his or her spouse. The vacation time used would be in addition to normally accrued vacation time. Salespeople who did not meet their quotas for three consecutive quarters would probably not be invited back for a fourth.

Someone who believes in Theory Y is characterized by the following example. A regional sales vice president might meet with the sales managers in his region to establish sales quotas for each year. Those meeting their quotas would receive a bonus according to the amount sold above the basic quota. The vice president would emphasize that high performance is an important factor when individuals are considered for management positions. In addition, keeping the product development department well informed of changes in consumer expectations is also considered to be an important part of the job.

More recent theories have gotten away from the notion that all rewards have to be of an economic nature. This is partly due to the research reported by McGregor and the simplicity of Theory X. It is unfortunate that many employers believe payment in and of itself is sufficient to motivate workers.

HERZBERG'S TWO-FACTOR THEORY

Building upon the two-theory McGregor model, Fredrick Herzberg theorized that some aspects of a job are considered to be low level. When these low-level aspects, called hygiene factors, are present, they simply result in nondissatisfied workers. Satisfaction with factors, such as company policies, relations with others, job security, and supervision, provide hygiene, but they do not result in improved job performance. Motivators, or satisfiers, are considered to be more powerful in their ability to meet worker needs. These motivators are things such as recognition, feelings of achievement, social interactions, and challenges. The heart of Herzberg's approach is that meeting hygienic measures will not markedly improve performance, but dissatisfaction with motivators may lower performance (Herzberg, 1966).

Herzberg tested his theory by asking workers to explain what job-related aspects made them feel exceptionally good or exceptionally bad about their jobs. His conclusion was that the presence of motivating factors, such as achievement and recognition, makes workers feel good and the absence of hygiene factors, such as adequate salary and security, makes them feel exceptionally bad.

In summary, Herzberg's theory is an oversimplified explanation of how needs influence motivation. Studies have shown that hygiene factors such as wages can satisfy needs and increase motivation. They have also shown that the absence of motivators, such as recognition, means that important needs are unsatisfied. The result is workers who are dissatisfied. However, his work helps to emphasize that lower-level needs are relatively finite and quickly satisfied, whereas higher level needs are rarely satisfied. As a result, building motivators into the work by making it more interesting and challenging should have a powerful and lasting effect on motivation, especially for employees whose lower-level needs are fairly well satisfied (Dessler, 2003).

VROOM'S VALENCE–INSTRUMENTALITY–EXPECTANCY THEORY

According to Vroom (1982), expectancy is the understood probability that a certain amount of effort will be instrumental in gaining a valued goal. Expectancy refers to the perceived relationship between a given level of effort and a given level of performance. This is the extent to which a person feels that his or her output at the job will actually lead to increased rewards or recognition. A person may think, "What are the chances of getting promoted if I work hard?" According to the worker's knowledge of the situation, the probability could be perceived as low, medium, or high. As an example, a female in a male-dominated organization may consider the probability of advancement to be low compared with her male counterparts.

The second component of expectancy is the valence, or value, that a particular outcome has for a worker. If promotion were not a valued goal, the valence of that goal would be low. Therefore, the person would not work hard for this goal.

In summary, Vroom postulated that motivation is a three-step process (Dessler, 2003). Does a person feel that the second-level outcome, such as promotion, is important or high in valence? Does an individual feel that high performance or a first-level outcome will be instrumental in getting a desired reward? Does a person feel that exerting effort will in fact result in a reward?

ADAMS' EQUITY THEORY

Equity theory is the idea that people compare how hard they work with what they get in return, and if they perceive a discrepancy, they are unhappy. The discrepancy may be between a person's internal standard for what an equitable return is for a certain amount of effort or it may be in comparison with some external reference (Adams, 1965).

This phenomenon frequently occurs when workers from different departments within the same organization compare their salaries. If differences exist as a result of external market forces, the result can be a degree of tension between individuals or between departments. What would happen if the worker in question was a female who was getting perceived low return for her effort compared with her male coworkers? She might reduce her output, she may quit her job, or she might consider filing a complaint under equal pay or fair employment laws. Perceived inequities produce unhappy workers.

LOCKE'S THEORY OF GOAL SETTING

Edwin Locke developed a theory that says that the goals set by a person's conscious intentions can ultimately affect performance. He proposed two major principles of goal setting. First, hard goals produce higher performance. Second, easy goals and specific goals produce higher performance than vague goals (Beck, 2000). An example of a vague goal is "Do the best you can."

The higher and more specific a person's goals are, the harder the person will try, and the higher the resulting performance or output. This finding was seen in a logging operation in Oklahoma. As part of a logging operation, truck drivers loaded cut logs and drove them to a mill. Their performance showed that they were often not filling their trucks to the maximum legal net weight. Traditionally, these drivers were simply encouraged to "do their best" when it came to loading to maximum weight. As part of the study, researchers arranged for a specific goal of 94 percent of the truck's net weight to be recommended to each driver. No monetary rewards were offered, and only verbal praise was given for increased performance. No special training was given to the drivers or the supervisors. The result was that performance (the weight loaded on each truck) increased dramatically as soon as the truckers were given specific, high goals. Performance also remained at an elevated level after the study was concluded (Dessler, 2003).

It was also shown that the more difficult the goal, the higher the level of performance. However, this assumes that the goals are accepted. Some studies in this area have analyzed the effects of goal setting in United Funds campaigns. Researchers found that goals must be perceived as attainable for higher performance to result. For example, productivity increased 25 percent when goals were set 20 percent higher than the previous year. When goals were set at 80 percent above the previous performance, productivity increased only 12 percent. In addition, when goals were doubled, to 100 percent of the previous performance, productivity actually decreased (Dessler, 1994).

EARLY REWARD RESEARCH

Over the years, many researchers have tried to predict the behavior of workers. With the arrival of the industrial revolution, vocations became more intricate and diversified. These diversified jobs brought with them the challenges of educating those workers and learning what motivated them to work and be productive. Productivity became more and more important as mass production and the industrial revolution changed the experiences of everyday workers and their workplaces.

Frederick Taylor, often named the father of scientific management, broke down jobs into their individual functions. By understanding the components of each job, management could plan every move and thus create an efficient flow of work. This was an extremely successful approach in the first half of the twentieth century. Rather than the haphazard, variable approach of the crafter, industry was well served by the predictable, efficient, consistent production of the assembly line (Cotton, 1993). As jobs became more complex, the limits of the scientific management method became apparent—such rigid methods do not lend themselves to complex jobs.

Since Frederick Taylor, many researchers have applied themselves to various theories. Kurt Lewin studied how employee involvement affected empowerment and productivity (Lewin, 1997). Eric Trist and Fred Emery built upon Lewin's ideas (Trist et al., 1997). They studied the employee social systems and the technical aspects of particular jobs. They discovered that productive, rewarding work occurs when the social system and the technical system are in harmony.

B.F. Skinner coined the term operant conditioning when he constructed a box to study the effect of rewards on learned behavior. The Skinner box enabled researchers to continuously record behavior patterns and the effect of reinforcers (rewards) on rats. As a result of Skinner's work, a general rule was established: The quicker rewards are given after an appropriate response, the more effective they are (Skinner, 1970). For example, if a child does something to please a parent and the approval is slow in coming, the child may not realize that the reward was for the earlier behavior. From the perspective of an employee, adults are able to distinguish a reward that may be late in coming, but managers should remember to be timely when attempting to reward employees.

Before particular rewards are discussed, it is beneficial to explain the difference between intrinsic and extrinsic rewards and motivation in greater detail. Early research focused on the existence of external rewards, relatively little work examined the internal factors that motivate people.

Extrinsic, or external, rewards are obvious and tangible. Examples of extrinsic rewards include pay, promotion, and benefits. Extrinsic rewards are easy to identify, but often difficult to provide. When an economy is shrinking, organizations look at ways to hold down costs. Recently, many employees were grateful to simply have a job, let alone receive some additional extrinsic reward in increased pay or benefit. This tolerance quickly dissipates when all employees do not forgo rewards or when some people receive very high levels of pay or other exaggerated extrinsic benefits.

Intrinsic motivators are those factors that make certain activities rewarding in and of themselves. These include achievement, challenge, self-actualization, games, puzzles, and creative endeavors. Additional intangible motivators include being appreciated for work that was done, being kept informed of organizational events, and having a sympathetic manager who takes time to listen. It is logical to expect that if external rewards are combined with intrinsic motivators, persons or groups should perform even better at the activities that they already like. This however, is not always the case.

Deci and Flaste (1996) concluded that intrinsic motivation and external rewards interact in the following way. External rewards facilitate behaviors when they primarily convey information that a person is competent, when the rewards are not perceived as controlling individual behavior, and when they are given for routine, well-learned activities. External rewards tend to impair performance when they are obvious and given for activities already of high interest and when they are related to such open-ended activities as problem solving. In most cases, people do not strive for predetermined rewards, but discover the rewards as they go along (Beck, 2000).

Turn-of-the-century scientific managers viewed motivation and productivity as a direct result of extrinsic factors. During the 1990s, most written work focused mainly on intrinsic factors. As with most concepts, ideas ebb and flow with time and in comparison to the most recent concepts. It is important to remember that both types of rewards have their place when rewarding employees. A savvy manager is aware of both types and employs them at the right time and in an appropriate measure.

The next section identifies specific rewards that can be used when limited funds are available to managers. This is not an exhaustive list, but rather a group of effective and proven methods that help to reward and motivate employees. The goal is to provide practical, creative ideas that readers can draw upon.

REWARDS AND RECOGNITION

Before we provide the list of rewards, it is vital that the following be understood. How managers and superiors present a reward or recognition is almost as important as what is being recognized. Arguably, it is more important than what is being given as a reward. If a manager simply drops off the best award that an organization is able to afford on an employee's desk and mumbles a "thank you" on the way out the door, money has been wasted. Indeed, more harm than good may actually result (CCH, 2003). Many good rewards have been wasted by bad deliveries. For example, a large boisterous celebration rewarding an employee who is shy and introverted will probably be wasted.

Creativity can often be the most difficult part of rewarding employees. When trying to reward employees, it is important to find out what motivates them. This requires taking the time to find out what specifically motivates each individual employee. **Table 16-1** provides some examples of rewards that do not require large sums of money.

Table 16-2 contains a list of suggestions for recognizing and motivating employees.

CONCLUSION

From pay raises and incentive plans to a simple note of thanks, employees want to be recognized and appreciated for their work. Managers are at the critical junction of matching employees' work needs with motivating their workforce to optimum efficiency. If done in an appropriate manner, motivating one employee results in motivation for more than one individual. The same approach is usually not effective for all employees. This is why knowing one's employees is so important. It requires hard work to motivate a department, a division, or an entire organization. Effective managers must expend time and effort to help identify those ideas that help motivate their employees. This is part of what it means to be a manager.

Returning to the long-term employees in the opening case study, not only is it important to understand what motivates each individual, but it is equally important to understand what motivational synergy exists. In other words, each individual in a group brings a set of abilities. When the abilities of all of the members of the group are combined, the group

Table 16-1 Low-Cost Rewards

1. Write a letter to the employee's family telling them about a recent accomplishment and what it means to the company or department.
2. Arrange for a vice president or upper manager to have lunch with the employee. The president of the company might call or meet with the employee to offer personal thanks for an effort or job that was well done.
3. Determine what an employee's personal hobby is and purchase a small gift that relates to that hobby.
4. Reserve a special parking space for an employee.
5. Wash an employee's car at work so that the task is completed before he or she leaves for home.
6. Write a personal note to the employee. Make sure that this note is handwritten. Personal notes mean much more than printed ones.
7. Put up a bulletin board. This board can be used to honor employees for excellent work. Letters, memos, pictures and thank-you cards can be placed here for employee recognition.
8. Have a Friday surprise. Surprise staff members with something nice on Friday, recognizing their hard work to complete a special project or just for hanging in there.
9. Make a grab bag of privileges. Print each privilege on a slip of paper and have the reward recipient draw or select one. Privileges may include the following: The manager will do one of the employee's job duties for a day; the manager will provide and deliver morning coffee and a bagel one day; the employee may be offered the choice of arriving late or leaving early for one day; the employee may be offered a work-at-home day.

Source: Mailleux & Associates (1997).

contributes more as a unit than what is individually possible. An understanding of each of the motivational theories provides a basis by which rewards can be considered that will actually encourage and foster improved or consistent performance.

Once supervisors better understand what motivates an individual or group, which reward is selected? What will actually be perceived as rewarding by the employees? Rewards can take two different forms, intrinsic and extrinsic. Intrinsic motivators are those that are rewarding in themselves, such as games, pastimes, and creative endeavors. External rewards are those rewards given to an individual as a result of a certain behavior. With regards to the case study, intrinsic motivators and creative extrinsic rewards must be tailored to specific situations.

Lastly, what specific rewards are available to this group that are timely, effective, and perceived in the proper manner? Supervisors and management can use employee recognition awards, other nonmonetary rewards, or other seemingly intangible acts to reward superior employees. Often it is more important to workers that they be recognized in nonmonetary ways rather than by more costly methods. Expanding the ex-

Table 16-2 Nelson's Ten Commandments of Recognition

1. Personally thank employees for doing a good job. Thank them face-to-face, in writing, or both. Do it early, often, and sincerely.
2. Take the time to meet with and listen to employees—as much as they need or want.
3. Provide specific feedback about performance of the person, the department, and the organization.
4. Strive to create a work environment that is open, trusting, and fun. Encourage new ideas and initiative.
5. Provide information on how the organization makes and loses money, upcoming programs or services, strategies for competing in the marketplace, and how the person fits into the overall plan.
6. Involve employees in decisions, especially as those decisions affect them.
7. Provide employees with a sense of ownership in their work and work environment.
8. Recognize, reward, and promote people according to their performance; deal with low and marginal performers so that they either improve or leave.
9. Give people a chance to grow and learn new skills. Show or help them to meet their goals within the context of the organization's goals. Create partnerships with employees.
10. Celebrate successes of the company, of the department, and of individuals. Take time for team and morale-building meetings and activities.

Source: Nelson (2003).

perience of rewards and understanding some of the practical ways to distribute those rewards provide a powerful arsenal in building or keeping a motivated workforce.

References

Adams, J.S. 1965. Inequity in social exchange. In L. Berkowitz (ed.), *Advances in Experimental Social Psychology.* New York: Academic Press.

Beck, R.C. 2000. *Motivation: Theories and Principles.* Upper Saddle River, NJ: Prentice-Hall.

CCH. 2003. *How to Reward and Recognize.* Riverwoods, IL: CCH Incorporated.

Cotton, J.L. 1993. *Employee Involvement.* Newbury Park, CA: Sage.

Deci, E.L., and Flaste, R. 1996. *Why We Do What We Do: Understanding Self-Motivation.* New York: Penguin.

Dessler, G. 2003. *Framework for Human Resource Management*, 3d ed. Upper Saddle River, NJ: Prentice-Hall.

Herzberg, F. 1966. *Work and the Nature of Man.* Chicago: World.

Lewin, K. 1997. *Resolving Social Conflicts and Field Theory in Social Science.* Chicago: American Psychological Association.

Mailleux & Associates. 1997. *Be creative when rewarding employees.*

Maslow, A.H. 1943. A theory of human motivation. *Psychological Review* 50 (5):370–396.

McGregor, D. 1960. *The Human Side of Enterprise.* New York: McGraw-Hill.

Nelson, R. 2003. Nelson's Ten Commandments of recognition. *Workforce*, April, pp. 50.
Skinner, B.F. 1970. *Science and Human Behavior.* New York: Simon & Schuster.
Trist, E., Emery, F., and Murray, H. 1997. *The Social Engagement of Social Science.* Philadelphia: University of Pennsylvania Press.
Vroom, V. 1982. *Work and Motivation.* Melbourne, FL: Krieger.

Resources

Periodicals

Benson, S.G., and Dundis, S.P. 2003. Understanding and motivating health care employees: Integrating Maslow's hierarchy of needs, training, and technology. *Journal of Nursing Management* 11(5):315–320.
Harmon, J., Scotti, D.J., Behson, S., Farias, G., Petzel, R., Neuman, J. H., and Keashly, L. 2003. Effects of high-involvement work systems on employee satisfaction and service costs in veterans' healthcare. *Journal of Healthcare Management* 48(6):393–406.
Ray, B. 2003. Reward cards motivate. *Occupational Health and Safety* 72(6):51–52.
Sims, B. 2003. In defense of incentives and recognition. *Occupational Health and Safety* 72(9):114–117.
Sourbeck, J. 2002. Incentive programs for the business office increase employee motivation. *Patient Accounting* 25(1):2–3.
Sumrow, A. 2003. Motivation: A new look at an age-old topic. *Radiology Management* 25(5):44–47.

Books

Belding, S. 2004. *Winning with the Employee from Hell: A Guide to Performance and Motivation.* Toronto, Ontario: E C W Press.
Gostick, A.R., and Elton, C. 2003. *Managing with Carrots: Using Recognition to Attract and Retain the Best People.* Layton, UT: Gibbs Smith.
Haasen, A., and Shea, G.F. 2004. *New Corporate Cultures that Motivate.* Westport, CT: Greenwood Publishing Group.
Kouzes, J.M., and Posner, B.Z. 1998. *Encouraging the Heart: A Leader's Guide to Rewarding and Recognizing Others.* New York: Wiley.
Richards, D. 2004. *The Art of Winning Commitment: 10 Ways Leaders Can Engage Minds, Hearts, and Spirits.* Chicago: AMACOM.
Smith, G. 2004. *Leading the Professionals: How to Inspire and Motivate Professional Service Teams.* London: Kogan Page.
Ventrice, C. 2003. *Make Their Day!: Employee Recognition that Works.* San Francisco: Berrett-Koehler Publishers, Inc.

Web Sites

- Employer–Employee:
  www.employer-employee.com/motivat.htm
- Foundation for Enterprise Development:
  www.fed.org/resrclib/subject.htm
- *Journal of Extension:*
  www.joe.org/joe/1998june/rb3.html

- Motivational Mecca:
  onlineconsulting.com/
- Nelson Motivation, Inc.:
  www.nelson-motivation.com/
- Small Business Information:
  sbinformation.about.com/cs/benefits/a/033003.htm
- U.S. Small Business Administration:
  www.sba.gov/

Organizations

American Management Association
1601 Broadway
New York, NY 10019
Phone: 212-586-8100
Fax: 212-903-8168
Web site: www.amanet.org/index.htm

Centers for Disease Control and Prevention
1600 Clifton Road
Atlanta, GA 30333
Phone: 404-639-3311
Public Inquiries: 404-639-3534 or 800-311-3435
E-mail: www.cdc.gov/netinfo.htm (Web form)
Web site: www.cdc.gov

Management Assistance Program for Nonprofits
2233 University Avenue West, Suite 360
St. Paul, MN 55114
Phone: 651-647-1216
Web site: www.mapnp.org/library/guiding/motivate/basics.htm

U.S. Chamber of Commerce
1615 H Street, NW
Washington, D.C. 20062-2000
Phone: 202-659-6000
Web site: www.uschamber.com/default

CHAPTER

17

Problem Employees

Timothy E. Horgan

Chapter Objectives

After reading this chapter, readers will:

- Appreciate the value of having written policies and procedures in place when attempting to resolve employee-related problems.
- Understand the importance of promoting positive norms among informal employee groups.
- Know that unlimited personal freedom is not in the best interest of organizations.
- Apply the process of progressive discipline, including employee discharge, in a competent manner.
- Acknowledge the absolute necessity and importance of documentation when processing employee problems.

Chapter Summary

Effective and successful organizations have written policies and procedures in place to help resolve employee-related problems. Managers of such organizations also try to instill positive values and norms among informal employee groups. Although they usually practice a style of management best described as being consistent with McGregor's Theory Y, they also appreciate the fact that unlimited personal freedom is not in the best interest of the organization. Progressive discipline, including employee discharge, is a process that must be applied in a consistent and competent manner. When dealing with problem employees, all activities must be documented. It is of paramount importance for all concerned—the organization, managers, and the affected employee.

Case Study

The mayor of a local community in your jurisdiction just called to tell you that your employees, along with a vehicle that has your department logo on the side, are at his city park playing Frisbee. You thank the mayor for calling and say that you will handle the situation immediately. This is not the kind of call you want to receive at two o'clock in the afternoon, but it happens. What actions do you take to address this situation? What can you do to prevent it from happening in the future?

INTRODUCTION

Every organization will encounter one or more problem employees. An effective and successful manager must recognize that there is a difference between problem employees and employee problems. Good organizational management and effective administration policies minimize employee problems that arise in the course of business. Of course problems will arise. It is management's responsibility to resolve them as best it can. This advice does not apply to employees who, for personal reasons, are unable or simply choose not to perform in a manner consistent with organizational policies. Consequently, all organizations must recognize the inevitability of problem employees. Further, prudent managers will create and put procedures in place to address such issues. At best, these procedures may deter or prevent problem situations from developing. At worst, they will provide a procedure that is fair and understood by all affected parties when problems do occur.

POLICIES AND PROCEDURES

An organization's operating rules must be clearly communicated to all employees, preferably during new employee orientation. These rules also must be consistently and rationally applied in a uniform manner throughout the organization. A prepared policy and procedural manual, authorized by the appointing board or council, should be provided to each employee. During new employee orientation and during the course of their employment, employees should be given opportunities for discussion with supervisors, upper managers, management representatives (ombudspersons), or others, either in groups or in one-on-one situations. The venues for these discussions should not be threatening to employees. Opportunities for discussion should be provided in a cyclic manner, usually every year, as well as any time that changes occur in basic policies or when updates are made to the policy manual.

A good policy manual contains enough detail about work times, benefits, ethics, duties, and evaluation to provide both clarity and direction to employees. The document also sets the tone of conduct, behavior, and expectations for the entire organization. A sample table of contents for an employee manual is contained in Appendix A at the end of this chapter. When establishing basic organizational requirements and benefits, care must be taken to strike an appropriate balance of expectations that employees can satisfy under conditions that management can provide. Excessive rules usually end up either being ignored by staff or inconsistently applied by managers. Benefits that appear in the policy manual but that are not actually available because of inconsistent application will eventually erode the meaning of the entire document for the staff. Essentially, a policy manual becomes both the contract and the code of conduct for an organization. These are the basic rules that the employee must follow and satisfy. In turn, the organization commits to provide a work environment and a benefits program that are fair and uniform.

Management must always be aware of established organizational policies when confronting personnel issues. This begins by managing personnel according to the manual; that is, managing in a consistent fashion. Many difficulties with personnel begin at the interface between staff and first-line supervisors. New managers are usually promoted based on their abilities to meet goals and objectives and to motivate people. They often manage to squeeze the system in a positive manner to move forward. Ignoring rules or bending policies or not applying the same standards to all staff members usually results in problems.

Learning to respond to negative situations is typically very difficult for new managers. Problem employees are among the most negative situations encountered in organizational life. New managers commonly react with anger due to the frustration associated with supervising a problem employee. Accordingly, upper management often first becomes aware of an employee performance issue when the problem employee files a grievance about an angry conversation that occurred with an inexperienced manager.

Effective and successful management should be an active and consistent process. Communication is required among individuals at different levels of management and between management and staff. Work status and progress reports should be relayed up through higher levels of management so that they can be assessed. Evaluation of that work should then come back down through the organization's regular channels of communication so that minor adjustments or corrections can be made.

PEER PRESSURE

Probably the most consistent method for shaping employee behavior in a positive manner and controlling potential employee problems is establishing and supporting strong work ethics and values within the organization. Consistently and frequently acknowledging and rewarding strong staff values empowers group values. These become very difficult for poor performers to ignore. The basic human need to fit in with a vital and active group of employees operating effectively and ethically is satisfied by better performance with a minimum of direction from management. This is a basic aspect of belonging to an informal group. It is also an example of McGregor's Theory Y (1967) being applied. (See Chapter 11 for additional information on informal group dynamics and Chapter 10 for more information on Theory Y.) Employees feel empowered by the responsibility delegated to them by management and by the accompanying sense of freedom.

Additionally, staff members usually have much more direct knowledge and exposure to problem employees. In an organization with strong values, problem employees get little support or shelter from their peers **(Table 17-1)**.

PERSONAL FREEDOM

Health agencies are filled with well-educated, professionally credentialed employees. High-quality staff members are normally expected to make professional judgments about their programs when considering activities such as inspections, client assessments, nuisance problems, and so on. However, decisions regarding items such as work schedules, legal requirements in programs, or positions in the organization are usually not left to staff members' judgment.

Every organization has to make decisions about how much personal freedom—the ability to exercise their own judgment over and in their jobs—employees can exercise. Unfortunately, there is no single formula for personal freedom that can be applied uniformly throughout an organization. Variations occur based on the nature of the tasks assigned and the level of the employee involved. The minimum requirements of

Table 17-1 Organizational Values: Shunning Slackers

Each year, the health district conducted an exercise on staff values. Staff members were divided into teams. Each team discussed organizational values. These values were then written down. Responses were then compared with those of other teams and also with those of the management team. The values of staff and the management teams were usually very similar. One year, staff teams included an additional item that management had not recorded: "Slackers are shunned." This brief statement was graphic and to the point! Not surprisingly, this was a very stable and successful staff with very few personnel problems. The value was internalized by staff members throughout the organization. It remains so to the present day, a testament to the power of strong group norms shaped by equitable management practices.

Source: Cuyahoga County Board of Health, 2000.

an organization should be referenced in the personnel policies document. When questions about items such as work time, vacation, and chain of command arise, the personnel policies document should be consulted to ensure that uniform interpretations are made for all employees. Any additional ability to exercise personal judgment must be worked out in different areas of the organization based on the types of staff and the different activities involved.

As an organizational policy, morale and performance typically improve when employees are given greater control. Organizations that are run on a Theory Y basis usually empower their employees to make decisions. Excessive restriction of personal freedom simply to guarantee control and make the job of management appear to be more simple—as with organizations that are run on a Theory X basis—may give the impression of success. In reality, this approach slows staff productivity and typically impedes progress. Most managers will find that open management, or empowerment, and closed management, or command and control, are style problems that arise between individuals in management. Maintaining clarity throughout an organization requires excellent communication. Reviewing and discussing day-to-day activities at multiple levels helps to blend differing personal styles of managing. By increasing communication, a more general organizational style is developed, which can promote personal freedom without compromising policy or other organizational requirements.

PROGRESSIVE DISCIPLINE

All employees and their managers are necessarily required to report their activities and to discuss them in enough detail to ensure that work requirements are met and organizational policies are implemented. These conversations typically occur on a daily or weekly basis and are a normal part of work. In particular, they are not part of a disciplinary approach to problem solving, although they may contribute to discovering a problem. When normal discussions, training, or mentoring are not adequate to resolve a problem, managers must make two decisions about disciplinary measures. The first decision centers on whether discipline is needed. The second involves the nature and severity of discipline that may be necessary.

Civil service rules require most public agencies to establish a policy of progressive discipline. A sample statement of such rules is contained in Appendix B at the end of this chapter. A progressive discipline policy helps managers resolve small employee problems by initiating modest disciplinary action, rather than letting minor issues develop into major problems requiring commensurate solutions. Progressive discipline is essentially a step-by-step process. It identifies an employee with a problem, documents the problem, describes an acceptable corrective action for the problem, and prescribes an appropriate level of discipline. The appropriate level of discipline prescribed for the initial problem gets progressively more severe if the problem continues to occur.

The key to progressive discipline is identification and documentation. Most employees make some mistakes or commit minor transgressions. If these are identified and documented early on, they can often be resolved by nothing more than an informal disciplinary discussion. Good employees usually learn from such an experience and typically do not experience any future serious problems. It is difficult for most managers, and especially new managers, to initiate these types of employee conferences.

For an average employee, missing an initial opportunity for addressing a problem does not result in damage either to the employee or to the organization. However, if the employee continues to have problems, and the problems get progressively worse, missing that initial opportunity to discuss problems is critical. It then becomes very difficult to satisfactorily resolve problems without major disciplinary action. Such delayed actions are often accompanied by a counter charge from the employee who has an artificially clean record and a legitimate claim that "Nobody said anything about this before." **Table 17-2** describes a progressive discipline model that can serve as a blueprint for most agencies. Minor adjustments may be required to accommodate organizational size, union contract agreements, or other local policies or rule requirements.

It is always prudent to ensure that, at each level of discipline, employees are treated fairly and within their rights. To ensure that the problem does not become a personal one between the employee and the different levels of management, no disciplinary discussion or hearing

Table 17-2 A Progressive Discipline Model

Problem	Action	Discipline
First documented problem	Informal hearing with supervisor	Verbal or written reprimand from supervisor
Second documented problem	Informal hearing with supervisor and section or division head	Written reprimand from upper management
Third documented problem	Formal hearing with division head	Job action, time without pay, reduction in pay; action authorized by appointing authority
Fourth documented problem	Formal hearing with division head and CEO	Significant job action, possible dismissal by appointing authority

should be conducted without a third party being present. In a disciplinary action, an overly aggressive manager or an overly defensive employee can make the situation worse than the problem originally warranted. A respected third party can help satisfy both entities and ensure that the disciplinary process is valid and effective.

■ DISCHARGE

When the progressive discipline process does not result in employee improvement or when the problem is so severe that progressive discipline is not an option (e.g., criminal activity, job abandonment, gross insubordination, and the like), discharge from employment may be the only solution. This is a very difficult legally precise response; it has no justification in public agencies for persons who simply "do not fit in" or "do not belong." Public agencies cannot dismiss someone without cause. This requirement can sometimes prolong the process of coping with a problem employee and usually forces management to provide *overwhelming* evidence for a dismissal. However, this is the basic protection provided to civil servants from adjustments in top management that are due to political changes after an election or from citizen perceptions that occasionally plague public agencies.

Discharging an employee as a result of a well-documented problem or series of problems is a final action conducted by the appointing authority. It is not the sort of action that should be threatened by lower levels of management to intimidate an employee, although managers can say that they are recommending dismissal.

Once dismissed, an employee normally has the right to appeal the process to local or state public employee review boards. Ultimately, an appeal can be made to the appropriate court system. The purpose of review by these boards and the courts is to ensure that the agency has been fair and that the dismissal is justified. Unfortunately, the appeals process is very expensive, very exacting, and very time-consuming. This is daunting for many agencies, especially small organizations that may not have or be able to fund adequate legal counsel. It is equally daunting to a dismissed employee. Complete documentation and a fair and thorough review by the appointing authority prior to a dismissal are absolutely necessary to ensure that an agency's action is justified and that the dismissal is the appropriate option.

Large organizations should consider retaining an inside agency counsel who has both background and experience in labor law to both prevent significant civil service and labor law problems and to effectively and legally resolve them when they occur. Smaller agencies normally have access to prosecutors or law departments in their jurisdiction. They are strongly advised to discuss any job dismissal prior to action by the appointing authority.

With legal support, many agencies include an additional step in the discharge process. After a formal disciplinary hearing during which the hearing officer or board recommends dismissal, the organization may attempt to reach an agreement with the employee to accept the employee's resignation rather than resort to discharge. Structuring such an agreement can prevent a drawn-out legal battle. The agreement also significantly improves an individual's opportunity to secure future employment somewhere else. This option is clearly in the best interest of the employee.

Despite the advantages of saving both money and time for an agency, some very critical ethical decisions must be made regarding the nature of the causes that led to the recommended dismissal and whether those causes should be hidden by some form of confidentiality agreement. This is especially true when there is evidence of criminal activities or when an obligation exists to report activities to a board or commission that may be related to maintaining a professional certification or license for the affected employee.

DOCUMENTATION

Throughout this chapter and the other chapters in this text, the importance of documentation is frequently discussed. The old adage "It's never done until the paperwork is done" is as timely and important now as it was when that phrase emerged in the distant bureaucratic past.

Documentation of employee problems is an absolute necessity. Agencies must clearly describe a problem and must also be able to document why it is a problem. The agency must be able to link the current problem back to the established policies and procedures of the organization, civil service rules, or criminal and civil laws.

An organization must have a valid tracking mechanism for employee activities and behavior. This system must be able to provide reports or documents that verify that activities, policies, and procedural requirements have been met. Although most organizations have such systems in place, problems can and will arise if they are not used. Management's correct use of these monitoring systems and the alertness of human resources personnel should be assessed at least every six months. These activities should become an integral part of an agency's work ethic and normal practices.

In addition to the basic records maintained by any organization, records regarding all discipline processes must be kept in an activities file or in personnel files. Documentation of any informal or formal hearings, or even very preliminary disciplinary discussions, should be memorialized. The records should be kept for some agreed-upon time (usually a year or more). Legal counsel should be asked for guidance in this area.

CONCLUSION

How should the Frisbee-playing employees be disciplined? Managers found out that this activity was being engaged in by a group of summer interns assigned to a vector control program. They had finished the work assigned to them for that day by the early afternoon. They chose to hide out in the city park rather than return to their work base or report back to the supervisor in the office. Management instituted changes to provide better tracking of the interns in the field. The interns themselves received an informal disciplinary hearing, resulting in verbal reprimands.

Documentation of the hearing was placed in the intern program file. The senior intern, who had four summers of experience in the program, received an additional verbal reprimand for his failure to act responsibly with the newer interns. He also lost his designation as the group leader. As a postscript, all of these interns were deeply embarrassed and chagrined by what happened. By all accounts, they have gone on to successful careers. One of the interns is presently employed and appreciated by the local health district. The mayor now serves as an officer of the health district's advisory council. He is also a supporter and proponent of an agency that, in his opinion, effectively manages and handles its problems.

Reference

McGregor, D. 1967. *The Professional Manager.* New York: McGraw-Hill.

Resources

Periodicals

Anderson, R. 2003. Stress at work: The current perspective. *Journal of the Royal Society of Health* 123(2):81–87.

Cryer, B., McCraty, R., and Childre, D. 2003. Pull the plug on stress. *Harvard Business Review* 81(7):102–107, 118.

Nicholson, N. 2003. How to motivate your problem people. *Harvard Business Review* 81(1):56–65.

Prussia, G.E., Brown, K.A., and Willis, P.G. 2003. Mental models of safety: Do managers and employees see eye to eye? *Journal of Safety Research* 34(2):143–156.

Sandberg, J. 2003. Office sticky fingers can turn the rest of us into Joe Fridays. *Wall Street Journal* 242(100): B1.

Books

Cloke, K., and Goldsmith, J. 2001. *Resolving Conflicts at Work: A Complete Guide for Everyone on the Job.* New York: Wiley.

DelPo, A., and Guerin, L. 2003. *Create Your Own Employee Handbook: A Legal and Practical Guide.* Berkeley, CA: Nolo Publishing.

DelPo, A., and Guerin, L. 2003. *Dealing With Problem Employees: A Legal Guide,* 2d ed. Berkeley, CA: Nolo Publishing.

Frost, P.J. 2002. *Toxic Emotions at Work: How Compassionate Managers Handle Pain and Conflict.* Cambridge, MA: Harvard Business School Publishing.

Hawley, C.F. 2004. *201 Ways to Turn Any Employee Into a Star Player.* New York: McGraw-Hill.

Web Sites

- Administrators of Internal Medicine: www.im.org/AIM/Meetings/AIMPastMeetings/21stAIMEducationalConference/antona.htm
- AllBusiness.com: www.allbusiness.com/articles/content/14672.asp
- Kottmann Consulting: www.dnaco.net/~bkottman/talking_technology/problem_employees.html
- Michigan State University: www.msue.msu.edu/msue/imp/modtd/33129602.html
- Soulwork Systematic Coaching: www.soulwork.net/Systemic/difficult_employees.htm

Organizations

American College of Healthcare Executives
One North Franklin, Suite 1700
Chicago, IL 60606-4425
Phone: 312-424-2800
Fax: 312-424-0023
E-mail: geninfo@ache.org
Web site: www.ache.org

American Management Association
1601 Broadway
New York, NY 10019
Phone: 212-586-8100
Fax: 212-903-8168
E-mail: customerservice@amanet.org
Web site: www.amanet.org/index.htm

U.S. Chamber of Commerce
1615 H Street, NW
Washington, D.C. 20062-2000
Phone: 202-659-6000
Web site: www.uschamber.com

U.S. Office of Personnel Management
1900 E Street, NW
Washington, D.C. 20415-1000
Phone: 202-606-1800
E-mail: er@opm.gov
Web site: www.opm.gov/er/poor/ceapp.asp

APPENDIX A

SAMPLE TABLE OF CONTENTS

Table of Contents

continues

Section 4. continued

Education Leave
Jury Duty
Employee Complaint Process

Section 5. Discipline

Employee Discipline

APPENDIX

Job Application
Guidelines for Handling News Media
Drug Free Workplace
Employee Assistance Referral Form
Request for Disciplinary Action
Notification of Results of Hearing
Employee Written Reprimand
Notice of Suspension
Personnel Board Order
Personnel Action Form
Employee Attendance Form
Employment Eligibility Verification
In-County Mileage Report
Out-of-County Travel & Expense Report
Discrimination/Harassment Complaint Form
Receipt of Personnel Policy

Source: Cuyahoga County Board of Health, 1999.

APPENDIX B

CUYAHOGA COUNTY BOARD OF HEALTH DISCIPLINE POLICY

The Board requires that all employees perform their duties in a competent and professional manner, and conduct themselves in such a way as to advance the goals of the Board and increase public confidence in the Board. This requires Board employees to refrain from behavior which might be harmful or which violates or conflicts with Board policies, practices or procedures.

In order to promote fair and impartial treatment of all employees subject to discipline, it is important that work rules be clearly understood, as well as penalties for unacceptable behavior. Discipline is never intended to be punitive. Discipline is intended to help employees to correct unacceptable behavior, and to ensure that the Board is staffed with competent, conscientious and concerned personnel.

The Board subscribes to the concept of progressive discipline. Progressive discipline is not intended to be punitive. The goal of progressive discipline is to help the employee recognize and correct certain unacceptable behavior before it becomes serious enough, or frequent enough to warrant termination. In applying progressive discipline, an employee"s prior work record and disciplinary record serve as a guide in prescribing the degree of discipline for a current infraction or work rule violation.

All employees of the Board shall retain their position during periods of good behavior and efficient service. Employees may be reduced in pay or position, suspended or removed, pursuant to the terms of section 124 et. Seq. of the Ohio Revised Code and for incompetence, inefficiency, dishonesty, drug and/or alcohol abuse, immoral conduct, insubordination, discourteous treatment to the public, neglect of duty, or any other failure of good behavior, or any other acts of malfeasance, misfeasance or nonfeasance in office.

Employees should be guided by Chapter 124 of the Ohio Revised Code for guidance in preserving their rights in the event discipline is imposed upon them.

Source: Cuyahoga County Board of Health, 1998.

CHAPTER

18

Union Management Issues

L. Fleming Fallon, Jr.

Chapter Objectives

After reading this chapter, readers will:

- Know some of the history of the labor movement in the United States.
- Appreciate the process of collective bargaining.
- Understand the due process clause of labor relations.
- Know common grievance procedures.

Chapter Summary

Unions evolved in the United States to restore balance to employer–employee relations. The American Federation of Labor was founded in 1886. The Congress of Industrial Organizations was formed in 1938. They merged in 1955. Unions interact with management through collectively bargained agreements. These contracts delineate dispute resolution procedures, pay rates, working conditions, benefits, and other issues specific to particular locations and occupations. Parties working under labor agreements are protected by a due process clause. At the present time, unions are uncommon in health departments. They are more prevalent in clinical health care settings.

Case Study

The following are excerpts from an arbitration case.

Issue: The parties agreed that the evidence and testimony would clarify the issue of smoking in a designated area.

Positions of the Parties:

- **Grievants:** Privileges enjoyed as a result of professional status were unjustly withdrawn.
- **Management:** It was complying with a 1981 Ohio statute.

Background: An Ohio law passed in 1981 addressed "nonsmoking areas in places of public assembly." It provided, in part:

> For the purpose of separating persons who smoke from persons who do not smoke for the comfort and health of persons not smoking, in every place of public assembly there shall be an area where smoking is not permitted, which shall be designated a no-smoking area . . .

Facts: The grievance arose after the passage of a board of education resolution on May 18, 1997. The resolution prohibited smoking in school buildings that were under the board's control. It was to become effective beginning with the 1997–1998 school year. Under a 1992 board resolution, smoking had been permitted in certain building areas. In 1996, the subject had been discussed at some length by representatives of the board and the teachers' association. Their September 1, 1996, to August 31, 1999, contract provided, in part:

> Article VI. Working Conditions, Teacher Rights, and Other Terms of Employment. This Agreement shall not be interpreted or applied to deprive employees of professional advantages heretofore enjoyed.
>
> Article V, Section E. The arbitrator shall be confined to consideration of the Contract and shall have no power to add to, alter, or subtract from the terms of the Contract.

Testimony: Testimony indicated that students, unlike teachers, had not been allowed to smoke "while on the Board's premises" either before or after September 1, 1996. Teachers and staff members had been allowed to smoke in the employee lounge. When faculty members voted to prevent smoking in the lounge, the principal of the building gave permission for smokers to go to the boiler room. This policy had continued during the time in which the dispute was reviewed by a court of common pleas and in arbitration. The president of the teacher's association attended the open meeting of the board, which was addressing "The Dangers of Primary and Secondary Smoke." He made it very clear that he was not speaking in his official position but as an individual when he urged the board to prevent any and all smoking inside school buildings.

How would you resolve this case? What recommendations would you make? Would you recommend binding arbitration?

INTRODUCTION

The term *labor relations* denotes dealings between representatives of a company and a union as they negotiate and comply with the provisions of their agreements. In *collective bargaining,* management and workers jointly determine the terms and conditions of employment. The former acts on behalf of a company whereas the latter function through a union. Central to this process is the labor relations agreement, or contract, in which mutually accepted terms and conditions are spelled out. Developing the specifics of a labor agreement and the application and enforcement of its terms comprise the core activities of the labor relations process.

HISTORY

Labor unions became a noteworthy political and economic force in the United States in the middle of the nineteenth century (Sloane and Witey, 2003). Although local craft-based associations of workers had been formed in the late 1700s (precursors of the movement may be seen in medieval craft guilds), these craft and trade unions remained scattered regional organizations. They did not have a significant national impact.

The Civil War was accompanied by mounting inflation. Encouraged by the short supply of labor, workers increasingly turned to trade unions to try to increase their wages to meet increasing costs. Between 1860 and 1865, the number of local craft unions tripled. The period between 1865 and 1905 was a time of widespread industrial expansion in this country. In addition, ownership of industries and companies became more concentrated. Workers foresaw the need for a strong united voice if they were to have any say in the wages and the conditions of their employment.

After several short-lived attempts, an enduring national association of unions, the American Federation of Labor (AFL), was formed in 1886. It was headed by Samuel Gompers. This loose association of craft unions had a goal of economic betterment of its members through collective bargaining with employers (Holley et al., 2000). It sought government protection and endorsement of collective bargaining, as well as labor's right to strike if necessary. This goal, however, was not easily won.

For many years, trade unions and collective bargaining were viewed with disfavor by those who believed that they were out of step with an independent and self-reliant national character. Although workers' rights to organize and bargain collectively had been upheld by some courts, these rights often seemed to run head-on into the rights of employers to conduct their business. Conflicts over established rights had to be adjudicated by the courts. A great majority of these cases were decided in favor of companies (Nicholson, 2004). Employers were often able to obtain court injunctions that forbade union organizing and strike activities even though they were not actually illegal (Barick, 1986).

There were bitter struggles as management and workers each sought control. Violence was common. Weapons such as strikes, lockouts, boycotts, blacklists, mass firings, and the use and misuse of injunctions were regularly employed with much economic damage and personal misery. Public opinion had come to favor strong unions as a counterbalance to large, powerful, and centralized corporations. Significant legislation was passed in an attempt to regulate interactions between labor and management (Nicholson, 2004).

The most important pieces of labor legislation are the National Labor Relations Act (NLRA; the Wagner Act of 1935) and the Labor–Management Relations Act (LMRA; the Taft-Hartley Act of 1947). These laws recognized the rights of workers to form unions and bargain on wages, hours, and working conditions with companies engaged in interstate commerce. They also set forth mechanisms to encourage, facilitate, and protect workers' rights. An NLRB administrative staff person investigated charges of unfair labor practices brought by craft and industrial unions and responded to their requests for representative elections.

In February 1938, the Congress of Industrial Organizations (CIO) was formed. John L. Lewis became its first president (Nicholson, 2004). The CIO and the AFL merged in December 1955 to become the AFL-CIO. At that time, more than one-third of all nonagricultural workers in the United States were union members (Farber, 1987). Union membership has steadily declined since the mid-1950s. Currently, approximately one worker in eight belongs to a union.

COLLECTIVELY BARGAINED AGREEMENTS

It is generally accepted that individuals join unions because they believe that the union will improve their work situation. By jointly dealing with their employer through their union representatives, workers expect to have a greater voice in terms of the bargain by which they sell their skills and efforts. Speaking with a stronger, collective voice, they expect to win some combination of the following: higher wages, improved benefits, protection against job loss, safer and more pleasant working conditions, and better chances for advancement (Holley et al., 2000).

The method most often used to form a union is a representation election conducted by the National Labor Relations Board using a secret ballot. The National Labor Relations Act sets forth the steps that may lawfully be taken by the organizing group in its pre-election campaign to persuade workers to join the union and the steps that may be taken by employers to discourage union membership. The latter usually oppose unionization because they believe that unions constrain business practices.

Once the NLRB recognizes a union as the sole bargaining agent for the workers in a group of related jobs known as a bargaining unit, it has the duty to represent all workers in that unit. The labor contract agreed to by the two parties applies to all bargaining-unit employees, union or nonunion. Management has the corresponding duty to bargain earnestly and in good faith with the union and not turn to any other agent with respect to bargaining-unit jobs.

Contract discussions or bargaining sessions between union representatives and management focus on the many issues involved in the what, where, when, and how workers shall perform their duties. They also focus on forms of compensation. Issues typically include the following: wages and benefits, work schedules, job-related health and safety, seniority, promotion, layoff, discharge, grievance procedures, union security, and management prerogatives. Virtually any subject can be considered during negotiations. Union security relates to a union's right to maintain itself as a viable organization. Management prerogatives refer to management's right to run a business or an agency.

Negotiation is a key element in this part of the labor relations process. A labor agreement is usually reached after negotiations take place and compromises are made. The provisions of a labor contract agreed to by the parties form a set of guidelines that delineate the rights and duties of management and those of workers with regards to job performance, working conditions, and compensation. Having settled upon an acceptable labor agreement, the parties are next faced with applying and administering its terms.

At the heart of contract administration is the method of handling grievances—allegations by an employee or a group of employees that management is not living up to the terms of the agreement. A *grievance* is distinguished from everyday complaints or gripes by the fact that it is usually in writing and formally presented for resolution through the grievance procedure specified in the contract. The collective bargaining agreement gives workers the opportunity to have grievances heard at two or three progressively higher levels in the management and union hierarchies in exchange for their pledge not to strike or otherwise interrupt the flow of work when problems occur. Most contracts specify that either management or the union can ultimately present the issue to a neutral third party, or *arbitrator*, for binding resolution if all lower-level steps outlined in the contract have been followed.

Employee discipline is considered by many to be the single most important issue in a labor contract. In a union environment, an employee may only be disciplined for just cause. Though the term *just cause* is somewhat nebulous, it conveys the idea that an employer may neither act capriciously nor in a discriminatory or unduly harsh manner. In short, management must be prepared to defend and justify any disciplinary action it takes as being both fair and reasonable.

Although management may discipline an employee in response to a violation of organizational rules, it must be able to prove that the violation occurred, demonstrate that the rule was known (or should have been known) to the affected employees, and show that punishment was both suitable and administered in an even-handed manner. Arbitrators hearing discipline cases have broad powers to decide whether just cause has been demonstrated by an employer and to modify, sustain, or revoke the penalty as appropriate. The concept of due process is taken very seriously by the arbitrator. In labor relations, *due process* means the strict observance of regular, established procedures in the course of any disciplinary action as well as during an employee's attempts to win relief from the action. It should be noted that discipline or any form of discrimination against an employee because of union membership or lawful union activity is strictly forbidden by statute.

A number of outside forces can significantly affect labor relations. The government affects labor relations through legislation and court decisions. Advances in technology can change job characteristics and the environment of the workplace and introduce entirely new operations and industries, as well as wipe out old ones. Changes in public opinion and public policy can drastically alter balances of power between employers and employees and can boost or depress, create or destroy, whole segments of an industry. Trends in national and international economic and trade patterns affect commerce at all levels.

The labor relations process as it has developed in this country has so far proved to be fairly adaptable (Holley, 2000). In general, the atmosphere surrounding union–management dealings has changed over the years. In some settings, the traditional adversarial stance of the parties is being replaced by more cooperative attitudes; both parties now recognize that most problems are shared. Two typical contemporary needs are to improve productivity and quality in order to compete for product markets and to control the cost of workers' health care benefits. Furthermore, leaders on both sides now recognize that solving mutual problems requires input from both managers and workers and that implementing solutions depends on mutual commitment and joint action.

THE DUE PROCESS CLAUSE OF LABOR RELATIONS

The Fifth Amendment to the U.S. Constitution states, in part, ". . . nor shall any State deprive any person of life, liberty or property without due process of law. . . ." For many years, U.S. courts have consistently held that a person's job is not a property right. Consequently, a 30-year-old, hourly employee who has property cannot be deprived of it without due process. However, the same individual who might have lifetime earnings in excess of a million dollars can be deprived of a job without due process of law. This cannot happen if the person is covered by a grievance procedure, the due process clause of labor relations.

A typical labor–management agreement contains many articles covering such items as wages, hours, and working conditions. Other articles specify how grievances are to be handled. An example of an article delineating grievance procedures is found in Appendix A at the conclusion of this chapter.

Ordinary gripes are not the same as grievances. A very high percentage of written grievances are resolved long before outsiders are called in to make final and binding decisions. Cases that are referred to a sole arbitrator or to a three-person board or committee usually involve policies or principles that are important to one or both of the parties.

When faced with a strike or slowdown or a dispute over the wages, hours, and working conditions, management often refers the matter to an arbitrator. This is especially true of federal, state, or local governmental bodies. Management may refer unresolved disputes about existing contract provisions to outside professionals. The mutual objective of organization and union representatives is to get a difficult controversy resolved so that they may get on with the delivery of programs and services.

CONCLUSION

It must be emphasized that collective bargaining is only one of many developments affecting relations between employers and employees. As organizations have evolved, so have issues between workers and management. Unions have emerged as one of several potential solutions to employer–employee conflict. Unions are uncommon in health departments. They are more likely to be found in clinical health care arenas. Well-prepared managers of public health agencies understand the history and concepts related to labor unions.

Returning to the opening case study in which both sides agreed to binding arbitration, the arbitrator ruled in favor of management, citing health concerns and recent trends relative to smoking. Supporting precedents included the fact that smoking is prohibited on domestic flights and that many domestic flights are longer than a typical school day. Among school employees, smokers were in the minority. The arbitrator noted that while all persons had personal rights, these did not supersede the rights of the majority or the right of the school board to regulate activity in the buildings under its control. The arbitrator added two stipulations. The first directed the school board to provide a sheltered location away from the school building in which staff members could smoke, but that students were excluded from. The second stipulation required the school board to offer smoking-cessation programs to all employees at no cost to the employees.

References

Barick, B.L. 1986. Occupational health programs: The ounce of prevention paying off. *Occupational Health and Safety* 54(9):38–45.

Farber, H.S. 1987. The recent decline in unionization in the United States. *Science* 238:915–918.

Holley, W.H., Jennings, K.M., and Wolters, R.S. 2000. *Labor Relations Process,* 7th ed. Mason, OH: South-Western Publishers.

Nicholson, P.Y. 2004. *Labor's Story in the United States.* Philadelphia, PA: Temple University Press.

Sloane, A.A., and Witey, F. 2003. *Labor Relations,* 11th ed. Upper Saddle River, NJ: Prentice-Hall.

Resources

Periodicals

Crow, S.M., and Hartman, S.J. 2002. Organizational culture: Its impact on employee relations and discipline in health care organizations. *Health Care Management* 21(2):22–28.

Epstein, D.G. 2003. Mediation, not litigation. *Nursing Management* 34(10):40–42.

Forman, H., and Powell, T.A. 2003. Union-management cooperation. *Journal of Nursing Administration* 33(12):621–623.

Forman, H., and Powell, T.A. 2003. Managing during an employee walkout. *Journal of Nursing Administration* 33(9):430–433.

Michael, J.E. 2003. Don't strike out in union negotiations. *Nursing Management* 34(11):15–16.

Palthe, J., and Deshpande, S.P. 2003. Union certification elections in nursing care facilities. *Health Care Management* 22(4):311–317.

Szczepanski, A. 2003. ANA/UAN defend charge nurses' right to organize. *Michigan Nurse* 76(9):8–9.

Books

BNA Editorial Staff. 2003. *Grievance Guide,* 11th ed. Washington, D.C.: BNA Books.

Fisher, G., Shaw, J.B., and Schoenfield, L.F. 2002. *Human Resource Management,* 5th ed. New York: Houghton Mifflin.

Hollinshead, G., Taiby, S., and Nicholls, P. 2002. *Employee Relations,* 2d ed. Boston: Pearson Higher Education.

Loughran, C.S.S. 2003. *Negotiating a Labor Contract: A Management Handbook.* Washington, D.C.: BNA Books.

Web Sites

- American International Mediation Arbitration and Conciliation Center for Dispute Resolution:
  www.aimac-adr.com
- Federal Mediation and Conciliation Service:
  www.fmcs.gov/internet
- National Academy of Arbitrators:
  www.naarb.org
- Office and Professional Employees International Union, AFL-CIO:
  www.opeiu.org/html/organizing_a_union_in_the_unit.html

Organizations

AFL-CIO
815 16th Street, NW
Washington, D.C. 20006
Phone: 202-637-5000
Fax: 202-637-5058
Web site: www.aflcio.org

Federal Mediation and Conciliation Service
2100 K Street, NW
Washington, D.C. 20427
Phone: 202-606-8100
Web site: www.fmcs.gov

International Brotherhood of Teamsters
25 Louisiana Ave., NW
Washington, D.C. 20001
Phone: 202-624-6800
Web site: www.teamster.org

National Labor Relations Board
1099 14th Street, NW
Washington, D.C. 20570-0001
Phone: 866-667-6572
Web site: www.nlrb.gov/nlrb/home/default.asp

National Right to Work Legal Defense Foundation
8001 Braddock Road
Springfield, VA 22160
Phone: 703-321-8510 or 800-336-3600
Fax: 703-321-9319
E-mail: info@nrtw.org
Web site: www.nrtw.org

U.S. Department of Labor
Frances Perkins Building
200 Constitution Ave., NW
Washington, D.C. 20210
Phone: 866-487-2365
Web site: www.dol.gov

APPENDIX A

GRIEVANCE ARTICLE

The following is an example of language from a contract in reference to grievances.

> *Adjustment of Grievances.* Should differences arise between the Company and the Union, or its members employed by the Company, as to the meaning or application of the provisions of this Agreement, or should any trouble of any kind arise in the plant, there shall be no suspension of work on account of such differences but an earnest effort shall be made by both parties to settle the dispute in the following manner.
>
> *Grievance Procedure.* First, between the aggrieved employee or employees with a member of the Grievance committee present and the Foreman and / or General Foreman. . . . Second, between members of the Grievance Committee as designated by the Union and Plant Superintendent and / or his designated representatives. . . . Third, between the committee with a designated representative. . . . Fourth, any difference or local dispute involving the meaning and application of any provision of the Agreement that has not been satisfactorily settled in the foregoing steps . . . shall be submitted to arbitration. . . . The decision of the Arbitrator shall be final and binding upon both parties. . . . The Arbitrator shall not be empowered to rule contrary to, to amend, or to add to or eliminate, any provisions of the Agreement.

PART IV

Relations with the Local Board of Health

CHAPTER

19

Daily Operations

Eric Zgodzinski
L. Fleming Fallon, Jr.

Chapter Objectives

After reading this chapter, readers will:

- Appreciate the importance of normality in daily operations.
- Recognize that clear and timely communications are essential for success.
- Understand that paperwork is an organizational necessity.
- See the value of benevolence and kindness in addressing minor mistakes and learning problems.
- Know some of the nonmonetary options that health department managers can use to motivate and reward their employees.
- Appreciate the concept of having some fun at work.

Chapter Summary

Normal operations are, by definition, routine. This is not synonymous with boring or uninteresting. Every organization must expend effort and use resources to pursue its missions, goals, and objectives. The rhythm of normal or typical operations offers employees a level of comfort. Maintaining a steady pace of operational activities, programs, and delivery of services requires skill. Communication, accurate recordkeeping, and maintaining employee enthusiasm on a day-to-day basis will largely determine organizational success over long periods of time.

Case Study

Pat walked into the office on a Monday morning and asked for clarification and assistance with filling out paperwork related to travel out of the county. Pat's supervisor said that the information was in the department policy manual. The supervisor also commented on the fact that Pat did not usually attend the bi-weekly staff meetings where the same information could have been obtained. What advice would you offer to Pat and the supervisor?

INTRODUCTION

Daily operations at local health departments can often be accurately described as organized chaos. Health departments can be very organized and structured during normal operations. For many departments, this may not be the majority of days. Local health departments often react to situations rather than plan ahead for them. Frequent calls come in regarding such diverse issues as a school with odor problems or concerns about a food-borne outbreak at a local restaurant. These issues tend to displace normal operations for a department. Daily operational routines differ from department to department. Many factors, including the region in which a department is located, its size, the programs offered, and the personalities of departmental staff members dictate the rhythm of daily operations.

DEFINING NORMALITY

A policy handbook should be in place for daily operations at a local health department. This helps to ensure that all employees understand what is expected of them. The handbook should have information on what time the normal working day starts and ends; how to properly complete routine paperwork, reports, and forms; what programs are offered and pertinent information about them; and contact numbers and other important information that the leadership of the department may decide to include.

The presence of a union is one factor that can affect normal operations. Departments may have time clocks to ensure that staff members are reporting and leaving as directed and to keep track of time off and pay. Other departments, with or without unions, may not have time clocks. Departments must adhere to set policies for operations. Whether these come from a handbook or from a union contract, all parties must know what is expected of them.

Reporting at a set time, whether in the field or to an office, is important for several reasons. Employees must be accountable to their departments. Members of the public expect and require services to be available at set times. Whether department leadership is flexible with starting or ending times depends on the type of management style, staff responsibilities, and the nature of the services being delivered.

Breaks and lunch are important aspects of the workplace. The Fair Labor Standards Act requires employers to set aside time for lunch as well as for breaks. How these requirements are implemented is up to the department. For example, an 8-hour working day may include two 15-minute breaks and a 45-minute lunch period. Management may allow one break to be taken concurrently with lunch to provide an hour-long lunch period instead of a 45-minute one.

COMMUNICATIONS

An important aspect of daily operations is communication with the general public. When members of the public call and require information of any type, such requests should be given priority. If the information is not readily available, personnel at the department should discuss the problem, complaint, or question and record the caller's contact information. Someone should then obtain the requested information in a timely manner. Timeliness in providing responses may vary, but for most requests it should not extend beyond a few minutes. However, if the desired information is difficult to obtain or beyond a department's control, a courtesy call should be made to inform the caller of the roadblock and to provide a time frame within which the requested information may be expected.

If the caller requests information that is beyond the scope of public health, assistance should be offered as to how such information may be obtained. The most impressive and best customer service that a health department can offer is taking a few extra minutes to locate a phone number or Web address for a caller. If a department relies on levies for funding, this small courtesy can return large dividends during funding renewal. Trained and knowledgeable staff should be on duty to answer questions quickly or have the ability to return calls in a timely manner. For larger departments, designated phone-duty personnel for environmental, nursing, or other programs can be on hand to answer calls. Excellence in customer service pays off in future endeavors.

Informational meetings are extremely important for several reasons. Designated days for division or departmental meetings are excellent venues for the exchange of information and ideas. During these meetings, philosophies of the department as well as proper implementation of rules and policies can be discussed. More importantly, these meetings offer employees the opportunity to come together either in groups or as an entire department. This develops camaraderie and a sense that everyone is working together for a common cause. Such meetings should be overseen by senior leadership persons and an agenda should be followed. Ground rules should be in place and adhered to within a structured approach. However, these meetings should be sufficiently flexible to permit a pathway for ideas to flow from the staff to management. This often produces a more efficient and productive department. The size of a department will dictate how these meetings are organized and how frequently they should be convened.

PAPERWORK

One aspect of local health department operations that all employees dread is paperwork. However, it is one of the most important functions of any department. Without proper documentation for travel, mileage, time off, overtime, services rendered, and consultation, a department has no way of confirming legitimacy or the proper reimbursement of funds. More importantly, documentation supports the activities of employees during the course of the day. Without this type of documentation, proper cost centers cannot be charged for work done. A major reason for requiring documentation is that many programs are funded based on the amount of time spent doing the work. Another important reason for documentation is if the department becomes involved in a court case. If proper and accurate documentation is not available, the health department may lose its case.

Filing of correspondence, inspections, and confidential information is both time- and space-consuming. However, keeping documentation is a prime function of any governmental agency. Some departments allow individuals to keep nonconfidential information at their desks. Although this may be easier for employees, it can produce concerns with regards to confidentiality and access. To offset these concerns, a central filing system is usually the best option. The advantage of a central filing system is that all files are kept in the same structured filing format. When a person requires a file generated by another individual within the organization, it can easily be located in the central filing system. Finally, with a central file system and common file format, there is less chance of inadequate documentation.

MISCELLANEOUS ISSUES

Overtime is another area that should be clearly delineated and understood by staff and managers. The provisions of the Fair Labor Standards Act dictate overtime policies and pay rates for all nonexempt employees. The policy manual should spell out how overtime is assigned—by whom and at what rate. Leadership in any department must be extremely diligent in tracking overtime usage. Unexpected overtime payments often create budget problems. Furthermore, if the department is unionized, improper assignment of personnel can lead to large payments to aggrieved union members who were higher on the seniority list. To offset budget concerns, the use of compensatory time instead of paid overtime should be considered. However, compensatory time is dependent on the department and its implemented policies. Compensatory time at overtime rates may be an option for nonexempt employees who work over 40 hours during one week.

Fun at work is one aspect that is missing from many agencies. Having fun at work does not mean that tax dollars are being wasted or that little work is getting done. On the contrary, when individuals have fun and want to come to work every day, efficiency, productivity, and overall customer service increase. Having fun at work does not always have to mean playing a practical joke or repeating the latest story at the water cooler. Leadership must figure out the best means for creating fun at work. Supervisors may decide to sanction birthday parties or occasional catered lunches. Other morale builders include activities such as annual golf outings, family picnics, clambakes, holiday parties, or other out-of-office functions. Encouraging individuals to attend education-related meetings or to join external committees is another way to improve employee satisfaction.

People are often resistant to change. A health department is no different. However, periodic changes, either wholesale or in smaller increments, can produce improved outcomes for a department. Stale employees become energized by new projects. Serving under different managers often improves daily operations. However, caution should be exercised when contemplating change. Change for its own sake can result in decreased efficiency.

Proper equipment is essential to accomplishing daily tasks. Improper, inadequate, or outdated equipment severely reduces productivity and decreases employee morale. Adequate equipment and supplies must be made available for the many different tasks of a health department. This does not mean that every individual requires the newest or most expensive piece of equipment on the market; however, proper equipment is a prerequisite for success.

Activity monitoring will differ from department to department. However, whether by hand or through a computer system, it is imperative that constant oversight of programs and services as well as allocation of money is accurately undertaken. By constantly collecting and filing data, employees and departments can access where they are relative to program goals and objectives. Such activities also help in the generation of proper reports and presentations.

Employee discipline was discussed in Chapter 17. For daily operations, benevolence regarding mistakes and minor actions should be the norm. Mistakes are part of the job, especially with new employees. However, depending on the nature and severity of a situation, benevolence may not always be an option. Major disciplinary issues or serious mistakes must be dealt with in a swift, proper, and deliberate manner. Most major disciplinary concerns are few and far between. However, if benevolence is not practiced and mistakes are not allowed to occur, two problems can develop. The first is that employees will not be learning. The second is that employees will be scared to take chances or move programs ahead. Another aspect of being benevolent is demonstrating support for employees when mistakes are made, both internally and outside of the agency. When individuals understand that their agency is behind them and that they do not need to be constantly concerned about losing their jobs due to mistakes, a healthier and more productive department is the result.

Safety and security are other important concerns of daily operations. Locks, cameras, security guards, and first aid kits are just the beginning of any agency's safety and security needs. Travel policies and use of company cars must be fully understood by all members of an agency. Driving license numbers and proof of insurance are a requirement for all employees who will use their own vehicles for agency activities. Health departments must maintain insurance protection for vehicles owned by the agency. Assurance of a nonviolent workplace and protection from unwanted or inappropriate conduct must be provided by all agencies. Every employee must understand evacuation plans and plans for sheltering in case of natural disasters or other emergencies.

Proper documentation of professional licenses and certifications as well as documentation of continuing education activities should be an ongoing task to ensure that all employees are credentialed and qualified for their specific duties and responsibilities. This does not mean that credentials must be checked on a weekly basis; however, they must be checked often enough to ensure that all employees carry them and that they are current.

All employees should have proper identification. Photo identification cards and business cards are a must. All employees should have and carry proper documentation of their employment by the health department. Identification cards should include a clear photograph with the appropriate wording and descriptions. They should be professionally produced and not appear to be homemade.

■ CONCLUSION

Ensuring the safety and health of the public is a fundamental goal of public health. All daily operations should directly or indirectly support this goal.

Returning to Pat, the employee seeking help in completing reimbursement forms, the supervisor provided a copy of the department's employee manual. He also instructed Pat to attend all future staff meetings. Routines must be established to ensure a baseline level of normality and similarity for operations of an organization. Pat attended the next two staff meetings but missed the third. The supervisor called Pat into his office for a conversation.

"Why did you miss the staff meeting?" he asked.

"I had other things to do," replied Pat.

"Everyone has job duties. Building and maintaining a strong employee team is one of my job responsibilities," replied the supervisor. He continued, "I schedule regular meetings to ensure that all of the people in the section have a basic level of knowledge about department procedures. This activity saves time because I have to explain things only once. I was planning to review the protocol for introducing ourselves to others while doing our jobs, including showing our departmental identification cards. Would you mind conducting that discussion, Pat?"

The presentation and discussion went well. Pat did not miss any more staff meetings. At the next annual review, Pat's supervisor complemented Pat on the change in behavior.

"You could have reprimanded me for missing a meeting," Pat said. "Instead, you showed some kindness and explained why the meetings were important. You also told me that I was an important employee when you assigned me to talk about identification. Thanks for your vote of confidence."

Resources

Books

Guo, K.L. 2003. An assessment tool for developing healthcare managerial skills and roles. *Journal of Healthcare Management* 48(6):367–376.

McClellan, M.B. 2003. Mission: Promoting, protecting the public health. *Food and Drug Administration Consumer* 37(2):12–17.

Mott, W.J. 2003. Developing a culturally competent workforce: A diversity program in progress. *Journal of Healthcare Management* 48(5):337–342.

Books

Byars, L.L., and Rue, L.W. 2000. *Human Resource Management*, 6th ed. New York: McGraw-Hill.

DeNisi, A.S., and Griffin, R.W. 2001. *Human Resource Management.* New York: Houghton Mifflin.

Noe, R., Hollenbeck, J.R., Gerhart, B., and Wright, P.M. 2000. *Human Resource Management: Gaining a Competitive Advantage.* New York: McGraw-Hill.

Rainey, H.G. 2003. *Understanding and Managing Public Organizations,* 3d ed. San Francisco: Jossey-Bass.

Web Sites

- Academy of Management:
  www.aomonline.org

- Governance Institute: www.governanceinstitute.com/home.aspx
- Management Sciences for Health: www.msh.org
- Society for Human Resource Management: www.shrm.org
- Workforce Management: www.workforce.com

Organizations

American Management Association
1601 Broadway
New York, NY 10019
Phone: 212-586-8100
Fax: 212-903-8168
Web site: www.amanet.org/index.htm

Centers for Disease Control and Prevention
1600 Clifton Road
Atlanta, GA 30333
Phone: 404-639-3311
Public Inquiries: 404-639-3534 or 800-311-3435
E-mail: www.cdc.gov/netinfo.htm (Web form)
Web site: www.cdc.gov

Management Assistance Program for Nonprofits
2233 University Avenue West, Suite 360
St. Paul, MN 55114
Phone: 651-647-1216
Web site: www.mapnp.org/library/guiding/motivate/basics.htm

National Association of County and City Health Officials
1100 17th Street, Second Floor
Washington, D.C. 20036
Phone: 202-783-5550
Fax: 202-783-1583
E-mail: naccho@naccho.org
Web site: www.naccho.org

The National Human Resources Association
P.O. Box 7326
Nashua, NH 03060-7326
Phone: 866-523-4417
Fax: 603-891-5760
E-mail: nhraadmin@humanresources.org
Web site: www.humanresources.org

CHAPTER

20

Accounting and Finance

L. Fleming Fallon, Jr.

Chapter Objectives

After reading this chapter, readers will:

- Understand basic accounting terms and concepts.
- Know how to read financial statements.
- Understand how financial transactions are recorded.
- Be familiar with accounting methods and management reports.
- Understand basic financial terms and concepts.
- Know how to process receivables.
- Recognize the importance of controlling and managing inventory.
- Know how to manage fixed assets.

Chapter Summary

This chapter provides an overview of accounting principles and financial concepts. It also explains some common accounting terms. The basic elements of finance include risk, the time value of money, receivables, inventory, fixed assets, and capital. Accounting and finance are interrelated, and their functions within an organization often overlap. Finance takes data that are generated through the accounting process and converts that data into meaningful information that can be used to make investment decisions.

Accounting may be likened to laboratory work. The raw values collected in the lab are similar to the raw data generated by an accountant. Some conclusions regarding the overall health of a person can be reached on the basis of individual lab results. Only in light of other related values can an accurate diagnosis be made. Finance is similar in that individual pieces of information are examined and compared with accepted standards. Finance professionals are then able to assess the health of a particular department or the overall organization and evaluate investment strategies.

Case Study

The new job seemed to be going well. Grant had technical competence and knew how to manage people. The pay increase that accompanied the new position was appreciated by his family. However, nagging in the back of his mind was one line of his job description: "Manages funds for the health department." In his youth, he had managed a paper route for over two years. He had counted money for his religious organization. Managing money for an entire organization was baffling. Other than offering him an adult beverage, what advice would you offer to this befuddled health department employee?

INTRODUCTION

Accounting impacts all organizational situations. Given the complexity of current tax and regulatory codes and accounting standards, most people managing a public health agency or employed by a large organization will use the services of trained accounting professionals. An informed person is less likely to make errors and will be in a better position to evaluate and monitor the accounting professionals engaged to assist in organizational, agency, or program management.

The essence of commerce is a transaction: Goods, services, or property are exchanged for other goods, services, property, or money. The operations of any organization, agency, or service are made up of a never-ending cycle of transactions. *Accounting* refers to the process of recording and summarizing these transactions and interpreting their effects on the affairs and activities of an organizational enterprise. The organization is also known as an *economic unit*.

A fundamental principle of accounting is that all transactions are recorded at their *original cost* (also known as the *historical cost*). The original or historic cost is the amount of money actually paid for a good or service. Accountants describe a transaction as the arm's length determination made by a willing buyer and a willing seller, neither of whom are required to buy or sell. Another way to describe a cost agreed upon for a transaction is impartial and not binding upon either buyer or seller. Original cost is usually a fair measure of the goods or services acquired. If an amount other than original cost, such as an estimate or appraisal, were used in recording business transactions, then accounting records and the information and reports derived from them would lose much of their usefulness. Accounting records would then reflect suppositions or fictitious data other than actual costs. This would create opportunities for fraud and deception of readers of financial summaries.

Accounting records serve many purposes. They summarize all of the financial activities and transactions of an organization or agency. Accounting records and the reports generated from this information provide much of the fundamental basis for management decisions. Financial statements, which are prepared from accounting records, form the basis upon which banks and other financial institutions lend money to an organization or business. An organization may be required to file its financial statements with regulatory agencies such as the Securities and Exchange Commission (SEC) or with investor groups or shareholders. The financial statements of a nonprofit agency are commonly required by the government entities that provide funding. Accounting records are the basis of the organization's income tax return. For most health departments, accounting records are used to justify continued funding. Accounting data are the final arbiter of success or failure of a program, service, or organization.

Established standards and conventions are applied in recording and presenting financial information to ensure that financial statements are meaningful to all readers. These standards and conventions are generated by the Financial Accounting Standards Board (FASB) and are known as Generally Accepted Accounting Principles (GAAP). The FASB requires that all accounting and financial statements follow GAAP. In some instances, the SEC also requires the use of GAAP. The FASB periodically amends these principles. GAAP is a set of technical rules that, when used, ensure a consistent and uniform methodology for financial reporting.

Public health agencies and departments use GAAP conventions. However, most also are required to use accounting conventions that have been developed by government units or agencies that provide support and funding. Although these systems share some basic similarities, there is no uniformity. Each state or territory has developed its own accounting conventions. The federal government uses a single system, but it is complex. Administrators of health departments are advised to learn basic accounting concepts and be prepared to learn slightly different procedures for the government units that provide financial support.

■ FINANCIAL STATEMENTS

Financial statements can be prepared at any point in time and can cover any period of time. It is common for financial summaries to be prepared monthly, quarterly, or annually. Accounting periods rarely exceed one year. Each business or organization selects a reporting period and prepares financial statements at the end of the designated reporting period.

The conventional minimum frequency for these reports is once a year. A 12-month reporting period that does not end on December 31 is considered a fiscal year rather than a calendar year. If not completed at the end of a calendar year, reporting period determinations should be made at a time that generally reflects the lowest inventory level, the end of a seasonal busy period, or the end of a funding or grant period.

When to end a fiscal year is an arbitrary decision. For example, the fiscal year of department stores typically ends on January 31. At that time, their inventories are generally at their lowest levels. This eases the task of counting inventory, because inventories are depleted after the holiday buying season. The fiscal year of health departments receiving government support often ends on September 30 to correspond with the end of the federal fiscal year.

There are three basic financial statements: a balance sheet, an income statement, and a statement of cash flow. Footnotes are integral components of financial statements and provide information needed to understand and analyze the financial statements, such as explaining the principles applied and the accounting methods used for different items.

The **balance sheet** summarizes the financial position of an entity at a given point in time by delineating its assets (amount it owns), liabilities (amount it owes), and equity (the difference between assets and liabilities). Equity in nonprofit organizations is more commonly referred to as *unrestricted net assets*.

The balance sheet depicts a balance (or equality) between total assets on one side and total liabilities and equity on the other. This equality is stated by the equation ASSETS = LIABILITIES + EQUITY. The first section of a balance sheet contains assets. These are considered *current assets*. Current assets are defined as cash or those assets that will be converted into cash within one year (cash, accounts receivable, inventories, etc.); property, plant and equipment; and other assets. The next section of the balance sheet contains liabilities and equity. These are classified as *current liabilities* (accounts payable, loans payable, taxes payable, etc.); *long-term liabilities* (loans not due or payable within one year); and *equity*. In for-profit enterprises, equity includes entries for common stock (ownership of the company), retained earnings (money put aside for future use), and net income for the period (how much money the company earned during the period covered by the balance sheet). In nonprofit arenas, the term *equity* is not used as it is related to ownership and profit. A corresponding term used in nonprofit accounting is revenue remaining after expenses. A balance sheet lists *net assets*. These typically include program materials, equipment, and the excess of revenues over expenses (any funds remaining at the conclusion of a program or budgeting cycle). Balance sheets are prepared on a regular basis on a specific date and provide a snapshot of financial conditions at midnight on that date. Comparative balance sheets representing different accounting periods are useful in assessing changes in an organization's financial condition.

An **income statement**, also referred to as the *statement of revenue and expense,* is a financial statement that delineates the profit or loss that a business or organization has incurred over a period of time. The income statement accumulates total revenue and expenses for a specific period. In preparing an income statement, all revenues, including sales, service revenues, and the like, are totaled. The *cost of sales* or *cost of services* is deducted. The result is the *gross profit*. Expenses are totaled and deducted from the gross profit. This results in the *net income or loss*. An income statement is prepared to summarize activity over a specified period of time, such as the fiscal year ending June 30 or for the three months ending on September 30. Comparative income statements can help in assessing a firm's profitability and identifying the components contributing to profitability over time.

Whereas the balance sheet summarizes the wealth position (equity) of an entity, an income statement provides information regarding revenue earned and total expenses incurred each accounting period and how an institution's wealth is affected through operations. These two statements are related in the following way: Revenues earned or support payments received (shown on the income statement) produce assets (cash on the balance sheet). Expenses incurred (shown on the income statement) reduce the assets (cash on the balance sheet).

If at the end of accounting period revenues exceed expenses, two things happen. First, the income statement will show a profit. In a nonprofit arena, the remaining cash is referred to as *excess of revenue over expenses*. This convention is used because nonprofit organizations cannot, by definition, earn a profit. Second, on the balance sheet, cash (or its equivalent) is increased. According to the accounting equation, if assets increase and liabilities remain constant, equity must also increase because ASSETS = LIABILITIES + EQUITY. Therefore, an increase in profit will increase equity and net worth. In contrast, a loss in operations, when expenses exceed revenue, will reduce equity and net worth.

A **statement of cash flow** provides information about cash received and cash paid out as well as data related to financial and investment activities during a particular period of time.

External auditors are people who review the transactions of an organization, check for compliance with accounting controls and relevant standards, and render an opinion concerning the accuracy of an organization's financial statements. External auditors are independent Certified Public Accountants who must be approved by supporting agencies and are paid as consultants. External auditors ensure that the financial statements of a health agency are prepared in conformity with generally accepted accounting principles.

RECORDING BUSINESS TRANSACTIONS

In any business or organization, each transaction that occurs is recorded and summarized as an activity or action of the agency. A department is treated as though it owns assets and owes creditors. A separate set of records is required to track a department's assets and liabilities.

A business or organization records its transactions in *journals*. Such journals are where data for similar types of transactions, such as all checks written by the organization, are recorded. Each transaction affects at least two ledger accounts and is entered into each one. This is the logic behind the so-called double-entry theory of accounting, in which debits must equal credits. Computerized accounting methods are now used by most public health agencies and departments, but the traditional methodology of using journals and journal entries has been retained. For example, if a department spends $500 to pay rent for the month of March, the cash balance is reduced by $500 and the rent expense is increased by $500. Ledger accounts, such as cash or rent expense, are established to accumulate similar expenditures that have been recorded and summarized in journals. This process is frequently referred to as *flow.*

ACCOUNTING CONCEPTS

All of an organization's transactions can be classified into one of the following overall categories: assets, liabilities, equity, revenues, and expenses.

An **asset** is an economic resource that is owned or controlled by an organization that has value. It is something that has a useful life extending beyond the current accounting period. Assets are tangible and intangible possessions. Examples of assets include cash, investments, inventory, accounts receivable, machinery and equipment, goodwill, and the like. Money or other potential income or accounts that are owed to a department or organization are frequently referred to as *receivables*.

A **liability** is a debt owed by an organization. Creditors have a claim against the assets, or a right to the assets of an agency, until all liabilities have been paid or removed. Examples of liabilities include accounts payable, taxes payable, and loans payable.

Equity, also known as *capital*, *net worth*, or *unrestricted net assets,* is the value of an organization or business (at historical or original cost) after all liabilities have been deducted from the assets.

Revenue is the earnings of an agency, whether from sales or provision of services to patients or customers. Revenue earned generally results in an increase in assets (primarily cash) through the operation of a program or delivery of a service.

Expenses are outflows of assets (generally cash) experienced during the operation of a business and in the production of revenue. Expenses are resources such as labor, supplies, and purchased services that are consumed in one year. Examples of other types of expenses are rent, interest, equipment repairs, and depreciation.

Profit, also known as *net income* or *excess of revenues over expenses,* in nonprofit facilities is what remains after expenses are subtracted from income. If expenses are greater than revenues, then the business is operating at a loss. Losses are indicated by the use of parentheses; ($200) indicates a $200 loss.

Depreciation

Certain tangible assets that have a useful life greater than one year are called *fixed assets.* For example, a CAT scan machine or other piece of equipment is a fixed asset. It is commonly accepted that a fixed asset is generally not worth as much as its purchase price after it has been used or installed. This difference in worth compensates for use, eventual obsolescence, or deterioration, and is called *depreciation.*

To alleviate this misrepresentation in financial statements, depreciation is recorded to reflect the gradual loss in the value of the asset when used in the course of business. Depreciation expense does not represent an outflow of cash. Rather, it is the recognition of expenses relating to a capital expenditure made in an earlier period.

Depreciation can be recorded in a number of ways: straight line, double-declining balance, sum of the years digits, and specific use. Each method gives different results. The depreciation method selected should closely mirror an organization's best estimate of the erosion in value of the asset. The method of depreciation should be used consistently over time unless the nature of the business changes and requires a change in the method of depreciation. Government entities often specify the method of depreciation that must be used by the agencies that they support.

Accounting Methods

Transactions can be recorded in one of two ways. The first method does not follow generally accepted accounting principles, but it is simpler and is sometimes used by small organizations or businesses. The second method is the more acceptable one for recording transactions.

The first method is the **cash basis** accounting method. With the cash basis method, transactions are recorded only when money actually changes hands, in other words, when cash is expended or received. Because a sale is recorded when cash is physically received, on the books it may not correspond to the time that the sale was actually made. When cash is actually expended, an expense is recorded. This may not correspond to the time the expense was, in fact, incurred.

The second method, the **accrual** accounting method, records revenue when the transaction takes place and revenue is earned. It does not have to correspond with the time the cash is actually received. Similarly, an expense is recorded when it is incurred, not when the cash is actually paid. Thus, accrual accounting uses specialized accounts such as accounts receivable, accounts payable, and accrued expenses to record all revenue transactions or expenses that have occurred but that have not been received or paid. The logical basis for the accrual method is the matching principle: Within an accounting period, all expenses and revenues associated with that time period are reflected.

Management Reports

An important reason for collecting and processing accounting data is so that managers can use the information to make informed decisions. Management reporting is one of the primary uses of accounting information. In addition to financial statements, management reports are prepared and used by managers at various levels to maintain or improve the fiscal control and profitability of a business or organization. Examples of management reports include budget reports, cash flow projections, profitability by product line reports, and ratio analyses. Budgets are discussed in Chapter 21. Readers are referred to accounting texts listed at the conclusion of this chapter for information on ratio analyses.

Cash flow reporting is the process by which estimates of cash payments and receipts are made to determine whether funds need to be borrowed on a short-term basis or if excess funds will be left at the end of a budget period. The figures generated by cash flow reporting are not always equal to those for revenues reported on an income statement, because the income statement is prepared using the accrual method of accounting. In contrast, cash flow reporting examines the anticipated collection of accounts receivable, the timing of satisfying accounts payable, and current levels of other debt, if any is allowed.

Profitability by product line reporting is an extension of the traditional income statement. In product line reporting, components of the income statement for an entire agency are allocated into product categories such as restaurant inspections, health promotion programs, and other clinical services. By specifically allocating both revenues and direct expenses incurred in the operation of each particular program, service, or department, the profitability of each individual unit can be determined. This information is useful when managing the overall fiscal health of the organization, targeting areas for growth and expansion, and determining the effectiveness of operating personnel.

Summary of Accounting

Accounting is inextricably linked with daily professional activities. No individual, department, or organization can survive without some understanding of the basic concepts of accounting. Having knowledge of fundamental concepts of accounting should relieve some of the pressures imposed by government regulatory agencies and legislative requirements. Public health professionals should understand the rationale and logic underlying accounting records.

FINANCE

The finance function should contribute to the process of determining the financial position of an organization or evaluating a specific planned investment. Planned investments may be as small as a single piece of equipment or as large as an entire product line. Finance is concerned with the use of funds within a business or organization, not just the supply of funds available.

Money is seldom available in unlimited quantities. Therefore, money has a cost. Evaluation of proposed projects that involve a need for funds should take into account the costs and other problems involved in getting needed funds. These factors should be balanced with the amount of added value (profits or other benefits) expected. A degree of uncertainty should be assigned to the expected profits or benefits, because most projects involve a degree of risk.

Receivables

Receivables represent the sale of goods or delivery of services on terms other than cash. Because most transactions are made on credit terms, an investment in receivables represents a major and continuous commitment of funds by a business or organization. The investment is increased as new credit sales are made and decreased as payment is received for previous credit sales.

The majority of credit sales are made on open account. With an open account, the seller keeps a book record of the obligation arising from the sale and does not ask the customer for formal acknowledgment of the debt or a signed promise to pay. With open-account selling, the obligation is not secured. This is in contrast with a receivable that is secured by an asset. With a nonsecured obligation, if the purchaser does not pay the bill, the seller must absorb the loss. In the case of a secured receivable, the seller can claim (or attach) the asset that was provided as security. The seller has the right to dispose of the asset to satisfy the debt owed.

The basic objective of managing receivables should be maximizing the return on investment. While receivables are outstanding, a company or organization does not have the money to invest or to use for its own purposes, such as the payment of debts and obligations.

Most credit departments have policies that stress short collection times in an effort to minimize bad-debt losses and the unavailability of funds in receivables. Factors that influence the size of an organization's investment in receivables are the terms of credit granted to customers deemed creditworthy; the payment practices of customers; the rigor of organizational collection policies and practices; the degree of operating efficiency in record keeping, billing, and adjustments; and the volume of credit sales.

Inventory

A portion of an organization or company's assets can be invested in inventory, which includes those assets available for direct sale in the normal course of business. This is often less of an issue for health departments than for profit-generating businesses. Manufacturers, wholesalers, and retailers typically maintain a large investment in inventory. Although the inventory investment is commonly published as a single figure, it is composed of raw materials, work in progress, finished goods, and minor supplies. The cost of inventory is more than just the price paid to acquire or manufacture the inventory. The cost of inventory also includes the costs of the land or storage space required for operations, the costs of insurance against damage, theft, and fire; and costs for security and heating or cooling (if necessary). Inventory can consist of large, durable goods with long shelf lives such as bicycle helmets, automobiles, or testing supplies. Inventory can be sensitive to time or styles, such as vaccines or newspapers that have short shelf lives.

As an industry, health care has inventory. Inventory may include supplies such as disposable instruments, blood products, and pharmaceuticals. Particular care must be maintained when balancing the availability of rarely used equipment and supplies and the fiduciary responsibility of providing health care services. For smaller health care organizations, either establishing agreements with health care equipment vendors or with a larger health care facility can minimize inventory costs and provide availability for any rare cases that may present themselves.

Obviously, inventory management is critical to the financial success of an organization. A product will not be a success if it is out of date, stale, unusable, ineffective due to the passage of time, or unavailable. Obsolete inventory is generally worth very little. In fact, its disposition can be costly.

Many department and retail stores have point-of-sales inventory methods whereby the sales register records a reduction in inventory. When the inventory of an item drops below a predesignated level known as the *order point*, an order for additional merchandise is generated. Optimum levels of inventory are dependent on factors such as the availability of raw materials, purchase economies (a larger order usually means a lower price per item), the outlook for changes in price, the time required to complete the manufacturing process, the availability of labor, and customer demand. Health care providers must often forecast disease patterns months in advance so that they can prepare for expected demands for vaccines, services, and products.

Fixed Asset Management

Fixed assets are those assets whose useful life to the organization or business exceeds one year. These include real property, buildings, equipment, and machinery. Some businesses are property intensive, such as utilities (large expenditures for land, generators, switching stations, poles and lines, and plants). Hospitals are both labor and property intensive. Large-property expenditures include land, buildings, and garages; laboratory equipment; hospital beds and furnishings; and state-of-the-art technological apparatuses such as MRI units, CT scanners, lithotripters, and equipment for surgical suites and intensive care units.

Once the initial outlay for an acquisition has been made, the fixed asset will then have ongoing support costs. Such support costs include, but are not limited to, building and equipment maintenance and upgrades, building staff, real estate taxes, and other costs relating to the occupation of space within the building. Hospitals and health departments also incur costs for staff and supplies to support advanced equipment for diagnosis and treatment.

With the advent of computer-controlled equipment, upgrades for software enhancements have increased the cost of equipment that heretofore may not have been necessary. The equipment itself may be fully functional, but software enhancements increase diagnostic or therapeutic efficiency. In some cases, consumers demand them. Health care organizations may then upgrade to maintain market share rather than to improve diagnostic accuracy or therapeutic efficacy.

Fixed assets are generally controlled through the use of a fixed-asset accounting system. In this system, each asset that is acquired by the organization or business is assigned a distinctive identification number and a responsibility or cost center. A tag with the asset number is secured to each item of property. The cost center is then responsible for the safeguarding and effective use of that particular asset. On a periodic basis, assets are counted or inventoried. This means that a review is made of the assets within an area of responsibility to check for their physical presence and review their condition.

Generating Cash

Borrowing is a way to secure cash for a short period of time. Lines of credit may be secured from commercial banks in advance of anticipated cash needs. Organizations typically repay these loans as expeditiously as possible, because their cost is usually high. Loans may be needed to pay obligations while receivables are being collected. Prudent planning and cash flow budgeting can minimize the use and cost of loans.

Nonprofit organizations may generate operating funds through grants, donations, or fund-raising efforts. Grants are outright gifts that are commonly designated for a particular use. Changing the initially designated use requires permission from the granting individual, agency, or foundation. Philanthropic donations are gifts that are given by individuals or foundations. The use of such donations may be restricted. Donations come in a variety of forms: cash, real estate, stocks, bonds, or life insurance policies. Fund-raising efforts can assume almost any form, from selling food or other products or services to raffles with huge prizes. Fund-raising efforts differ from grants or donations in that a product or service is usually involved. Organizations are not restricted in how they may spend the funds raised.

■ CONCLUSION

Finance is concerned with the generation and use of funds to support organizational objectives, whereas accounting records transactions and summarizes how funds are expended. Money has costs associated with its procurement and use. Costs are associated with maintaining equipment and inventory. Health department managers often become involved in financial matters. Knowledge of the techniques used should improve their understanding of organizational funding, limitations, resources, and resource allocation.

Returning to the case study, a reasonable first step would be for Grant to read a book that provides material on both accounting and finance. He must understand accounting conventions and procedures whether or not he actually keeps the books for the department. Having an understanding of accounting and finance will help him to manage the department's funds.

As a second step, he should meet with the department's external auditor to learn about the audit process. Becoming familiar with the requirements of an internal audit will help him prepare for one.

Meeting with the financial heads of the organizations that provide support to the health department is an important aspect of the new job. Each funding source will require an annual report that summarizes how its funds were spent. Unfortunately, each agency will have its own accounting rules and presentation format. This is simply part of the territory for nonprofit organizations that are funded by other agencies or government units.

On a day-to-day level, accounting is similar to learning to play a musical instrument. Practice and experience are the keys to learning and becoming proficient in the language and conventions of accounting and finance. Asking questions is a good habit to acquire. Finance and accounting require scrupulous honesty and openness.

Resources

Periodicals

Healthcare Financial Management Association. 2004. Credit balances. Spotlighting a little-known area of risk and opportunity. *Healthcare Financial Management* 58(1 suppl): pp 1–8.

Kaplan, R.S., and Norton, D.P. 2004. Measuring the strategic readiness of intangible assets. *Harvard Business Review* 82(2):52–63.

Kosmin, E.A. 2003. Get the money! Excuses you can expect when your debtors don't pay their invoices on time—and what you can do about them. *Contemporary Long-term Care* 26(9):43–46.

Larkin, H. 2004. Finances. Denials into cash. *Hospital Health Networks* 78(1):20–22.

Lowes, R. 2003. Collect from patients online? *Medical Economics* 80(23):23–24.

Stenklyft, T.A. 2004. To collect debts, look in the right places. *Texas Dental Journal* 121(2):168–170.

Books

Baker, J., and Baker, R.W. 1999. *Health Care Finance: Basic Tools for Non-financial Managers*. Sudbury, MA: Jones & Bartlett.

Cleverley, W.O. 2004. *Essentials of Health Care Finance,* 5th ed. Gaithersburg, MD: Aspen Publishers.

Finkler, S.A. 1999. *Issues in Cost Accounting for Health Care Organizations,* 2d ed. Gaithersburg, MD: Aspen Publishers.

Gapenski, L.C. 2001. *Healthcare Finance: An Introduction to Accounting and Financial Management,* 2d ed. Chicago: Health Administration Press.

Kaufman, K. 2002. *Finance in Brief: Six Key Concepts for Healthcare Leaders,* 2d ed. Chicago: Health Administration Press.

Neumann, B.R., and Boles, K.E. 1998. *Management Accounting for Healthcare Organizations,* 5th ed. Dubuque, IA: Kendall Hunt.

Nowicki, M. 2001. *The Financial Management of Hospitals and Healthcare Organizations,* 2d ed. Chicago: Health Administration Press.

Zelman, W.N., McCue, M., Millikan, A.R., and Glick, N. 2002. *Financial Management of Health Care Organizations: An Introduction to Fundamental Tools, Concepts and Applications*. Malden, MA: Blackwell Publishers.

Web Sites

- American Accounting Association:
  www.aaahq.org/index.cfm
- Association for Accounting Administration
  www.cpaadmin.org
- CPA Associates International:
  www.cpaai.com
- Financial Accounting Standards Board (FASB):
  www.fasb.org
- Healthcare Financial Management Association:
  www.hfma.org

Organizations

American College of Healthcare Executives
One North Franklin, Suite 1700
Chicago, IL 60606-4425
Phone: 312-424-2800
Fax: 312-424-0023
E-mail: geninfo@ache.org
Web site: www.ache.org

American Institute of Certified Public Accountants
1211 Avenue of the Americas
New York, NY 10036-8775
Phone: 212-596-6200
Fax: 212-596-6213
Web site: www.aicpa.org/index.htm

Association of Government Accountants
2208 Mount Vernon Ave.
Alexandria, VA 22301
Phone: 703-684-6931 or 800-242-7211
Fax: 703-548-9367
Web site: www.agacgfm.org/homepage.aspx

Financial Managers Society
100 West Monroe, Suite 810
Chicago, IL 60603
Phone: 312-578-1300 or 800-275-4367
Fax: 312-578-1308
E-mail: info@fmsinc.org
Web site: www.fmsinc.org/cms

National CPA Health Care Advisors Association
One Valmont Plaza, Fourth Floor
Omaha, NE 68154
Phone: 888-475-4476
Fax: 402-964-3811
E-mail: info@hcaa.com
Web site: www.hcaa.com

CHAPTER 21

Budgets

Virginia Cogar
L. Fleming Fallon, Jr.

Chapter Objectives

After reading this chapter, readers will:

- Appreciate the importance of budgets.
- Recognize that budgets are planning, control, and audit documents.
- Understand that budgets are used to evaluate operating performance.
- Know the four components of a complete budget package: a statistics budget, an expense budget, a revenue budget, and a cash budget.
- Know how to use budgets to make informed fiscal decisions.
- Know how to formulate a comprehensive budget.
- Understand options in the budget process.

Chapter Summary

Budgets are key planning, control, and audit documents. A complete budget package has four components: a statistics budget, an expense budget, a revenue budget, and a cash budget. Options are available when formulating budgets. These topics are discussed in this chapter.

Case Study

Lou Smith, the health department's senior sanitarian, was drinking coffee and playing with his bagel rather than eating it. The department's fiscal officer had directed program heads to submit requests for next year's budget. Lou had been promoted seven months ago. His only prior experience with budgets was being told "No, there is no money in the budget" when he requested a new computer two years ago. Nothing in his training had prepared him for this. Luckily, the budget numbers are not due for another week. What advice would you give to Lou?

INTRODUCTION

Budget preparation and budget oversight are usually considered to be managerial duties. Managers should expect to prepare a budget for their area of responsibility. A basic understanding of accounting is helpful because information pertaining to costs must be extracted from accounting data for both revenue and expenses. Managers must examine and understand the information about historical costs, how they have changed over time, and how service volume has changed over time. Managers also must understand sources and timing of revenues. When developing a budget, managers must consider the goals of the organization for which they work and the programs and services for which they are responsible.

Nationwide, health outcomes have improved only minimally over the past decade although overall spending on health has increased (Centers for Medicare and Medicaid Services, 2004). This suggests that managers must focus on cost control and efficiency. Health department directors develop and manage larger, consolidated budgets. Heads of subunits participate in decisions on acquiring equipment and supplies and on the expenditure of resources, and thereby also contribute to budget preparation. Public health agencies generate cash flows, acquire assets, and put those assets to work, as do most organizations and businesses. The decision-making rules that public health agencies should use are based on the same economic principles as those governing any other type of enterprise. Most managers consider developing a budget and adhering to it during the fiscal year to be their basic financial tasks. Managers who fully understand budgets realize the power of budgets as planning and analytical tools.

ROLE OF THE BUDGET IN EVALUATING OPERATING PERFORMANCE

A budget is a plan for the use of funds. Most budgets cover a 12-month period, but this is not an absolute requirement. A budget is not merely an allocation of funds. An allocation imposes overall spending constraints. A budget is not a bank account from which funds are taken. In the context of planning for a department of health, a budget provides a plan for the use of funds to meet the objectives and goals of an agency for the interval of one operating or fiscal year. Changes in plans at program or service levels should be incorporated into an overall budget. Information should flow from lower levels of management to higher ones.

The budget should transition an operating plan into a program for the expenditure of funds. Preparing the budget is a critical step in planning. It designates portions of the available funds for predicted, expected, or anticipated expenses. These are identified as specific category-by-category line items in the budget document. This process translates an operating plan into a plan for financial action. Making decisions as to how an agency will use its resources (funds, equipment, supplies, and personnel) is part of this planning. The operating plan becomes reality as the budget is spent.

The budget should be considered to be a working document for all levels of an organization. Once a fiscal-year budget is completed, it should not be considered to be final—filed and promptly forgotten. Efficient managers will use the budget as a tool to help them succeed in their job responsibilities. Account spending and balances for each budget category should be periodically reviewed. From this analysis, managers can gauge progress toward accomplishing program and overall agency objectives. Throughout the year, these assessments can uncover the need for immediate financial adjustments to ensure that all remaining tasks for the year are completed. This information will be timely in so far as planning for the next fiscal year's budget should begin long before the end of a particular budget period.

The original category-by-category expenditure plan is compared with actual spending. This is done periodically and at the end of the budget period. This is a method for evaluating how well the organization is meeting its operating and financial goals. Spending, revenue, cash flows, and service volume should be evaluated in this manner. Meaningful evaluation is possible only if expenses are correctly entered in the categories for which they were incurred. Valid entries must be made so that the true amount of funds spent or required for that category is known. This comparison reveals if categories were overfunded or underfunded for the fiscal year. This comparison enables better budget planning for subsequent fiscal years. The results of this comparison make the budget a useful evaluation tool for auditing and evaluation purposes.

Budgets serve four roles. The budget is a one-year plan for the use of funds. It is a tool by which an agency's operating plan becomes the program for the expenditure of funds. The budget is a working document to keep each component of the larger agency running smoothly during the year and between years. Finally, a budget is a tool for evaluation. Budgets provide one of the most powerful planning and analytical tools available to any organization.

■ COMPONENTS OF A BUDGET

A complete budget has four major components: the statistics budget, the expense budget, the revenue budget, and the cash budget. A capital budget is a minor component that is normally developed separately but in conjunction with an expense budget. It is a subset of projected expenditures for items that have useful lives or expected periods of service that exceed one year. Overall agency operating plans are used to prepare the statistics budget for the agency. A similar process is used to compile budgets for program or service areas. The **statistics budget** includes items that can be forecasted. These include utilization by type of service, payer mix, acuity level, and capital acquisitions. It also includes items such as staffing levels that are determined as matters of policy. The statistics budget may be written in a very detailed manner. The expense, revenue, capital, and cash budgets are subdivisions of the statistics budget, and are the transaction records of an agency. These records should also be reviewed periodically throughout the budget period. At the end of the fiscal year, all budgets will be evaluated as part of an assessment of how successfully an organization met its objectives.

The **expense budget** is a prediction of the total expenses or debit accounting entries of an organization based on its operating plan to meet the goals and objectives established by a board of health. These goals and objectives may be determined from information gathered from a local needs assessment or survey. Other expense categories stem from government mandates. Recent Centers for Disease Control and Prevention directives on bioterrorism provide an example of this type of government mandate. Federal, state, or local laws and statutes may mandate other items in an expense budget.

The **revenue budget** is a prediction of how much revenue or credit accounting entries will be generated during the budget period. Revenue sources for a health department include anticipated funding allotments from the general tax base, block grants, special levied taxes, grants from other sources, license fees, and payments for other services provided. Revenue budgeting becomes complicated when sources of income are variable or unpredictable.

The **cash budget** summarizes the amount and timing of anticipated flows of cash into (revenue) and out of (expenses and capital acquisitions) an agency. It is a prediction or forecast of an agency's ability to meet its expenses. A cash budget is usually presented in a spreadsheet format. Past experiences of an agency, documented in accounting records, provide the basis for preparing a subsequent cash budget.

The **capital budget** is a plan for acquiring new, long-lived assets and is developed separately from an expense budget. Capital acquisitions are included in the overall budgeting process because they require cash, although they may not involve an expense during the current budget period. Asset selection and operation are the basic problems of capital budgeting. Agencies that cannot access external sources of capital to finance the acquisition of new technology and equipment are likely to fall behind in providing services. Organizations select and operate assets so as not to require external subsidies. It is desirable to avoid depending on external subsidies because they may change or be lost over time. Such reliance also distracts an agency, redirects expenditures of time and energy, and interrupts its efforts to secure subsidies that may be required for future operations.

MAKING INFORMED BUDGETING DECISIONS

When formulating the statistical budget for a future fiscal year, the expense, revenue, capital, and cash budgets of an agency for the previous fiscal year are examined. Budgeted allocations are compared with actual amounts used. This is how agencies evaluate how well they fulfilled their operating and financial goals during the budget period. Specific attention is given to the originally projected and actual expenditures on a category-by-category basis. This is done for all planned spending, revenue, and cash flows of various subunits of a public health department. Planned amounts are compared with the reality that emerged during the budget period.

Budgetary review and analysis should seek to identify categories that were over funded and those that were underfunded. Look for changes in funding needs and service volume that have occurred over time. Evaluate the success of the budget in enabling employees to meet health department objectives. Taking the time to make these comparisons yields valuable information that can improve budget planning for the following fiscal year. Successful organizations learn from the events of the past so as to be better prepared for the future.

FORMULATING A COMPREHENSIVE BUDGET

An annual reassessment of the goals and objectives of an agency should precede the budgeting process. The mission, goals, and objectives of the agency should be aligned with the best information available from the local service area. If the results of a needs assessment are available, they should be referenced when reviewing the agency's goals and objectives. If the needs assessment is dated or is lacking, conducting an assessment in the near future should become an agency goal. Survey information from in-house or external sources should be sought to obtain the most recent information. The justification is simple. An agency cannot serve the needs of the local area unless these needs are identified and prioritized. Keep in mind that needs and priorities will shift over time. A reevaluation of the appropriateness of agency goals and objectives should precede the beginning of the budgeting process by several months.

Several sets of information are required for the budget planning process to be successful. One of these is a clear and accurate statement of current agency goals and objectives. Another required data element is the results of a completed examination of the budgets from the previous fiscal year. Any changes in programs, services, or staffing that have or will be made must be known. Also needed are budget requests from each manager and program or service head. These requests should be tempered by the need to focus on cost control and efficiency as well as optimum program delivery. The statistics budget of the fiscal year must meet the objectives and goals of all programs and services areas as well as the entire department. Remember that a statistics budget is the operating plan that is being prepared as a guide for the use of funds for the interval of the next operating year.

BUDGETING PROCESS OPTIONS

Before initiating the budgeting process, the health officer, deputy, or fiscal officer will want to consider the budgeting process options that are frequently used. When making budgeting decisions, it is usually helpful to answer the following questions. Should the justification for line items in the expense budget be incremental or zero based? What detailed information is needed for each program or service area? Who or what are the best sources for this information? Is the desired process for input of information from the bottom up, top down, or a mix? Is it best to operate with a fixed expense budget? Should some programs or service areas have flexible expense budgets?

Incremental versus Zero-based Budgeting

The process of incremental budgeting uses the previous fiscal operating plan, expense budget, and revenue budget to guide and justify the operating plan, expense budget, and revenue budget for the next fiscal period. Most agencies, organizations, and health departments use the incremental budgeting process.

Zero-based budgeting is an alternative process that requires a complete item-by-item annual review of the operating plan. Every proposed item in the expense budget must be justified on its own merit each year with its own budget package and without reference to previous years. Zero-based budgeting requires that each activity and expenditure be justified by a program or service need. The intent is to increase agency efficiency; however, zero-based budgeting requires a great deal of work.

Bottom-Up versus Top-Down Budgeting

The bottom-up budgeting process starts with information provided by the lowest level of personnel. This information is then relayed up the administrative chain of command to senior managers. Information from program or service employees often interfaces with the public and is vital for making the budget an effective planning tool. Proposed expense and revenue budgets from the lower levels are good starting points for developing a composite budget. To the extent that more input is received from these employees, the process is increasingly bottom-up budgeting.

However, senior managers must enforce cost controls in order to stay within the agency's financial constraints. Top-down budgeting occurs as senior managers influence and control the budgeting process. The most effective organizational budgeting occurs with some degree of balance between bottom-up information flow and top-down control. Budget hearings between individuals of various levels provide opportunities for feedback, negotiations, and adjustments. In the end, senior managers make the final budget allocations because they are responsible for monitoring fiscal activities and ensuring a balanced budget. Libby (1999) reported a significant increase in employee performance when subordinate voices in the budgeting process are followed by communicating the rationale for the subordinate's lack of influence over the final budget. Suggestions made by lower level personnel may have to be modified or eliminated by upper level managers as a budget is developed. Providing feedback to employees who make suggestions during the preparation of a budget acknowledges their suggestions and contributions. Such comments from senior managers are rewarding to those people making them. Employees who have a sense of involvement are likely to be more productive than are employees who feel that their comments and suggestions are not valued.

Fixed versus Flexible Expense Budgeting

Fixed expense budgeting assigns a specific dollar amount to every line item. Flexible expense budgeting enables variable costs to be adjusted as the service load varies. Flexible budgeting does not provide free access to unlimited funds. It may be appropriate to have some fixed and some flexible components in a department's expense budget. It is appropriate to set up a flexible expense account for program or service units having a high proportion of variable costs. As a guideline, flexible expense accounts should be reserved for units whose revenue increases as its service volume increases. A unit with fixed revenues cannot increase its level of service. Unless flexible revenue budgets are available, a flexible expense budget is not justified. A department of health that is operated with local tax appropriations and provides free services cannot have a flexible expense budget. In that circumstance, the department of health must use fixed expense budgeting.

CONCLUSION

This chapter has provided a brief overview of budgets and the budgeting process. Budgets are essential control documents. Budgets make significant contributions to the success of any organization. Budgets are used to plan, execute, and audit organizational plans and activities. A complete budget package has four major components: a statistics budget, an expense budget, a revenue budget, and a cash budget; and one minor component: a capital budget. Budgets should be reviewed at periodic intervals. Budgets are comprehensive documents with several options with regards to the budgeting process and the document type.

Returning to the initial case study, Lou should use last year's budget as a guide. He should read budget printouts on a periodic basis so that he will be familiar with the documents. Lou asked the department's fiscal officer for a copy of the general budgetary guidelines. Wisely, Lou asked for help. At the same time, he admitted that this was his first budget. He decided that he would admit his lack of experience rather than try to bluff his way through the process and possibly make an otherwise avoidable error.

After reviewing budgets for the past two years, Lou scheduled a training session with the fiscal officer. He asked for assistance as a first time budget compiler. The fiscal officer was pleased to help and sent Lou to a two-day seminar on budgeting. Lou now reviews his budget every month and has started compiling data for the next budget cycle. Due to his reduction in budget-related job stress, Lou no longer plays with his bagel in the morning. He has learned to dunk his bagels in his morning coffee.

References

Libby, T. 1999. The influence of voice and explanation on performance in a participative budgeting setting. *Accounting, Organizations, and Society* 24(2):125–137.

Centers for Medicare and Medicaid Services. 2004. Health accounts. Available at www.cms.hhs.gov/statistics/nhe.

Resources

Periodicals

Browning, P., von Cube, A., and Leibrand, H. 2004. Minimum public health standards as a basis for secure public health funding. *Public Health Management and Practice* 10(1):19–22.

Diez, C. 2004. Dollars and sense: Maximizing your budget. *Biomedical Instrumentation and Technology* 38(1):19–24.

Fedor, F.P. 2004. Changing views about "usual charges." *Healthcare Financial Management* 58(1):32–36.

Vastag, B. 2004. States' health care budgets faltering. *Journal of the American Medical Association* 291(9):1057–1058.

Books

Baker, J., and Baker, R.W. 1999. *Health Care Finance: Basic Tools for Nonfinancial Managers*. Sudbury, MA: Jones & Bartlett.

Cleverley, W.O. 2004. *Essentials of Health Care Finance*, 5th ed. Gaithersburg, MD: Aspen Publishers.

Gapenski, L.C. 2001. *Healthcare Finance: An Introduction to Accounting and Financial Management*, 2d ed. Chicago: Health Administration Press.

Neumann, B.R., and Boles, K.E. 1998. *Management Accounting for Healthcare Organizations*, 5th ed. Dubuque, IA: Kendall Hunt.

Zelman, W.N., McCue, M., Millikan, A.R., and Glick, N. 2002. *Financial Management of Health Care Organizations: An Introduction to Fundamental Tools, Concepts and Applications*. Malden, MA: Blackwell Publishers.

Web Sites

- American Accounting Association: www.aaahq.org/index.cfm
- American Association for Budget and Program Analysis: www.aabpa.org
- Association for Budgeting and Financial Management: www.abfm.org
- Healthcare Financial Management Association: www.hfma.org
- Maryland Association for Nonprofit Organizations: www.mdnonprofit.org/INDEX.htm

Organizations

American College of Healthcare Executives
One North Franklin, Suite 1700
Chicago, IL 60606-4425
Phone: 312-424-2800
Fax: 312-424-0023
E-mail: geninfo@ache.org
Web site: www.ache.org

American Institute of Certified Public Accountants
1211 Avenue of the Americas
New York, NY 10036-8775
Phone: 212-596-6200
Fax: 212-596-6213
Web site: www.aicpa.org/index.htm

Association of Government Accountants
2208 Mount Vernon Ave.
Alexandria, VA 22301
Phone: 703-684-6931 or 800-242-7211
Fax: 703-548-9367
Web site: www.agacgfm.org/homepage.aspx

Financial Managers Society
100 West Monroe, Suite 810
Chicago, IL 60603

Phone: 312-578-1300 or 800-275-4367
Fax: 312-578-1308
E-mail: info@fmsinc.org
Web site: www.fmsinc.org/cms

National CPA Health Care Advisors Association
One Valmont Plaza, Fourth Floor
Omaha, NE 68154
Phone: 888-475-4476
Fax: 402-964-3811
E-mail: info@hcaa.com
Web site: www.hcaa.com

CHAPTER

22

The Health Officer's Role in Board Development

Vaughn Mamlin Upshaw

Chapter Objectives

After reading this chapter, readers will:

- Know the responsibilities of the board of health.
- Identify the role of the health officer in developing the board of health.
- Know specific guidelines that health officers can use to improve the effectiveness of their boards of health.

Chapter Summary

This chapter briefly reviews why local boards of health exist and outlines the benefits they provide to public health at the community level. In order to appreciate the importance of a board of health's contribution to its local public health department and facilitate the board's development, it is important for health officers to understand the scope of a board of health's work and its primary responsibilities. The chapter describes the core responsibilities of the local board of health to ensure that health departments establish the necessary legal basis, policies, resources, collaborative efforts, and accountability systems to protect and promote public health at the local level. Following a review of board responsibilities, the role of the health officer in guiding and developing the board of health is examined. The chapter offers specific examples and guidelines for health officers who are interested in improving their local board's work.

Case Study

Chris Andrews, the local health director, is frustrated because the monthly board of health meeting is coming up and too many issues are on the board's agenda. The board meetings always follows a standard agenda. The board approves the agenda and the minutes, reviews old business, attends to new business, and then adjourns. Sometimes there are just too many things to cover in a 90-minute meeting. Chris is getting ready to present a number of topics to the board chair. Chris also wants to see if they can agree on what to include on this month's agenda.

A number of issues will be discussed at the upcoming meeting. The budget must be presented and approved by the board. The health department is initiating a new community health improvement process, and board members should be briefed on upcoming activities. The board's policy subcommittee members have proposed revisions to the tobacco-control policy and are scheduled to present their recommendations to the board for adoption. A citizen is scheduled to address the board and ask for a more stringent leash law. The health department division directors are scheduled to give their quarterly program reports.

Chris is concerned about the board's ability to get its work done because, last month, during the discussion of old business, a new board member spontaneously asked the board to reconsider its recent decision to establish a school health center. This side-tracked the board's discussion and postponed important issues until this month's agenda. The budget must be presented and approved this month so that new funding requests can be made during the county's upcoming fiscal allocation process. Chris knows from experience that the board members will have many questions about the budget, and the discussion will require much time on the agenda.

In addition, the upcoming community health improvement initiative was on last month's agenda. About six months ago the board heard a brief presentation about this initiative. The process is now getting started, and the board members are expected to be involved. It is important that the board members be given details about upcoming activities and be prepared for their role in this community-wide process, especially because elected and community leaders will attend the meeting. Chris wants the board of health to be visible and participate in the community health improvement initiative.

With changes in the state law regarding tobacco-control authority for local boards of health, the board chair directed the board's policy committee to update the local tobacco-control policy to reflect the revised law. Chris does not expect a lot of controversy on this topic, although the board chair has hinted that the two newest board members might raise concerns about the tobacco policy.

A citizen has requested time on the agenda to talk about strengthening the current leash law. Chris knows that this individual has a reputation in the community for being talkative. As a result, Chris is eager to limit the time for the board to consider the individual's request, but is uncertain about how to raise this concern with the board chair.

Finally, the program directors have a number of things to report. The board chair recently asked that the program directors attend board meetings on a quarterly basis and provide summaries of their recent activities. The chair thought that this would help board members become more familiar with the management team and with the health department's programs. This is the first time the program directors are attending the board of health meeting. Chris knows that many of these people have been working on their presentations for the board all week.

As Chris pulls into the board chair's driveway, it is clear that the board has more issues to consider than can be covered in a 90-minute meeting. It would help to extend next week's meeting, but the board has agreed to meet at 7:00 P.M. and adjourn at 8:30 P.M., because some board members have a long drive home. People leave prematurely if the meeting is longer than 90 minutes.

Chris feels as though the board is not sufficiently responsive to the health department and the community. Chris lacks confidence in the board chair's ability to keep the meeting focused on the agenda, making sure that the major issues are addressed. "Yikes!" Chris thinks getting out of the car, "What can I do to get my board of health to function more effectively?"

What issues do you think the board and the health officer should address? How would you prioritize the items on the board's agenda? What actions would you recommend Chris and the board take to improve their effectiveness?

INTRODUCTION: WHY HAVE A BOARD?

The author of a magazine article offered advice on how to start a business. He advocated starting a sole proprietorship because, in his view, the only thing worse than a partnership was a board of directors. This is understandable for small business owners who want to run their businesses according to their own visions and preferences. However, in the public and nonprofit sectors, executives neither own the organizations nor can they exclusively pursue their own visions and preferences. The public or community owns the organization. Members of the public exercise their ownership of public and nonprofit organizations by having community representatives serve on the organizations' governing boards. Executives in public and nonprofit organizations require knowledge and skills to work effectively with these boards to ensure that community owners get the results they seek.

In the United States, local health departments are overseen by and are accountable to a wide variety of different boards (U.S. Department of Health and Human Services, 1997). There are an estimated 3,200 local boards of health in the United States. Most of these are directly associated with overseeing a local health department. The governing structures of boards of health vary. Some local board of health members are elected, whereas others are appointed. Some members serve exclusively on a health board. Others are responsible for local government oversight, such as a county commission or city council, but also have responsibility for overseeing the health department. Because of this variation, it is difficult to make definitive statements about how boards of health look or how they operate.

For the purposes of this chapter, however, it is important to make some basic assumptions about the relationship between a board, its executive, and the agency being run. In this chapter, a governing local board of health is an entity that has responsibility for making policy and financial decisions for the local public health department and is responsible for hiring and firing the local health officer.

DUTIES OF A BOARD OF HEALTH

Figure 22-1 illustrates a framework for board of health responsibilities developed by local board of health members and public health leaders

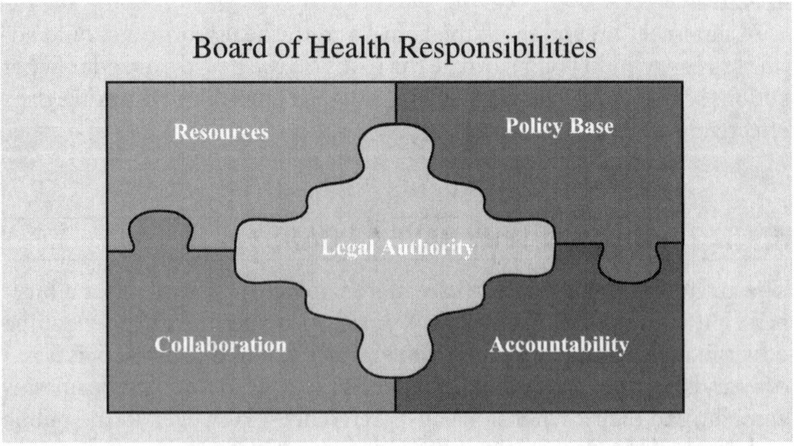

Figure 22-1 Local Board of Health Responsibility Puzzle

Source: Centers for Disease Control and Prevention (2003).

from across the country. This framework reflects their common understanding of the responsibilities of public boards of health. They agree that regardless of their structure, all local boards are responsible for ensuring legal authority, a policy base, adequate resources, collaboration, and accountability for public health at the local level. In some circumstances, boards of health may share these responsibilities with other local government entities, but every local government must guarantee that these governing functions occur for public health.

Legal Authority

Boards of health may perform a variety of functions. They may be authorized by state law to adopt public health policies; issue rules and ordinances; enforce regulations; hire, reward, and fire personnel; and adjudicate appeals. For example, if a health board adopts a local environmental ordinance, it is responsible for enforcing the new rules, making sure adequate resources and personnel are available to implement the rules, and serving as an adjudicatory body in instances where citizens want a variance or wish to appeal a decision. State laws may direct elected boards and commissions to govern local public health. In other situations, these functions may be delegated to appointed boards. In any event, local government is obligated to fulfill responsibilities under federal, state, or local laws to promote and protect community and environmental health. In instances where legal authority is absent, a local board of health must decide whether to pursue its policies independently or to seek additional authority through the legislative process.

Policy Base

A local board of health is responsible for adopting local public health policies, setting directions, and establishing strategic priorities. Well-informed boards ensure that organizational priorities are consistent with community needs and local concerns. Boards are most effective when they understand and promote a common vision for a healthy future and when all members of a board agree on how to achieve the goal. The central policy question that a local board of health must ask is: "What services do we provide to what people, at what quality, and at what cost?" (Carver, 1997). Using this question as a litmus test, a board can determine whether a particular issue is sufficiently important for the board to address. If, for example, a board is deciding the best approach to help local teenagers to stop smoking, it is involved at the implementation level. It should reiterate its support for programs that help people avoid smoking or stop smoking, but refrain from telling the staff how this should be accomplished.

Having access to appropriate and current community health information is essential if a board seeks to ensure that health department policies, programs, and initiatives promote and protect a community's health. Once a policy is adopted, the board must speak with a united voice in support of the decision (Carver, 1997). Even if individual board members oppose the policy before it is adopted, once the policy is approved, every member of the board must agree to support the decision (Oliver, 1999).

Resources

A board must ensure that the health department has the resources it needs to provide essential public health services and ensure that the resources are appropriately allocated to accomplish key public health objectives. With regards to providing resources, the board of health may be involved in approving grant applications, contracts, and budgets or in setting fees and issuing tax levies. In each case, the board should be certain that sufficient resources are available to support essential public health programs, that the resources are used to address key priorities, and that resources have been disbursed in an equitable manner.

Collaboration

Boards of health may collaborate with a variety of different groups in various ways. A board that wants to establish a school-based health clinic may have to work with the local board of education to develop guiding principles and establish goals for such a center. A health department may seek support from a local hospital and medical society to conduct a community health assessment. Board of health members may be asked to contact persons on other boards to ask for their help.

Even when board of health members are not calling or meeting with other community leaders, they should be thinking about how to improve collaboration throughout the community to achieve local public health goals. Board of health meetings provide a public forum where citizens may observe and participate in the democratic process (Houle, 1997). Local health departments use board of health members to act as the eyes and ears of the community and to serve as bridges to key constituencies. As local citizens, board of health members are well positioned to engage the community and represent local concerns, needs, and expectations for community health. Because they are community members, they are likely to be seen as legitimate spokespersons and have the ability to promote community dialogue and engage key stakeholders in the public health mission. They represent the organization, its mission, and its programs in their formal duties at community functions and public meetings. Board members strengthen the link between a health department and the community it serves.

Board of health members often are community leaders with ties to key stakeholder groups in the community and beyond. For example, health board members often have relationships with local and state elected officials, business and professional leaders, and other influential groups. As professionals and citizens, these members can use their networks to engage key partners and facilitate collaboration. By bringing diverse individuals and groups together to address public health priorities, board of health members fulfill their responsibility to ensure collaboration.

Accountability

Some government entity must assume accountability for public health at the local level. The board of health is the body usually vested with this responsibility. A board of health becomes accountable for public health primarily by hiring, evaluating, and discharging its health officer. The health officer is usually the only employee directly supervised by a local board of health. The health officer assumes responsibility for all other personnel decisions within a health department.

Local boards of health also ensure accountability through regular reviews of program activities and accomplishments as well as progress toward key priorities. On a regular basis, a health board should revisit its vision and mission and assess how well its programs are addressing major issues. By establishing measurable goals and objectives and using them to monitor agency performance, a board of health maintains a system of accountability that can be communicated back to the community and to other important stakeholders.

In summary, local health boards perform a variety of functions. Though their size and shape differ considerably throughout the country, they have an important role in protecting and promoting community health. Local health boards serve as the government's presence at the local level, carrying out legally mandated functions on behalf of the public's health. Acting as community trustees, local board members are responsible for developing a compelling vision and mission for community health and establishing policies that promote these goals. A board of health is responsible for ensuring that resources are available, adequate, and wisely used in accomplishing key public health objectives. The board serves as an important link between a health department and community and is able to engage key partners in addressing public health needs and issues. Accountability for accomplishing public health objectives at the community or municipal level ultimately rests with the local board of health. It must establish appropriate and relevant mechanisms to ensure that public health programs are effectively operated.

THE HEALTH OFFICER'S BOARD WORK

Maintaining a relationship with the board is among the most important activities of a health officer. Few programs educate public health executives on the topic of working with their governing boards. Because the quality of an executive's relationship with the governing board will be reflected in the success of both the executive and the board, it is essential that executives learn how to work with and develop their boards.

Many issues can affect the relationship between a health officer and the local health board. Organizations that consistently achieve strategic goals and objectives establish trust, open channels of communication, and mutual respect among their leaders (Herman and Heimovics, 1991). Building trust is something that occurs over time, as people keep promises, show respect for each other, foster positive relationships, and consistently make meaningful contributions. Modeling these characteristics in one's own behavior and helping to build trust throughout an organization, board, and community is fundamental for a health officer's own long-term success.

Together, a local board of health and its health officer work as a team to chart a course for community health. By having a board that is fully engaged in its responsibilities, a health officer gains board members' support and advocacy for public health issues; benefits from the board serving as a buffer between the department and community in controversial situations; and has access to interested citizens who have insight and connections within the community. The board of health, in turn, benefits from having a health officer who is a member of its team. A health officer is instrumental in accomplishing local goals and in providing leadership for public health at the local level. For these and other reasons, it is critical that board of health members and health officers recognize and value the contribution that each makes to building an effective leadership team.

Staying Focused on the Mission

To help the board of health remain focused on priorities, the health officer must reinforce the meaning of the department's work by continuously linking public health policy proposals, program activities, and program results with the organization's mission, vision, and key goals. Health officers can create contexts for their boards by ensuring that board members understand the history of public health in their community and how it has evolved over time. Orienting board members and new staff with a historical review of the organization and describing events can help board members understand the importance of the issues they face in the present and provide them with a strong foundation to develop strategies and a vision for the future. Elements to include in such a review include identifying different organizational and community leaders who have influenced the organization; noting major external influences on the department, such as new government initiatives or legislative changes; highlighting significant crises and their associated consequences for the agency; chronicling how local initiatives and programs were established; reviewing the development and change of community and organizational partnerships; and identifying key organizational successes and accomplishments.

Public health departments are government agencies that operate within a complex political environment. Within this environment, local health officers and their boards are responsible for ensuring an open and democratic process for public health decision making and policy development. Health officers can improve their board's effectiveness by making sure that board members design and follow an explicit process for reviewing, adopting, or changing policies and understand their legal responsibilities for conducting meetings and public hearings. The health officer helps the board operate most effectively by keeping people focused on core public health values and the local public health vision. By framing decisions and policy proposals so that they clearly address the public health mission and key goals, a health officer establishes a consistent framework for board deliberation and decision making.

Educating the Board

In order to stay focused on policy and make the best decisions, a board must educate itself about the organization's programs and health-related activities at the local, state, and national levels. Health officers can improve the effectiveness of board policy making by helping board of health members identify knowledge gaps and organizing educational opportunities. In developing educational programs or offering external educational options, it is important that board members be exposed to information targeted at a high level of policy making. Such in-depth information will help the board of health to shape the organization's vision, mission, and goals and to identify strategic opportunities and key priorities. Programs focusing on low-level operations and administrative details are not as useful. For example, it is appropriate for board of health members to attend a statewide meeting focused on establishing health objectives for the next decade. It would be inappropriate for them to attend a workshop to learn about how to conduct soil tests.

A health officer can help the board to stay focused on high-level policy and strategy by ensuring that the board of health designs and follows a process by which its members learn and progress through board committees and leadership positions (Chait et al., 1996). New members must understand their roles and responsibilities. Orienting new board members to the board, the public health organization, and their individual responsibilities is essential. To take full advantage of their expertise and creative capacity, every board member should have an opportunity to contribute to the work of the board as a member of a committee, as a committee chair, or as an officer. These leadership roles should be clearly defined and their terms limited to ensure that individuals do not become entrenched in particular positions.

Setting a Strategic Direction

A board's primary function is to establish the strategic direction for the health department on behalf of the community (Chait et al., 1996). A board should focus on the future and the direction in which the health department should be moving, not on where the organization has been. A board should use policy to move toward its vision of the future (Carver, 1997). By making sure that issues coming before the board are strategic in nature, the health director can help the board perform this important role. Too often, boards focus on what the health department has done and not on what the organization should do. The board's agenda should be forward-looking.

Creating Accountability Systems

At the same time, the health officer must ensure the board that the organization indeed produces the intended results. Through standardized reporting formats, the health officer can provide the board with meaningful information that it can use to ensure that policies and programs are progressing as expected (Chait et al., 1996). Some health officers may be hesitant to provide such information to their board because the performance of the organization is often equated with executive performance. If the organization performs poorly, the board may assume that it is the health officer's fault. In some cases, this may be true. In other cases, failure to achieve expected results may be due to factors outside of the health officer's control. To help the board understand such complex issues, health officers can summarize their own efforts in particular areas, describe how the organization is committed to continuous improvement, and provide the board with evaluative reports that show how the agency is progressing toward stated goals and objectives.

Fostering Collaboration

Public health results from partnerships between the local health department and a complex web of health and human service providers, schools, businesses, and other community-based groups. To improve the board's understanding and ability to represent the interests of the community, opportunities should be provided for members of the board to interact with others in the community and to meet with key stakeholders on public health issues. The health officer plays an important role in identifying strategic issues and organizing appropriate forums for such interactions.

Encouraging collaboration between the health department and its community partners and other stakeholder groups is an important board responsibility. Depending on its legal authority, composition, and jurisdiction, the board may have links with multiple constituencies. Fostering and developing relationships will increase board members' understanding and appreciation for public health issues. Health officers can encourage this process by getting individual board members involved in community events or inviting representatives of other boards and organizations to attend activities sponsored by the health department.

Guiding and Managing Board Processes

Local health officials can facilitate board development by initiating and helping to maintain structures for the board to accomplish its work. One of the most important tasks is to arrange the board's agenda so that it focuses on high-level policy issues. Time at board meetings should be spent on strategic decision making or exploring future directions toward which a health department should strive in the future. Much board time can be wasted on issues that must be approved by the board, but that do not require substantial discussion. For instance, accepting grant dollars or approving routine contracts, if considered independently, can use up a substantial amount of board meeting time. For such issues, it is appropriate to use a consent agenda. If board members have received and reviewed background information in advance, standard contracts and similar items can be approved early in a meeting, using a single vote, leaving time for discussion of more important issues.

It is common for boards to get bogged down in the discussion of old business by reviewing what has been previously discussed and, in many cases, approved and implemented. Rather than talking about what has already occurred, the health director should provide the board with brief written updates on key activities, including program director reports, and place major discussion items early on the agenda. The health officer performs a key role in ensuring that the board has sufficient time to consider issues in advance, to understand its responsibility for a particular issue, and to be well informed about the matters on which it must act.

It can be difficult for a health officer to know what and how much information should be provided to the board. It will help the board and the health officer if they develop criteria for governance information and focus board-related materials on items that will strengthen the board's strategic decision-making ability. Criteria for governance information include a number of items, such as using executive summaries to update board members on important information, events, and current issues; establishing standard formats for all program reports; focusing on progress toward key objectives, major events (good and bad), and areas for additional work and improvement; providing illustrations of how programs and activities support the organization's mission and the delivery of essential public health services; and reporting numbers in comparison, where possible, with similar data (e.g., comparing the number of people seen in a family planning clinic during the current month with previous months or with forecasted numbers or against data from the same months in previous years).

The location, time of day, and duration of board meetings influences the way a board operates. Most local health boards are organized by law as public bodies and thus must operate under open-meeting laws. The time and location of meetings must be announced, in advance, in papers circulated within the jurisdiction. Boards of health must establish a regular schedule for their meetings, making sure that they meet frequently enough to address major issues in a timely manner. For example, it is unlikely that quarterly board of health meetings are adequate to provide oversight of the health department, evaluate the health director, and ensure a strategic direction for the public health in the community. The time of day for board meetings will affect their length and accessibility. Evening meetings are usually the easiest for working board members and the general public to attend, but some boards prefer to meet during work hours, before work, or during an extended lunch hour. If funds are available, providing a meal in conjunction with a board meeting is a positive way for board members and senior management to get to know one another. Conducting meetings in settings that are accessible for people helps improve attendance by both board members and the public. In large jurisdictions, it may be beneficial to rotate the location of meetings so that no group of board members or the public is always burdened with driving a long distance.

Periodically holding a longer-than-normal board meeting, for example, an annual retreat, is a good way to engage board members in discussions of more complex and strategic issues. The health director should arrange for the board to hold special strategic planning meetings to ensure that the entire board supports the major goals for the organization and that the board has time to perform an annual self-assessment. The board must take time annually to assess how well it is carrying out its roles and responsibilities and progressing with its governance processes, codes of conduct, and leadership development. Such self-assessment can assist the board in setting clear goals and objectives for its work, help identify areas where the board can improve its effectiveness, and uncover new areas of interest for board activity.

■ PUTTING IT ALL TOGETHER

There is no single or best way to improve board of health governance. Making governance issues a priority for both the health officer and the board is an important first step in increasing everyone's capacity. Health directors perform important roles in making sure that board members understand their roles and responsibilities; the history, traditions, and culture of the organization; and major issues for public health in the community. The health officer has a responsibility to help the board clarify its governing processes and make certain that explicit structures are in place to cultivate and build informed and responsive board of health leadership.

The health officer can use an annual agenda and a standardized system for providing governance information to involve board members in strategic and high-level policy issues. Clarifying how the health department is accomplishing major priorities through timely and regular presentations and written reports provides board members with a stronger understanding of public health problems and programs. As knowledgeable representatives of the community, board members can be instrumental in building, fostering, and maintaining collaborative relationships within the community and with key stakeholder groups. Health officers can support collaboration by actively creating opportunities for board members to interact with the community and political leaders.

CONCLUSION

The local board of health is responsible for ensuring that public health at the local level has the appropriate legal basis, policies, resources, collaborative relationships, and accountability systems in place to protect and promote the public's health. The health officer performs a critical role in developing and guiding the governance process, creating structures and processes that support the board of health's core responsibilities, and providing perspectives that illustrate the complexities and opportunities related to improving community health.

Returning to the health officer in the opening case study, Chris met with the board chair. They agreed to extend meetings to two hours beginning next month, giving members ample time to make necessary arrangements. They also agreed to establish a schedule so that only one department head presented at each meeting. This rotating approach will provide members of the board with a steady flow of information. It also reduces the burden and anxiety levels of health department personnel. These changes will be announced at the next board meeting.

Having made structural changes to the agenda, they prioritized items for the next meeting. Old business does not improve with age and should be addressed in an expedited manner. The postponed item was scheduled to be first. The chair will allocate five minutes to discussion of the decision to establish a school health center. If additional discussion is needed, the matter will be referred to a board committee. If a second vote is requested, it will be taken. The chair will ask the board's legal counsel for an opinion about this procedure. The chair will also admonish the board that revisiting concluded business wastes time. Members receive materials in advance and are responsible for coming to meetings fully informed.

The budget is the most important item of new business. Without a budget, the operations of a health department must cease. The proposed budget will be discussed and then the chair will seek a motion for its approval. Chris and the chair agreed that most substantive issues in the budget had been resolved in the preparation process.

As a courtesy to members of the community, the citizen proposing a more stringent leash law was scheduled next. The chair planned to hear the proposal and then refer it to a board committee for review and recommendations. This will save meeting time.

They decided that the new community health improvement process would require the most time for discussion. While important, the tobacco-control policy recommendations are not time-sensitive. These items were scheduled for the end of the meeting and will be discussed if time permits. Chris and the chair expect the items to be deferred until next month due to time constraints.

They also decided to schedule a four-hour board training session outside of the regular meeting time. New members will be oriented during the first hour. Chris and the chair will spend the remaining time discussing board duties, responsibilities, and expectations. They agreed that this training should become an annual event. Lunch will be provided to underscore the importance of the board's activities in relation to improving the health of the community.

References

Carver, J., and Schrader, A. 1997. *Boards That Make a Difference: A New Design for Leadership in Nonprofit and Public Organizations.* San Francisco: Jossey-Bass.

Centers for Disease Control and Prevention. 2003. *The National Public Health Performance Standards.* Atlanta, GA: Public Health Practice Program Office, Centers for Disease Control and Prevention.

Chait, R., Holland, T., and Taylor, B. 1996. *The Effective Board of Trustees.* Phoenix, AZ: Oryx Press.

Herman, R., and Heimovics, R. 1991. *Executive Leadership in Nonprofit Organizations: New Strategies for Shaping Executive–Board Dynamics.* San Francisco: Jossey-Bass.

Houle, C.O. 1997. *Governing Boards.* San Francisco: Jossey-Bass.

Oliver, C. 1999. *The Policy Governance Fieldbook: Practical Lessons, Tips and Tools from the Experiences of Real-World Boards.* San Francisco: Jossey-Bass.

U.S. Department of Health and Human Services. 1997. *National Profile of Local Boards of Health.* Atlanta, GA: Centers for Disease Control and Prevention.

Resources

Periodicals

Boutin, C.C. 2003. Responding to governance challenges: The audit committee. *Trustee* 56(4):29–38.

Coid, D.R., Williams, B., and Crombie, I.K. 2003. Partnerships with health and private voluntary organizations: What are the issues for health authorities and boards? *Public Health* 117(5):317–322.

DeMuro, P.R. 2002. Telltale signs your board of directors may be providing ineffective governance. *Healthcare Leadership and Management Report* 10(11):1–8.

Peregrine, M.W., and Schwartz, J.R. 2003. Taking the prudent path. Best practices for not-for-profit boards. *Trustee* 56(10):24–27.

Stack, R.T., and Pointer, D.D. 2003. Beyond good: Improving governance means not settling for what's merely adequate. *Modern Healthcare* 33(32):28–35.

Weil, T.P. 2003. Governance in a period of strategic change in U.S. healthcare. *International Journal Health Planning Management* 18(3):247–265.

Books

Carver, J. 2004. *Board Leadership*. New York: Wiley.

Chait, R. 2002. *How to Help Your Board Govern More, Manage Less.* Washington, D.C.: National Center for Nonprofit Boards.

Floyd, R.A. 2003. *Courage to Lead: Reflections on Authentic Leadership for Non-profit Volunteers and Boards of Directors.* Austin, TX: 1st World Library.

Poiner, D.D., and Orlikoff, J.E. 1999. *Board Work: Governing Health Care Organizations.* San Francisco: Jossey-Bass.

Web Sites

- Charity Channel:
  www.charitychannel.com/nbgr.shtml
- CompassPoint Non-profit Services:
  www.compasspoint.org
- Internet Nonprofit Center:
  www.nonprofits.org/npofaq/03/02.html
- *McKinsey Quarterly:*
  www.mckinseyquarterly.com/article_abstract.asp?ar=1407&L2=18
- Progressive Business Publications:
  www.pbp.com/nbreport.html

Organizations

American Public Health Association
800 I Street, NW
Washington, D.C. 20001-3710
Phone: 202-777-2742
Fax: 202-777-2534
E-mail: comments@apha.org
Web site: www.apha.org

BoardSource
828 L Street, NW, Suite 900
Washington, D.C. 20036-5114
Phone: 202-452-6262 or 800-883-6262
Fax: 202-452-6299
Web site: www.boardsource.org

Center for Nonprofit Management
606 S. Olive St., Suite 2450
Los Angeles, CA 90014
Phone: 213-623-7080
Fax: 213-623-7460
E-mail: main@cnmsocal.org
Web site: www.cnmsocal.org/index.html

Centers for Disease Control and Prevention
1600 Clifton Road
Atlanta, GA 30333
Phone: 404-639-3534 or 800-311-3435
E-mail: www.cdc.gov/netinfo.htm (Web form)
Web site: www.cdc.gov

National Association of County and City Health Officials
1100 17th Street, Second Floor
Washington, D.C. 20036
Phone: 202-783-5550
Fax: 202-783-1583
E-mail: naccho@naccho.org
Web site: www.naccho.org

National Association of Local Boards of Health
1840 East Gypsy Lane Road
Bowling Green, OH 43402
Phone: 419-353-7714
Fax: 419-352-6278
E-mail: nalboh@nalboh.org
Web site: www.nalboh.org

CHAPTER

23

State and National Associations

Hans Schmalzried

Chapter Objectives

After reading this chapter, readers will be able to:

- Recognize the value of membership in national and state public health associations.
- Describe the organizational structure and governance of a typical public health association.
- Explain the primary differences between a national association and its affiliates.
- Know some of the specific benefits associated with membership in the National Association of County and City Health Officials.

Know some of the specific benefits associated with membership in the National Association of Local Boards of Health.

Chapter Summary

Public health professionals need all the help they can get to keep up with rapidly occurring changes in the field. Joining and becoming actively involved in a public health association offers many benefits. A number of associations, both at the state and national levels, are organized specifically for the purpose of advancing and enriching the careers of public health professionals. By and large, professional public health associations serve to improve professionalism. The goals of these associations include improving standards of membership performance and encouraging advocacy, research, and innovation. This chapter describes and discusses some of the more typical professional associations that leaders in public health may want to consider joining.

Case Study

Almost 70 percent of local public health agencies serve populations fewer than 50,000 people. In these smaller agencies, resources are often not available to address certain public health issues, such as supporting and passing secondhand-smoking regulations. Agencies serving larger populations usually have greater resources to address pervasive public health issues. A local public health agency was concerned about the large number of smokers in its jurisdiction, but lacked the resources to implement substantive education or advocacy efforts. The health board president described his department's dilemma: "The smoking rate in our community is greater than the average for this state. This is unacceptable. I'd like the board and health department to address this issue but we have no extra funds to allocate to the task." What advice would you offer to the board president?

INTRODUCTION

Administration of day-to-day operations at a local health department can be both time-consuming and demanding. Public health leaders are expected to be knowledgeable and prepared to address new and emerging health issues and concerns. They help health commissioners and local health officers stay current with the latest developments in the field of public health so as to respond quickly and appropriately to public health events. Peer networking and collaboration offer many benefits no matter what an individual's particular discipline or profession.

Professional organizations assist health professionals in meeting and networking with peers. Many public health associations in the United States are looking for new members. Public health professionals in all positions should determine which association will best meet their needs.

ASSOCIATIONS FOR PUBLIC HEALTH PROFESSIONALS

Professional associations are organizations that people join to connect with others who have similar interests. Professional associations provide a powerful resource for building and expanding peer network opportunities and keeping members up-to-date on relevant developments at the state and national levels. Professional associations work to promote the best possible practice among members of the profession. Individuals practicing public health may have memberships in several professional associations depending on their specific interests or discipline. In fact, one of the missions of most public health associations is to promote high standards of professional practice for their discipline or occupation (McKenzie et al., 2001).

Professional associations vary widely with regards to their size. Professional associations generally retain the services of an executive director. Larger associations have numerous support staff, whereas some smaller ones may have none. In fact, some smaller state associations have no offices and employ only a part-time executive director who works out of his or her home.

Professional associations commonly generate their largest share of funding through membership dues, charges for educational and training workshops, and registration fees for annual meetings and conventions. At many annual association meetings, companies will pay the association for space to set up booths to display their goods and services to members. Funds raised from these different sources are used for association operating expenses, which include executive director and staff salaries, office space, lobbyists, and office supplies.

Membership dues are probably the most reliable source of income for associations. Many organizations have different categories of membership and membership dues. Some professional associations charge dues based on the population of the jurisdiction served or the number of individuals employed by the member's agency. When an association uses a membership fee schedule based on population or agency size, agencies serving larger populations or those that have many staff members pay higher membership fees. Without this graduated membership fee schedule, members serving smaller agencies or those serving less-populated jurisdictions might not have the means to afford membership fees. Some professional associations incorrectly assume that membership fees are paid by the member's agency. Many agencies do not provide membership fee payment as an employment benefit. A common underlying concern is that agencies lack resources to pay for association memberships. When this is the case, health professionals should consider paying their association membership fees out of their own pockets. Students interested in careers in public health are encouraged to become members of associations. Most professional associations offer a greatly reduced membership fee rate for students.

It is important for agency decision makers to understand and recognize the importance of their public health professionals' involvement in professional associations. Although each professional association is unique, most provide similar services for their members. These include providing continuing education programs for professional certification or registration; hosting annual conventions where members share research results and interests with colleagues; publishing professional publications and legislative updates; publicizing policy development issues; and advertising career opportunities.

Political lobbying is another important activity provided by some professional associations. Some of the larger professional associations support powerful lobbying efforts both nationally and in some state legislatures. The purpose of these lobbying efforts is to benefit the association's membership and profession. The ultimate goal of lobbying efforts, of course, is to positively influence the public's health.

There are many professional associations in the United States. It is the purpose of this chapter to describe those typically joined by public health professionals. Many professional associations at both the state and national levels that might be of value to people working in or associated with public health will not be discussed. Readers are encouraged to search out and explore those professional associations that might be the most professionally helpful or personally rewarding (Scutchfield and Keck, 2003).

PROFESSIONAL ASSOCIATIONS FOR HEALTH COMMISSIONERS AND HEALTH OFFICERS

Public health is a multidisciplinary field; public health leaders emerge from a variety of occupations or disciplines. The primary leaders of public health agencies in the United States are the local health commissioners. In some jurisdictions, they are referred to as health officers. Individuals serving in these capacities can have training in any one of several disciplines, including medicine, environmental science, sanitation, veterinary medicine, nursing, dentistry, and health education. Despite public health's multidisciplinary nature, health commissioners and health officers must speak with a unified voice. The profession of public health must take precedence over the particular educational backgrounds and disciplines of health commissioners and health officers (Rowitz, 2003).

The **National Association of County and City Health Officials (NACCHO)** is considered the national voice of local public health administrative professionals. NACCHO's mission is to be the national organization that represents local public health agencies. NACCHO members serve over 75 percent of the population of the United States. NACCHO represents and serves nearly 3,000 local public health agencies throughout the United States. A relatively large association, NACCHO is located in Washington, D.C. and supported by approximately 45 staff members and an executive director. It is governed by a 32-member board of directors composed of health officials from around the country elected by their peers. NACCHO members have opportunities to serve on a variety of committees (National Association of County and City Health Officials, 2004a).

NACCHO has been at the forefront of research conducted on behalf of local public health agencies. Their work has kept federal policymakers informed at critical times to ensure that the concerns of local public health agencies are being addressed. NACCHO ensures that national policy holders hear the voice of local public health officials. This is accomplished through member guidance, involvement in legislative efforts, and partnerships with other public health advocates (National Association of County and City Health Officials, 2003).

Through its members, NACCHO has created a strong network of public health leaders connected through e-mail lists and city, county, and metro forums. NACCHO has brought together ever-growing numbers of local, state, and federal stakeholders to learn from and support each other's work at its annual conference.

NACCHO has been successful at developing innovative tools such as the Protocol for Assessing Community Excellence In Environmental Health (PACE EH), the Indoor Air Quality Tool for Schools Training Program, and numerous publications and training programs. Strong member involvement ensures a practice-relevant approach. NACCHO serves as an information clearinghouse to national and state community partners through its monthly *Public Health Dispatch* and quarterly *NACCHO Exchange. The Public Health Dispatch* has a regular section entitled "News from Washington" that keeps members informed on emerging issues. NACCHO also maintains an online Legislative Action Center that enables members to participate in grassroots advocacy efforts (National Association of County and City Health Officials, 2004b).

The **American Public Health Association** (APHA) is the oldest and largest organization of public health professionals in the world, representing more than 50,000 members from over 50 occupations of public health. It actively serves the public, its members, and the public health profession through its research and practice programs, publications, annual meeting, awards program, educational services, and advocacy efforts. Health commissioners and health officers should consider joining the APHA. However, APHA has a much broader public health focus than NACCHO, which caters to health commissioners and is specifically focused on the needs of local public health agencies (American Public Health Association, 2004a).

APHA represents all segments of the professional public health workforce. It is subdivided into Sections, Special Primary Interest Groups (SPIGS), and Caucuses that encourage members' active participation. These subdivisions serve to shape APHA's expertise into tightly organized units, providing a wealth of knowledge in all areas of public health. APHA uses its annual meetings to influence national public health policy trends (Rowitz, 2003).

APHA has 53 state public health affiliates, including every state and the District of Columbia. Although APHA is considered to provide the national voice for public health, it could not succeed without the complementary efforts of its state affiliates. State affiliates champion the same goals as APHA—to promote, protect and advocate for the public's health. The state public health associations are independently established, often having different memberships and focuses (American Public Health Association, 2004b).

NATIONAL ASSOCIATIONS FOR OCCUPATIONS OR DISCIPLINES

Many health commissioners and other public health officials desire and need a connection to their particular occupation or the discipline in which they were originally trained. A number of national associations are available to provide public health officials with these opportunities. The National Association of Environmental Health (NEHA), the Society for Public Health Education (SOPHE), the American Nurses Association (ANA), the American Association of Public Health Physicians (AAPHP), the American Association of Public Health Veterinarians (AAPHV), and the American Association of Public Health Dentistry (AAPHD) represent specific public health occupations or disciplines most typically joined by public health professionals.

The **National Environmental Health Association (NEHA)** is the logical association for health officials who want to remain connected to their environmental science or sanitarian education and experience backgrounds. NEHA offers a variety of programs that are in keeping with the association's mission of serving environmental health and protection professionals for the purpose of providing a healthful environment for all. NEHA has approximately 5,000 members (National Environmental Health Association, 2004).

NEHA's philosophy is to promote cooperation and understanding among environmental health professionals, to contribute to the resolution of worldwide environmental health issues, and to collaborate with other national professional associations to advance the cause, image, and professional standing of environmental health. NEHA is committed to fostering efforts to improve the environment in cities, towns, and rural areas throughout the world to create a more healthful environment and quality of life for everyone.

NEHA sponsors a variety of programs. The association offers seven national credential programs. These include the Registered Environmental Health Specialist/Registered Sanitarian (REHS/RS), the Certified Environmental Health Technician (CEHT), the Registered Hazardous Substances Professional (RHSP), the Registered Hazardous Substance Specialist (RHSS), the Registered Environmental Technician (RET), the Certified Food Safety Professional (CFSP), and the NEHA Radon Proficiency Program. In addition, NEHA conducts an annual conference and exhibition along with a number of technical workshops throughout the year.

NEHA publishes the *Journal of Environmental Health,* a widely respected, peer reviewed journal. The journal is published and distributed monthly to the membership. It provides current environmental health articles and information for members.

NEHA has about 27 paid professionals and several contract staff. A full-time chief executive carries the title of executive director. The association is governed by a 15-member board of directors that is chaired by the association's president. Officers are elected by the membership.

The majority of NEHA's members work in the public sector. Many are employed by local public health agencies. The only qualification to be a regular active member is that an individual be a professional who is employed in the environmental field.

NEHA has affiliates in 47 states, plus Jamaica and the District of Columbia. It also has three special affiliates: one for industry, another for those in uniformed service, and one for administrators. Affiliations help to promote the strength and diversity of NEHA.

The **Society for Public Health Education** (**SOPHE**) is a membership option for health officials who have an interest or specialization in health education. SOPHE has a diverse membership of health education professionals and students from across the nation. SOPHE promotes healthy behaviors, healthy communities, and healthy environments through its membership, network of local chapters, and its partnerships with other associations. SOPHE's primary focus is on health education. It provides leadership through research and practice, professional development, and public outreach (Society for Public Health Education, 2004).

SOPHE is governed by a house of delegates, with one delegate from each of its 24 chapters, and a board of trustees. The house and board hold two business meetings each year. Chapters must meet SOPHE requirements, although they are autonomous with regards to their governance and financial structure.

SOPHE has an active Advocacy Committee that includes representation from each of the 24 chapters. Rapid responses to national legislative issues are facilitated through a communication phone tree and fax system. SOPHE is similar to other national associations that adopt resolutions to provide an organizational foundation for action on selected issues of interest.

SOPHE promotes professional development by offering two continuing education conferences annually, each attracting 300 to 400 health professionals. SOPHE provides distance-learning opportunities such as video teleconferences and self-study journal articles to enhance continuing education opportunities for health professionals at the local level. Members are encouraged to get involved in one of the six special interest groups, which are focused on topics ranging from community health to worksite health.

Public health officials with nursing backgrounds stay current with their discipline on the national scene through membership in the **American Nurses Association** (**ANA**). ANA is a very large professional association, representing the nation's 2.6 million registered nurses through its 54 state associations and 13 organizational affiliate members. ANA advances the nursing profession by fostering a high standard of nursing practice, projecting a positive and realistic view of the profession, and providing advocacy efforts at the state and national level on health care issues affecting nurses and the public (American Nurses Association, 2004).

ANA members receive free subscriptions to the ANA's award-winning bimonthly newspaper, *The American Nurse,* and its highly respected monthly magazine, *American Journal of Nursing*. These publications provide detailed, current news and research for the nursing profession. ANA also maintains a popular Web site, *Nursing World*. The Web site provides instant access to nursing-specific information and activities.

ANA's biennial national convention and the state nurse association's annual conventions provide excellent opportunities for members to network with their peers, learn more about their profession, and earn continuing education units.

Physicians who become public health officials stay connected to their peers through membership in the **American Association of Public Health Physicians (AAPHP)**. AAPHP is open to licensed active physicians, retired physicians, and resident physicians. One major objective of AAPHP is to serve as the voice of public health physicians in the American Medical Association (AMA), sister public health associations, the government, and the public. AAPHP helps to keep public health on the agenda of the AMA (American Association of Public Health Physicians, 2004).

Veterinarians who enter the public health field have the opportunity to connect with colleagues with similar interests by joining the **American Association of Public Health Veterinarians (AAPHV)**. Membership is open to veterinarians who are, or who have been, engaged in formal activities related to public health and who are current members of the American Veterinary Medical Association (AVMA). The AAPHV supports programs to promote and improve the professional education, communication, and collaboration of public health veterinarians in order to reduce human illness, animal illness, and promote public health (American Association of Public Health Veterinarians, 2004).

The **American Association of Public Health Dentistry (AAPHD)** is composed of public health officials with oral health or dentistry backgrounds. AAPHD has embraced the challenge of improving the total health for all citizens through the development and support of effective programs for oral health promotion and disease prevention (AAPHD, 2004).

STATE ASSOCIATIONS

Many professional public health associations at the national level have connections with associations organized at the state level. A state association with a connection to a national association is commonly referred to as an *affiliate*. The strength of the connection between a national association and its state affiliates varies. Some state associations are established independently from the national organizations and may have different goals. State public health associations focus primarily on state and local issues affecting public health.

State associations offer opportunities for involvement and leadership by public health professionals. Logistically, state-level associations offer members more opportunities for communication and involvement than national ones. Statewide issues and legislation have more profound and direct effects on the day-to-day operations of local health agencies.

State associations assume important roles in the organization of health affairs in states and localities. State associations, similar to their national counterparts, function as sources of relevant information for their memberships. They typically provide regular publications, including journals and newsletters of special interest to the respective fields. Annual meetings serve as forums to discuss current issues and ongoing research and also act as employment exchanges. Furthermore, many state associations maintain regular contact with legislators and government officials, the media, and allied organizations to represent member interests and further the cause of public health.

One tangible benefit of membership offered by many state-level associations is an annual salary and benefit survey of all the local public health agencies in the state. Results of such surveys are collated and distributed to the membership to help guide them in crafting annual wage schedules and benefits for their staff and administration.

Public health associations in some states have considered merging their organizations into one large state federation. Economics and the notion that one voice in a state can more effectively represent public health primarily drive the trend for state associations to merge and form federations. In states where federations are being considered, some associations are reluctant to enter such mergers for fear of losing their identities. Hybrid federations may be an option in these situations. One hybrid model involves associations pooling their resources to share office space and staff while still maintaining separate identities.

ORGANIZATIONAL ASSOCIATIONS FOR VOLUNTEER HEALTH BOARD MEMBERS

At least 70 percent of the estimated 3,186 local health departments in the United States are governed by boards of health. Boards of health serve as policy makers for most of these local health jurisdictions. The **National Association of Local Boards of Health (NALBOH)** was formed in 1992 by several state local health board associations to provide a national voice for concerns of local boards of health. Prior to NALBOH, there was no organized public health advocacy activity at the national level on behalf of local boards of health (Scutchfield and Keck, 2003).

Few who assume a seat on a board of health truly understand the complexity and responsibility of the position. In addition, few board members have any training or experience in public health. Health boards oversee large numbers of public health services and the resources made available to deliver them. They have a large domain of authority. In the past, training and orientation of board members was left to the local health department they represented and sometimes assistance was provided by the state health department. There was little, if any, interaction among board members in neighboring jurisdictions. It wasn't until the late 1980s that boards of health in some states formed their own state associations of local boards of health. NALBOH was a major product of the state board of health associations (Scutchfield and Keck, 2003).

NALBOH continues to grow and has become an increasingly important player in public health at the local, state, and national levels. NALBOH is establishing itself as a significant voice for local boards of health on matters of national public health policy. A satellite office is maintained in Washington, D.C.; however, its main office is in Bowling Green, Ohio, in recognition that the majority of health boards are located in rural areas of the country.

NALBOH supports its members in many ways, including sponsoring an annual educational conference and producing a nationally televised public health lecture series. To keep current on national public health issues, each NALBOH member receives a quarterly newsletter entitled *NewsBrief*. Members also receive information and educational programs designed specifically for persons serving on local boards of health. Grant opportunities are available to the membership along with technical assistance in policy and organizational development. NALBOH advocates for policy and resources to benefit healthy communities (National Association of Local Boards of Health, 2004).

CONCLUSION

The importance of membership in state and national associations cannot be overstated. Professional associations help public health professionals to maintain professional competency and to learn about new developments and research in various fields. National and state associations provide support for professionals and board members. The dictum that there is strength in numbers is very true in the field of public health.

Returning to the board of health meeting that opened this chapter, small local public health agencies can benefit directly from membership in professional associations. Using membership benefits available from NACCHO and NALBOH, the small public health department implemented an advocacy program. This had a profound effect on preventing secondhand-smoke exposure in workplaces and businesses throughout the community.

Through NALBOH's Tobacco Control Conference Call program, the local public health agency received advice and technical assistance from other local public health agencies that had already implemented such control measures. NALBOH also provided a listing of local public health agencies that had successfully enacted smoke-free business and workplace regulations. The local public health agency joined the Smokeless Locals e-mail list-serve, a collaborative project sponsored by NACCHO and NALBOH. The e-mail list-serve provided a forum for the local public health agency to learn more about promoting tobacco prevention and control initiatives through peer exchanges. Through this forum, a small grant opportunity became available that helped the local public health agency purchase videos, displays, and other educational materials.

The local public health agency also secured a very informative and helpful document entitled *Program and Funding Guidelines for Comprehensive Local Tobacco Control Programs* from NACCHO. The *Guidelines*, along with all the other resources made available through the two associations, provided a solid foundation for the local public health agency to structure its local tobacco-control efforts. (This case study is a true account of the actions of a local public health agency in Ohio serving a population of 27,000 people.)

References

American Association of Public Health Dentistry. 2004. Available at www.aaphd.org.

American Association of Public Health Physicians. 2004. Available at www.aaphp.org.

American Association of Public Health Veterinarians. 2004. Available at www.avma.org/aaphv/default.htm.

American Nurses Association. 2004. Available at www.nursingworld.org.

American Public Health Association. 2004a. Structure. Available at www.apha.org/about.

American Public Health Association. 2004b. State affiliates. Available at www.apha.org/state_local.

McKenzie, J.F., Pinger, R.R., and Kotecki, J.E. 2001. *An Introduction to Community Health,* 4th ed. Sudbury, MA: Jones & Bartlett.

National Association of County and City Health Officials. 2004a. Service. Available at www.naccho.org/membership.cfm.

National Association of County and City Health Officials. 2004b. Products and tools. Available at www.naccho.org/tools.cfm.

National Association of County and City Health Officials. 2003. Annual Report. Washington, D.C.: National Association of County and City Health Officials.

National Association of Local Boards of Health. 2004. Available at www.nalgon.org.

National Environmental Health Association. 2004. Available at www.neha.org.

Rowitz, L. 2003. *Public Health Leadership: Putting Principles into Practice.* Sudbury, MA: Jones & Bartlett.

Scutchfield, F.D., and Keck, C.W. 2003. *Principles of Public Health Practice.* Albany, NY: Delmar Publishing.

Society for Public Health Education. 2004. Available at www.sophe.org.

Resources

Periodicals

Conger, J.A., and Fulmer, R.M. 2003. Developing your leadership pipeline. *Harvard Business Review* 81(12):76–84.

Price, J.H., Akpanudo, S., Dake, J.A., and Telljohann, S.K. 2004. Continuing education needs of public health educators: Their perspectives. *Journal of Public Health Management and Practice* 10(2):156–163.

Web Sites

- American Association of Public Health Veterinarians: www.avma.org/aaphv/default.htm
- Association of State and Territorial Health Officials: www.astho.org

Organizations

American Association of Public Health Dentistry
1224 Centre West, Suite 400B
Springfield, IL 62704
Phone: 217-391-0218
Fax: 217-793-0041
E-mail: natoff@aaphd.org
Web site: www.aaphd.org

American Association of Public Health Physicians
1300 West Belmont Avenue
Chicago, IL 60657-3200
Phone: 773-832-4400
Fax: 773-880-2424
E-mail: judic@ncchc.org
Web site: www.aaphp.org

American Medical Association
515 North State Street
Chicago, IL 60610
Phone: 800-621-8335
Web site: www.ama-assn.org

American Nurses Association
600 Maryland Ave., SW
Suite 100 West
Washington, D.C. 20024

Phone: 202-651-7000 or 800-274-4262
Fax: 202-651-7001
Web site: www.nursingworld.org

American Public Health Association
800 I Street, NW
Washington, D.C. 20001-3710
Phone: 202-777-2742
Fax: 202-777-2534
E-mail: comments@apha.org
Web site: www.apha.org

Association of State and Territorial Health Officials
1275 K Street, NW, Suite 800
Washington, D.C. 20005-4006
Phone: 202-371-9090
Fax: 202-371-9797
Web site: www.astho.org

Centers for Disease Control and Prevention
1600 Clifton Road
Atlanta, GA 30333
Phone: 404-639-3534 or 800-311-3435
E-mail: www.cdc.gov/netinfo.htm (Web form)
Web site: www.cdc.gov

National Association of County and City Health Officials
1100 17th Street, Second Floor
Washington, D.C. 20036
Phone: 202-783-5550
Fax: 202-783-1583
E-mail: naccho@naccho.org
Web site: www.naccho.org

National Association of Local Boards of Health
1840 East Gypsy Lane Road
Bowling Green, OH 43402
Phone: 419-353-7714
Fax: 419-352-6278
E-mail: nalboh@nalboh.org
Web site: www.nalboh.org

National Environmental Health Association
720 S. Colorado Blvd., Suite 970-S
Denver, CO 80246-1925
Phone: 303-756-9090
Fax: 303-691-9490
E-mail: staff@neha.org
Web site: www.neha.org

Society for Public Health Education
750 First Street, NE, Suite 910
Washington, D.C. 2002-4242
Phone: 202-408-9804
Fax: 202-408-9815
E-mail: info@sophe.org
Web site: www.sophe.org

PART V

Interactions with Colleague Health Commissioners

CHAPTER

24

Interagency Cooperation

Timothy Horgan
Eric Zgodzinski

Chapter Objectives

After reading this chapter, readers will:

- Appreciate the importance of interagency cooperation.
- Understand how to conduct negotiations that will lead to interagency cooperation.
- Identify weaknesses resulting from lack of interagency cooperation.
- Know how to implement interagency cooperation.

Chapter Summary

Interagency cooperation is essential for public health to succeed. Many essential resources are controlled by agencies other than public health departments. Trust must be developed among stakeholders. Access to resources must be negotiated and formalized. Interagency cooperation is an ongoing need and activity for health departments.

Case Study

Murphy's Law always seems to accompany outbreaks of infectious disease. Bacterial meningitis provides an acute illustration of problems associated with an outbreak of disease if no preceding groundwork has been laid for interagency cooperation. One Friday afternoon, just before the closing time of a local public health department, a call was received from an infectious-control practitioner at a local hospital. The caller said that a 19-year-old male college student had died from bacterial meningitis. His girlfriend had just been admitted for headache and fever. At the local college attended by the two individuals, rumors of the death and illness had begun to circulate among the students. Within 10 minutes, the media began to call the public health department to find out what was occurring at the local college. The media wanted a confirmation of the deaths of two male students from the college. To make matters worse, it was found that the two individuals in question spent last night at the male parent's house in an adjacent county.

About an hour after the start of the crisis, the media was still calling the local health department and had begun to make contact with the hospital and with the adjacent county's health department. The two health departments spoke to the media and stated similar facts but were not truly delivering the same message. The doctor who first treated the individuals took it upon himself to discuss the public health implications of bacterial meningitis and the proper treatment protocols. The hospital physician told members of the public that they should be receiving drug prophylaxis.

Just before midnight, more than 100 people were at the hospital wanting prophylaxis. By 6:00 A.M. the next day, over 3,000 individuals were demanding treatment. No communications between any of the agencies had occurred for more than seven hours after the first call was received. Even with people lining up at the door of the hospital and health department, the media still had no single message to tell the public. The state health department was called at noon on the second day. How would you have handled this situation?

INTRODUCTION

For many people in public health, *interagency cooperation* is a foreign term with diverse perceived outcomes. The reluctance of public health officials to fully embrace the notion of cooperation with many different agencies is not only somewhat naïve, but also a potential liability. If a health department does not cooperate and interact with other agencies, it cannot fully protect the public's health. Agencies cannot ignore the fact that they have a responsibility to protect the health of the community in which they work. Departments must build relationships and understand the various resources that they may call upon.

Some of this lack of interagency cooperation stems from the fact that agencies have a limited view of the world. This makes it difficult for individuals to allow others into their territory or agency. Many individuals do not want to share money, ideas, or power with others. Sometimes individuals have difficulty reaching out to other organizations or recognizing the validity of the outcomes that result from interagency cooperation. This chapter addresses some basic ideas and concepts of interagency cooperation for public health officials. It does not discuss detailed theories or processes; it does review basic ways and processes to reach a minimal level of interagency cooperation.

BARRIERS TO COOPERATION

For years, public health departments have not worked well with each other. The record is not much better with agencies outside of the public health arena. The problem of not working well with other agencies stems from individuals who seek to protect their department's territory.

Territoriality is the result of a number of factors. The first is that most leaders of public health agencies feel that they know what is best for their jurisdiction and do not feel that they should allow outsiders within their circle. Another reason for territoriality is finite resources. Competition with other agencies for money tends to create a protective, territorial type of atmosphere. Finally, a set jurisdiction with boundaries creates a restricted way of working. Lines on maps often create a hostile attitude among those who work inside those lines.

Local and regional health districts often are configured to reflect political boundaries. In many cases, patterns of commerce do not respect political boundaries. Arbitrary boundaries may contribute to dysfunction in terms of interagency cooperation. Such boundaries create specific areas to which public health jurisdictions must adhere. Health issues more commonly exist along geographic and regional lines, following political boundaries. When public health operates within a relatively confined political area and a problem requires attention outside of a single jurisdiction, the public's health is inadequately protected. To truly ensure public well-being, health departments and personnel must cooperate and function as a team.

The foundation of a true cooperative approach is to identify community partners and regional stakeholders. Building relationships with these individuals and organizations is the first step to building a productive atmosphere that can improve public health and protect entire communities.

IDENTIFYING PARTNERS

Face-to-face meetings contribute significantly to the building of positive relationships. To start the relationship-building process, meetings should be scheduled among senior managers from the various organizations. During these meetings, it is imperative that those attending have the ability to make decisions and direct workforces. This will create a solid foundation for long and beneficial relationships.

The senior managers of each organization should identify areas where coordination is necessary and where resources can best be utilized. Leibs (1997) discussed the role of culture in communications. Applying Leibs' comments to public health interagency cooperation, when identifying partners, one must take different cultures into account. Culture includes areas of the state or county in which agencies are located or the type of agency involved, such as law enforcement or hospitals.

Use existing forums such as hospital infectious disease meetings, terrorism strike force meetings, or any other venue that is attended by multiple agencies to initiate discussions among representatives of different agencies. Such encounters provide useful forums to build relationships and generate interagency cooperation.

Once relationships have been created, trust has been established, and areas of common interest have been identified, a memorandum of understanding should be developed. Sharing of staff, resources, and, quite possibly, budgets may be necessary and will require documentation to ensure proper use and reimbursement as needed. Memorandums of understanding have been used for other services, such as fire and law enforcement. Memorandums of understanding permit competing agencies to share equipment, personnel, and other resources that may be needed. A prime example in public health is a regional commitment to infectious disease control. City and county health departments often work in cooperation with other suburban health departments to track and understand infectious diseases within regions that cross political boundaries. Cooperation among many different partners must be undertaken to ensure the success of such an effort.

In one location, many different partners came together to effectively create and maintain a regional infectious control group. Public health epidemiologists as well as public health staff, hospital infectious-control practitioners, laboratory personnel, academics, and other regional health district personnel were all involved in the regional infectious control group. This group created an interagency approach to a problem. The focus of the interagency cooperation was community health. Nagel (1997) discusses the importance of having a team that is committed to working together, communicating, and sharing information and techniques. The team must be ready to act on short notice. He also discusses a parallel concept of a web organization that also fosters interagency communication largely through e-mail. The communicating agencies are not necessarily physically adjacent to each other.

The regional infectious-control group provides one example of how the future of public health depends on interagency cooperation for success with new programs as well as revamping older ones. Agencies of organizations that work alone do not benefit from the experience of others with similar problems. Links with distant agencies simply multiply the opportunities for learning and benefiting from the experiences of other organizations. Other programs may require different groups or individuals. When public health analyzes a watershed's water quality, it must involve public health agencies from multiple jurisdictions, political leaders, business and community leaders, academics, environmental agencies, citizen groups, and people from various human service agencies to properly conduct such an analysis. Other examples of programs that benefit from a multiple-agency approach are solid waste, food protection, air pollution, and most other environmental programs whose effects extend beyond a single jurisdiction.

BALANCE

How are all of these groups actually brought together, assembled, and their resources managed? First, identify all operational groups and delineate their responsibilities. This is accomplished by deciding what problem will be addressed and then bringing together the applicable resources. Once appropriate individuals are assembled, they must identify policies and clearly articulate the purpose of the group. A group leader must foster creativity while retaining focus on the reasons for the group. Do not stray from the general purpose of the group but facilitate free thinking.

To have a successful group, all members must respect the political and other positions of each person in the group. Exercising power or restraint on an individual basis will become extremely important as the group begins to coalesce.

Workloads should be distributed in a manner that mirrors the distribution of the group members. A convenient example is a multijurisdictional regional board of health. Not every community will have its own representative, but geographic representation should be employed. For example, the largest community will have the most work to do, but also the most representation.

However, one community should not have so much representation that it can dominate a discussion or direct an outcome. By-laws should be implemented to ensure that no dominant block of voters or representatives can consistently overwhelm the various interests. The by-laws should ensure a balance of power. For example, will a simple majority or plurality be required when making decisions? Remember that the choices made will dictate how outcomes are achieved and often influence the outcomes themselves. Maguire (1996) sums up the discussion by noting the dual importance of effective by-laws and ongoing communications.

TRUST

The price of cooperation is trust. Effective interagency cooperation can only be achieved if trust is shared among all parties. For many, this is the most difficult portion of the process of building cooperative efforts. Trust does not come easily or quickly. Trust must be earned. In a recent study, approximately one-third of all U.S. employees surveyed felt that management is trustworthy (Draper, 1996). Since employees perform the work of agencies, the notion of trust extends to other agencies. Clearly establish group goals and strive for fairness among all involved parties. Expect differences within the group. However, do not allow this to disrupt the trust-building process or hinder the attainment of the final goals that have been established for the group. Mistakes are inevitable. Agencies are not infallible. When mistakes occur, do not dwell on them, but try to see how the error improves the process and what must be addressed so it does not occur again. More importantly, do not allow groups or individuals to chastise the agency that made the mistake. Take the opportunity to build stronger bonds with that group. Keep the goals in view.

RELATIONSHIPS WITH LOCAL, STATE, AND FEDERAL AGENCIES

Public health should develop relationships with several different types of organizations. The first of these are local agencies. These organizations may be political or service-related but have programs that are related to public health. Many of these agencies directly serve members of the community. Public health's contribution will most likely center on these agencies' programs.

Working with state agencies can be both rewarding and challenging. State agencies are large and bureaucratic. Receiving information from these entities may require patience, and building relationships can be difficult. However, once relationships are established, large amounts of work can be accomplished. For the most part, state agencies set the tone for public health, write model programs and legislation, audit local agencies, and act as conduits for information from local departments to the federal government.

Many state and local agencies look to the federal government only as a source of funding. This is unfortunate, because federal agencies can offer a wealth of support and information. Local agencies often have similar attitudes toward state organizations. Federal public health agencies develop policies and have some oversight over state health departments. Managers in federal government agencies often have a difficult time forming relationships with people in state agencies. They are less likely to form relationships with local entities.

The local public health department's contact with a federal agency is usually through the Centers for Disease Control and Prevention during an investigation of a food-borne illness or disease. Tension among groups often emerges when the Centers for Disease Control and Prevention is involved in tracking or solving a problem. It is the duty of local health departments to build relationships that will accomplish the tasks at hand.

The U.S. Environmental Protection Agency and state-level environmental protection agencies have firm mandates. Local agencies must have the capacity to perform tasks requested by the Environmental Protection Agency such as inspecting home septic systems to identify a source of ground water contamination or inspecting exhaust ventilation systems of local industries to identify a source of air pollution. If the local agency has the capacity, that agency is responsible for ensuring compliance with environmental regulations. Local agencies lacking the equipment or expertise to address environmental problems must request such services from the state or federal EPA. In some instances, such as air pollution, only the state or federal EPA has the legal authority to act. The federal agency stands behind local health agencies and drives enforcement. Relying on a non-local agency for enforcement can be troublesome when attempting to build local relationships. Local entities understand the political and community concerns within their jurisdictions. The enforcement agency may require a different method of accomplishing a task than a local agency had planned.

CONCLUSION

Cooperative training programs and collaboration between agencies have not been actively promoted over the last 50 years. The events of September 11, 2001 have prompted local agencies to reconsider this approach Since then, public health has improved due to interagency collaboration. Future improvements are likely to come from agencies and public health departments working together. With public health being in a state of flux as a result of concerns over biological terrorism and emerging pathogens within a shifting society, the rate of increased interagency cooperation is not likely to diminish.

In the opening case study, interagency communication was lacking. No prior discussions among the agencies had been convened to discuss these types of crises or concerns. No health department spokesperson was decided upon. The hospital took it upon itself to direct public health efforts with regards to the situation. No sound or proper media release was prepared because no communications were being undertaken. The state health department was contacted much too late.

When it was finally over, about 15,000 individuals received prophylaxis and approximately $50,000 was spent on the crisis. Much of the money was wasted. Having emergency plans prepared in advance saves time and provides a script that can be followed. Press releases for many situations can be prepared in skeleton form in advance. Protocols for soliciting help should be prepared in advance. Over the next year, the health departments and the hospital worked together and with other agencies in the community. All were determined that the events of the meningitis case would never be repeated.

References

Draper, J. 1996. The cynical work force. *Communication World* 13(7):24–30.

Leibs, S. 1997. Ready to integrate the enterprise. *Industry Weekly* 246(13):46–50.

Maguire, B. 1996. How to walk the talk. *Journal for Quality and Participation* 19(3):20–26.

Nagel, R.N. 1997. Scratching the surface. *Industry Weekly* 246(13):54–56.

Resources

Periodicals

Hudson, B. 1998. A joint working. Take your partners. *Health Service Journal* 108(5590):30–31.

Polgar, M.F., Johnsen, M.C., Starrett, B.E., Fried, B.J., and Morrissey, J.P. 2000. New patterns of community care: Coordinated services for dually diagnosed adults in North Carolina. *Journal of Health and Human Services Administration* 23(1):50–64.

Secker, J., and Hill, K. 2001. Broadening the partnerships: Experiences of working across community agencies. *Journal of Interprofessional Care* 15(4):341–350.

Smith, W., and Dowell, J. 2000. A case study of co-ordinative decision-making in disaster management. *Ergonomics* 43(8):1153–1166.

Books

Calder, M.C., and Horwath, J. 1999. *Working for Children on the Child Protection Register: An Inter-agency Practice Guide.* Burlington, VT: Ashgate Publishing.

Roaf, C. 2002. *Coordinating Services for Included Children: Joined-up Action.* Berkshire, UK: Open University Press.

Organizations

American Public Health Association
800 I Street, NW
Washington, D.C. 20001-3710
Phone: 202-777-2742
Fax: 202-777-2534
E-mail: comments@apha.org
Web site: www.apha.org

Centers for Disease Control and Prevention
1600 Clifton Road
Atlanta, GA 30333
Phone: 404-639-3311, 404-639-3534, or 800-311-3435
E-mail: www.cdc.gov/netinfo.htm (Web form)
Web site: www.cdc.gov

National Association of County and City Health Officials
1100 17th Street, Second Floor
Washington, D.C. 20036

Phone: 202-783-5550
Fax: 202-783-1583
E-mail: naccho@naccho.org
Web site: www.naccho.org

National Association of Local Boards of Health
1840 East Gypsy Lane Road
Bowling Green, OH 43402
Phone: 419-353-7714
Fax: 419-352-6278
E-mail: nalboh@nalboh.org
Web site: www.nalboh.org

U.S. Environmental Protection Agency
1200 Pennsylvania Ave., NW
Washington, D.C. 20460-0001
Phone: 202-272-0167
Web site: www.epa.gov

CHAPTER

25

Sharing Resources

Hans Schmalzried

Chapter Objectives

After reading this chapter, readers will:

- Understand the value of sharing various resources among local health departments.
- Recognize how local health departments can enhance public health's infrastructure through sharing and affiliation.
- Know the methods that local health departments with limited resources can use to enhance their capacity to address the 10 essential public health services.
- Describe how local health departments with limited resources can address the increased demand for accountability.
- Describe examples of how local health departments, particularly those serving small populations, have increased program delivery and efficiency through sharing resources.
- Describe one model where an agency director is shared between two local health departments.

Chapter Summary

Tighter budgets and increased responsibilities are requiring many local health departments, especially smaller ones, to become more creative about the administration and delivery of services. Another challenge is the increase in specialization and the need for highly skilled staff to effectively carry out the primary public health functions. Some local health departments are finding that they can meet these challenges through sharing resources with other local health departments. This chapter describes and discusses some of the experiences of local health departments that share resources. The sharing methods described include sharing personnel, joint programming, affiliations, and even sharing an agency director.

Case Study

The consolidated school district superintendent was looking for help. She wanted to conduct vision-screening programs in the fall and seminars on eating habits during the spring. Even though the consolidated school district included five counties, financial resources were not available to conduct the programs she envisioned. She called the health officer of the county health department. After exchanging pleasantries, she made her request. The health officer replied that the department had access to a part-time nurse with training in prevention. However, the time available would not be enough to meet the superintendent's program goals.

"Are any options available?" asked the superintendent.

"Possibly," replied the health officer, "there are four other health districts within the area served by the consolidated school district. I'll check with my colleagues."

Should the health officer have offered to help? If so, what proposals could he have made?

INTRODUCTION

Most local public health agencies are small and minimally staffed. Given their limited resources, how can such agencies improve their surge capacity to respond to public health emergencies? Operational policies and procedures among local health departments are often inconsistent. These inconsistencies can make it difficult for neighboring local health departments to work together during emergencies that affect multiple health districts. How can affiliations among local health departments improve effectiveness in responding to public health emergencies? Many smaller local health departments lack the administrative capacity to either develop or maintain updated operational policies and procedures. How might an affiliation of local health departments help foster the development of up-to-date policies and procedures, especially those addressing public health emergencies? This chapter addresses these key questions.

SHARING PERSONNEL AMONG LOCAL HEALTH DEPARTMENTS

Nationwide, there are nearly 2,900 local health departments (National Association of County and City Health Officials, 1995). Populations served by local health departments range from approximately 9 million in Los Angeles County to communities with as few as 100 to 200 people. Almost 70 percent of local health departments serve populations fewer than 50,000, and about 50 percent of all local public health departments serve fewer than 25,000 people (National Association of

County and City Health Officials, 2001). Local health departments serving small populations are likely to have a small tax base, few personnel, and offer a limited scope of services. Many smaller local health departments may have the desire to increase staffing capacity, but cannot justify or fund a full-time position. Sharing personnel is one option for them to consider (Scutchfield and Keck, 2003).

Through the sharing of personnel, local health departments can create additional capacity relative to their size. For example, some professional positions (e.g., physician, epidemiologist, sanitarian, health educator, nurse practitioner) are commonly shared among multiple jurisdictions. In many instances, local health departments have found that by sharing personnel they are able to secure the expertise needed to ensure that capacity is available in a quantity that matches local needs but that is within local budgetary constraints (Milne, 2000). Following are two examples of how local health departments were able to increase capacity through sharing personnel.

The first example involves two neighboring local health departments in need of additional sanitarian staffing for their food-service inspection programs. Newly adopted state rules had increased the minimum number of inspections to be performed for food-service operations. More staffing time was required for inspections, but not enough to justify or pay for a new full-time sanitarian in each of the respective jurisdictions. One option was for each local health department to recruit a part-time sanitarian.

Recruitment efforts for a part-time employee by both of the respective local health departments were unsuccessful. The pool of candidates available for employment as a part-time sanitarian was very small. In this particular situation, the few candidates who were attracted by part-time positions were more interested in the training and experience that would be provided. The training would qualify them for full-time positions elsewhere. In such circumstances, the local health departments would become revolving doors and training grounds for other agencies offering full-time employment.

The two local health departments decided to share a full-time sanitarian. The two local health departments agreed that the sanitarian would work 60 percent of his time at one health department and 40 percent at the other. The sanitarian was hired as a full-time employee by one of the local health departments. A contract was negotiated with the other local health department stipulating that the cost of benefits, wages, and other expenses would be split according to the agreed upon proportion of time the sanitarian works at each respective local health department. The sanitarian received a paycheck and the same benefits package as other employees at the local health department that hired him. Each respective local health department provided appropriate supervision for the sanitarian as well as office space and clerical support.

In the second example, an epidemiologist was hired by one local health department and shared with five other neighboring local health departments. Under a federal public health infrastructure grant administered by the state health department, local health departments are required to retain the services of an epidemiologist so that there is a minimum of one epidemiologist for every 200,000 people. The six local health departments in this example identified their region as an area with a combined population of 200,000. Each of the six local health departments committed one-sixth of the epidemiologist's salary, benefits, and other expenses including supplies, equipment, travel, and training.

Having access to all of the necessary high-technology equipment, the epidemiologist works from the office of the local health department that is his direct employer. He easily conducts monitoring and surveillance activities in the six-department area. Occasional travel to the other neighboring jurisdictions is necessary when the epidemiologist's expertise is needed to assist in the coordination of disease outbreak investigations. Annual performance evaluations for the epidemiologist are conducted with representatives from each of the six local health departments. This particular arrangement for an epidemiologist has become a model for providing epidemiological monitoring and surveillance in other regions of that state.

Many local health departments are inadequately funded and have very small staffs. Maintaining a competent and well-trained workforce is a great concern for public health professionals. Furthermore, staff size is directly correlated with the ability to provide the 10 essential public health services (Public Health Foundation, 2004). Sharing personnel can provide some local health departments with competent staff that they could otherwise not afford.

■ JOINT PROGRAMS AT LOCAL HEALTH DEPARTMENTS

Some local health departments have found it advantageous to form joint programs between two or more health agencies. This can be an effective method to save on administrative costs. The savings from reduced administrative costs can be invested into providing more services for the participating health districts. Some local health departments have found success when they take a regional approach toward grant proposals for new programs.

Grant agencies are more apt to fund a proposal for a population serviced by multiple local health departments as opposed to awarding several grants to multiple local health departments to service the same population. In most instances, the chances for successful grant proposal awards are increased when local health departments adopt a regional approach. Joint programs usually make sense only when the local health districts involved are contiguous to one another and share some of the same population characteristics, such as size, population dispersal (rural or urban), age distribution, and ethnicity. The needs among jurisdictions in a particular region often are similar; public health issues do not stop at an arbitrary line drawn on a paper map.

Local health departments serving counties with the greatest needs are often those having the fewest available resources. Local health departments with more abundant resources can benefit from helping less economically solvent neighboring health districts in a region. For example, more affluent departments may offer epidemiology services to other area departments who cannot afford to hire an epidemiologist of their own. Enhancing the public health infrastructure of local health departments results in improvement in health status throughout an entire region.

Local health departments considering joint programming should begin slowly by working with a single local health department on a time-limited program. The magnitude of joint programming should be increased only after the relationship has had a chance to develop and solidify. Mutual trust must be established. Initial limited successes with joint programming can build confidence among the participants and provide motivation for more ambitious subsequent accomplishments. A joint program among more than two local health departments should be considered only after evaluating the experience of program collaboration between just two local health departments.

One example of joint programming involves two local health departments combining to conduct a Women, Infants, and Children (WIC) program. WIC is a federally funded nutrition education program designed to promote good health for pregnant, breastfeeding, and postpartum women and their children from birth to age five (U.S. Food and Drug Administration, 2004). Two local health departments located in contiguous rural counties agreed to submit their grant proposal to operate WIC as one joint program.

As proposed, the joint WIC program was to be administered and staffed by one of the local health departments. The other local health department's responsibilities were to provide clinic space, make referrals, and promote the program. This worked well for the second local health department, because it did not have space for additional administration and staff offices. A single program director manages staff serving the two local health departments. Dieticians and support staff split their time between the two different jurisdictions. This particular program has been recognized as one of the most cost-effective and efficient WIC programs in its state.

Joint programs among local health departments can be structured in a number of ways. They may be formal or informal. In the WIC program example, the arrangement was simple and informal. Simplicity is a powerful criterion when choosing an appropriate structured arrangement (National Association of Local Boards of Health, 1997). However, jurisdictions considering joint programs also should consider creating a memorandum of understanding to provide guidance in the unlikely event of a program-related problem.

LOCAL HEALTH DEPARTMENT AFFILIATIONS

Many local health departments have limited capacity to provide or ensure the provision of the 10 essential public health services in their communities. Many factors hamper their capacity, including limited financial resources and personnel. In addition, the demand for accountability continues to increase at all levels within local health departments. Organizations of public health professionals are trying to improve the profession by increasing training requirements and introducing certification of individuals, programs, and organizations (Cioffi et al., 2003; Lichtveld and Cioffi, 2003). Although these actions are positive for public health, they impose proportionally greater burdens on local health departments, especially smaller ones, to provide needed or mandated services (Milne, 2000). Local health departments are able to meet higher expectations and have additional opportunities for growth through the formation of affiliations that enable the sharing of both resources and responsibility.

In recent years, it has become clear that an increasingly important aspect of strengthening the public health infrastructure is enabling local health departments to work together on a collaborative basis. The formation of affiliations among groups of local health departments is one method to facilitate this collaboration. It should be noted that different terms can be used to describe such affiliations, and the distinctions are often blurred. Affiliations can be formed for short-term efforts or established to address ongoing problems on a long-term basis. In general, affiliations are formed to achieve specific goals according to a common plan. The rationale for forming affiliations is that the goals are beyond the capacity of any single participating local health department. In order to thrive, an affiliation among a group of local health departments must undertake activities that are important to all members. The alliance must benefit the individual members as well as the group (Turnock, 2004).

Local health departments who form affiliations reap many benefits. Such formal relationships among local health departments can ensure a broader range of inputs and perspectives from which to consider problems and possible solutions. A detailed example of an affiliation is provided in Appendix A at the conclusion of this chapter. Once the decision to form this affiliation was made, an important question had to be addressed, namely, who should represent each of the local health departments in the affiliation? In this case, it was desirable to include agency leaders and some lower-level staff members who were more familiar with the issues. There is no single, best response to the question of representation. Each situation is different.

Early decisions in the formation of an affiliation are important. The decision makers should consider issues such as the partnership's expected life span, criteria for membership, and expectations for participation, both during and between meetings. Constant vigilance is necessary to identify operational problems. A common problem is lack of participation by some members. A variety of different strategies can be implemented to include the few members who are not contributing to the process. For example, members who are not contributing may be given specific assignments. They should be closely monitored to ensure that they are participating. Careful assessment of the combined group's strengths and weaknesses is necessary to maintain the vitality and momentum of the affiliation (Thompson et al., 2002).

Keys to successful affiliations include strong and informed leadership, trust, a shared vision, good communication, and knowledge of the affiliation process. Having a positive attitude toward affiliation and the perception that the benefits of the alliance outweigh the costs are also helpful in fostering affiliation efforts. Barriers to achieving successful affiliations include a lack of guidance about how to form such associations and a lack of time or energy to commit to the effort (Thompson et al., 2002).

Strong affiliations among local health departments can lead to consolidations. Reports going back 50 years have proposed extensive consolidation of small local health departments (Turnock, 2004). Supporters of consolidation argue that the advantages afforded to local health departments include more efficient administration, broader financial resources, improved personnel management, less duplication of services, and improved physician reporting (Turnock, 2004). The disadvantages suggested by those opposed to local health district consolidation include a fear that home rule may be endangered by loss of local control, the possibility that wealthy health districts might pay disproportionately more to support health services than surrounding poorer areas, and a loss of status by some agency directors.

Some states have required local health departments to consolidate. Approximately 8 percent of local health departments serve districts that include more than one county (National Association of County and City Health Officials, 2001). Idaho provides a convenient example. The 44 counties of Idaho are organized into seven local health districts. This arrangement created larger population and tax bases for the new health departments. In turn, this allowed them to enhance staffing and personnel skills, thereby strengthening the public health infrastructure.

LOCAL HEALTH DEPARTMENTS SHARING A SINGLE AGENCY DIRECTOR

In some cases, the agency director of the local health department has medical training. In many departments, the responsibilities of administrator and medical director reside in two different individuals. Agency directors (also commonly referred to as the health commissioner or the health officer) have the responsibilities of providing leadership and resolving administrative issues within their departments. Agency directors who are not licensed physicians may rely on medical advisors to make medical decisions (Scutchfield and Keck, 2003). Budgetary restrictions within many smaller local health departments make it difficult for them to recruit and retain appropriately trained agency directors. One method that has been successful for recruiting and retaining professional agency directors is the sharing of a director between two neighboring local health departments.

Recruiting an agency director for a local health department is heavily dependent on issues such as salary, the pool of candidates with the needed skills, the reputation of the organization, and the skills of those in charge of recruiting. The agency director is usually the most difficult person for a local health department to recruit. Attracting appropriately qualified candidates for a full-time position is challenging. Local health departments determined to hire a qualified part-time agency director are faced with an even greater challenge.

Over 20 percent of local health departments are served by a part-time agency director. The smaller the population of the jurisdiction served, the more likely the agency directorship will be a part-time position (Gerzoff et al., 1999). Half of the local health departments in the United States have fewer than 20 full-time equivalent staff, and 25 percent of these departments employ fewer than eight staff members. Local health departments are sparsely staffed in comparison with many other types of organizations with comparable scope and range of activity. They also operate with modest levels of financial resources (Gerzoff et al., 1999).

Sharing an agency director is a viable option for smaller local health departments to consider. Local health departments that do not have the funds to hire a full-time agency director will likely have greater success in attracting a more suitable candidate if they share a full-time person among them. Such an arrangement has many benefits, both tangible and intangible. If a single local health department can only afford to hire a part-time agency director, two neighboring departments that cooperate can both have the advantage of a full-time director. This increases the frequency of the agency director's public health interactions. Public health interactions and better performance have a positive correlation (Lovelace, 2000).

In one example, two local health departments have shared the same agency director for almost two decades. Seventeen years ago, two local boards of health from neighboring counties met and agreed to share one full-time agency director between them. At the time, physicians who were preparing to retire headed both of the health departments. Because each physician had a full-time private practice, each spent only a few hours each week at their local health departments. It was their suggestion that a full-time agency director be hired and shared between the two counties. They felt that there was just too much activity at a health department for a physician with a private practice to oversee. Furthermore, many issues were not of a medical nature. Because neither of the local health departments could afford to employ a full-time agency director, they decided to pursue a shared arrangement.

The single (shared) agency director has a joint contract between the two local health departments. In the contract, the agency director promises to divide his time between the two local health departments, spending equal time in each county. Attending all board meetings of both jurisdictions is a contractual obligation.

Both local health departments pay the agency director the same salary. In essence, he has two part-time positions with two separate agencies. The contract makes provisions for full-time benefits, the costs of which are split between the two local health departments. The agency director has the choice of any personal health insurance plan offered by either local health department. Each local health department pays 50% of the health insurance cost per month or year, whichever applies. Holiday, vacation, and sick leave benefits are established in the contract and split evenly between the two local health departments. Training, travel, and meeting expenses are divided evenly between the two departments. When an expense benefits only one department, the jurisdiction that benefits pays the cost.

The agency director in this example has a basic schedule for evenly dividing his time. The schedule has enough flexibility so that the director can be present wherever he is needed at any particular time. In many respects, each of the departments has the availability of a full-time agency director.

One key to the success of this model is a strong management team and office manager or administrative assistant working at each respective local health department. These individuals are empowered to make many of the necessary day-to-day operational decisions. The shared agency director does not have time for unproductive micromanagement.

It is difficult to determine the point in organizational evolution when a local health department reaches the level of programming or staffing where a part-time shared agency director is no longer effective. The decision to make the change from a part-time to a full-time agency director is probably driven more by the ability to fund such a position than any other factor.

CONCLUSION

Jointly funded programs provide an alternative to health districts that have limited resources. This chapter has presented several examples of affiliation agreements. Open communications, trust, and a willingness to think creatively are requirements for a successful affiliation involving two or more health districts.

In the case study, the health officers all knew each other and agreed that the superintendent's proposed programs could have significant impacts on the health of children in the area. They could also result in considerable cost savings over the next few decades. They convened a special meeting to consider the problem. After discussion, the health officers drafted a proposal for consideration by the five local boards of health. The five health departments would contribute equal amounts to hire a full-time nurse with expertise in school health. One district would provide office space for the nurse. Travel costs would be equally divided among the districts.

A formal agreement was drafted and approved by the five health boards. A suitable candidate was then identified and hired. In her first year, 72 students were referred to local optometrists for eye examinations. Seventy-one of them now wear corrective lenses. One case of juvenile diabetes was diagnosed. Later in the school year, classes on nutrition were held. During the second year, an additional 31 children were referred for eye examinations. The products in school vending machines were changed. Students may now purchase a variety of fresh fruit and juices instead of chips and soda. In the third year, a team of board members, the superintendent, the nurse, and a local optometrist described the collaborative program to attendees of the annual convention of the National Association of Local Boards of Health. Three local boards in other states have written to the superintendent for details about the collaborative program.

References

Cioffi, J.P., Lichtveld, M.Y., Thielen, L., and Miner, K. 2003. Credentialing the public health workforce: An idea whose time has come. *Journal of Public Health Management and Practice* 9(6):451–458.

Gerzoff, R.B., Brown, C.K., and Baker, E.L. 1999. Full-time employees of U.S. local health departments, 1992–1993. *Journal of Public Health Management and Practice* 5(3):1–9.

Lichtveld, M.Y., and Cioffi, J.P. 2003. Public health workforce development: progress, challenges, and opportunities. *Journal of Public Health Management and Practice* 9(6):443–450.

Lovelace, K. 2000. External collaboration and performance: North Carolina local public health departments. *Public Health Reports* 115(4):350–357.

Milne, T.L. 2000. Strengthening local public health practice: A view of the millennium. *Journal of Public Health Management and Practice* 6(1):61–66.

National Association of County and City Health Officials. 1995. *1992–1993 National Profile of Local Health Departments.* Washington, D.C.: National Association of County and City Health Officials.

National Association of County and City Health Officials. 2001. *Local Public Health Agency Infrastructure: A Chartbook.* Washington, D.C.: National Association of County and City Health Officials.

National Association of Local Boards of Health. 1997. *National Profile of Local Boards of Health*. Bowling Green, OH, National Association of Local Boards of Health.

Public Health Foundation. 2004. Essential public health services. Available at www.phf.org/essential.htm. Retrieved February 16, 2004.

Scutchfield, F.D., and Keck, C.W. 2003. *Principles of Public Health Practice,* 2d ed. Albany, NY: Delmar.

Thompson, D., Socolar, R., Brown, L., and Haggerty, J. 2002. Interagency collaboration in seven North Carolina local public health departments. *Journal of Public Health Management and Practice* 8(5):55–64.

Turnock, B.J. 2004. *Public Health: What It Is and How It Works,* 3d ed. Sudbury, MA: Jones & Bartlett.

U.S. Food and Drug Administration. Women, Infants and Children Program. Available at www.fns.usda.gov/wic. Retrieved February 16, 2004.

Resources

Periodicals

Bashir, Z., Lafronza, V., Fraser, M.R., Brown, C.K., and Cope, J.R. 2003. Local and state collaboration for effective preparedness planning. *Journal of Public Health Management and Practice* 9(5):344–351.

Gebbie, K., Merrill, J., Hwang, I., Gebbie, E.N., and Gupta, M. 2003. The public health workforce in the year 2000. *Journal of Public Health Management and Practice* 9(1):79–86.

Griffith, J. 2003. Establishing a dental practice in a rural, low-income county health department. *Journal of Public Health Management and Practice* 9(6):538–541.

Hajat, A., Stewart, K., and Hayes, K.L. 2003. The local public health workforce in rural communities. *Journal of Public Health Management and Practice* 9(6):481–488.

Mete, C., Cioffi, J.P., and Lichtveld, M.Y. 2003. Are public health services available where they are most needed? An examination of local health department services. *Journal of Public Health Management and Practice* 9(3):214–223.

Potter, M.A., Barron, G., and Cioffi, J.P. 2003. A model for public health workforce development using the National Public Health Performance Standards Program. *Journal of Public Health Management and Practice* 9(3):199–207.

Veazie, M.A., Teufel-Shone, N.I., Silverman, G.S., Connolly, A.M., Warne, S., King, B.F., Lebowitz, M.D., and Meister, J.S. 2001. Building community capacity in public health: the role of action-oriented partnerships. *Journal of Public Health Management and Practice* 7(2):21–32.

Books

Green, L., and Ottoson, J.M. 2001. *Community and Population Health,* 8th ed. New York: McGraw-Hill Higher Education.

McKenzie, J.F., Pinger, R.R., and Kotecki, J. 2002. *An Introduction to Community Health,* 4th ed. Sudbury, MA: Jones & Bartlett.

Miller, D., and Price, J.M. 1997. *Dimensions of Community Health,* 5th ed. New York: McGraw-Hill Higher Education.

Novick, L.F., and Mays, G.P. 2000. *Public Health Administration: Principles for Population-Based Management.* Sudbury, MA: Jones & Bartlett.

Web Sites

- American Public Health Association: www.apha.org
- City and County: The Voice of Local Government: www.americancityandcounty.com
- National Association of Counties: www.naco.org

Organizations

Association of State and Territorial Health Officials
1275 K Street, NW, Suite 800
Washington, D.C. 20005-4006
Phone: 202-371-9090
Fax: 202-371-9797
Web site: www.astho.org

Centers for Disease Control and Prevention
1600 Clifton Road
Atlanta, GA 30333
Phone: 404-639-3311, 404-639-3534, or 800-311-3435
E-mail: www.cdc.gov/netinfo.htm (Web form)
Web site: www.cdc.gov

National Association of County and City Health Officials
1100 17th Street, Second Floor
Washington, D.C. 20036
Phone: 202-783-5550
Fax: 202-783-1583
E-mail: naccho@naccho.org
Web site: www.naccho.org

National Association of Local Boards of Health
1840 East Gypsy Lane Road
Bowling Green, OH 43402
Phone: 419-353-7714
Fax: 419-352-6278
E-mail: nalboh@nalboh.org
Web site: www.nalboh.org

Public Health Foundation
1220 L Street, NW, Suite 350
Washington, D.C. 20005
Phone: 202-898-5600
Fax: 202-898-5609
E-mail: info@phf.org
Web site: www.phf.org

APPENDIX A

AN AFFILIATION OF SIX COUNTY LOCAL HEALTH DEPARTMENTS

Six contiguous county local health departments in a rural area agreed to initiate a formal affiliation in an effort to be better prepared to respond to suspected food-borne disease outbreaks in the region. The six counties cover over 2,565 square miles and serve a population of approximately 205,000 people. Prior to this affiliation, personnel from the six county local health departments communicated among themselves, but each agency was, for the most part, very independent. When suspected food-borne outbreaks occurred within a particular county, normal procedures prevailed. A suspected outbreak that crossed county lines was a very different matter. Local health departments in the affected counties would muddle through, but there was no formal structure in place to facilitate combining the resources available among the various departments in the region. Of equal importance, no formal protocols for communication were in place.

The six-county affiliation took on the name "Six-pact." The Six-pact created a mission to provide it with clear guidance and direction for its first initiative. The Six-pact's mission was to create and implement a model of the public health process by increasing collaboration and decreasing inconsistencies in environmental health policies and procedures (i.e., food safety, campgrounds, private water, etc.) among the rural Six-pact health districts.

Through this affiliation, the Six-pact decided its first project would be to develop standardized investigation procedures for suspected outbreaks of food-borne illness. Agreeing that there was a real need for this initiative, Six-pact members made it their first priority. The Six-pact counties chose this particular initiative at the beginning of their affiliation because bolstering preparedness for suspected outbreaks of food-borne illness would strengthen their individual and collective public health infrastructures. Media attention to disease outbreaks was increasing. This was accompanied by public demands for accountability. Existing departmental procedures were both outdated and inadequate. The event that catalyzed the effort was a *Salmonella* outbreak. Migrant farm workers were being treated at three hospital emergency rooms located in three different Six-pact counties.

Frequent meetings were convened and many hours were spent in collaboration among the local health department administrators and environmental health directors. In all, approximately a year was required for the Six-pact group to complete its initiative. To accomplish their goal, they focused on a series of objectives, including the development of a common procedural manual for investigations of suspected food-borne illnesses. The manual includes flow charts, communications templates, and standardized reporting forms for use when conducting investigations of suspected outbreaks of food-borne illness. Tabletop exercises were conducted to test and fine-tune the new Six-pact response system.

In the event of a suspected food-borne illness outbreak in the six-county area, a system now exists to pool resources, most importantly, manpower. This is an important benefit the Six-pact affiliation. As individual local health departments, each of the Six-pact departments has, at most, one full-time equivalent sanitarian who is regularly assigned to conduct food-service inspections. Before the Six-pact was formed, an influx of experienced manpower would be needed to appropriately respond to a major suspected food-borne illness outbreak. The most likely source would have been the state health department. Now, locally knowledgeable resources are available in less than an hour. Instead of each local health department responding alone to suspected food-borne illness outbreaks in their respective jurisdictions, through the Six-pact affiliation they are now prepared to take it on as a group following a well-designed and tested system. As many as 16 sanitarians are poised to mobilize and act in the event of a suspected outbreak of food-borne illness in the six-county area.

PART VI

Emergency Preparedness: Terrorism, Accidents and Natural Disasters

CHAPTER 26

Emergency Preparedness

Ronald Burger
L. Fleming Fallon, Jr.
Jay MacNeal
Diana Wilde
Eric Zgodzinski

Chapter Objectives

After reading this chapter, readers will:

- Understand emergency-preparedness planning.
- Develop relationships with other local agencies that contribute to emergency preparations.
- Recognize the importance of conducting an inventory of potential threats, including so-called high-profile targets.
- Identify needed resources locally and in neighboring jurisdictions and organizations.
- Know how to craft formal written agreements that will ensure the availability of resources.
- Know how to create an emergency plan of action.
- Understand how to conduct tabletop exercises.
- Train team members to respond to emergencies.
- Know how to stage and evaluate full-scale practice drills.
- Understand the public health Incident Command System (ICS).
- Recognize the need for formal and informal communications networks.

Chapter Summary

Emergency-preparedness planning is critical to successfully responding to a public health threat. Establishing relationships is the first step to creating trust among emergency team members. Potential threats must be identified and the likelihood of being involved in an event estimated. Resources must be identified and secured. Formal plans to address emergency situations must be developed and evaluated. Scenarios must be created; the emergency team's responses to such scenarios must be tested and evaluated. Formal and informal communications networks must be established. The public health Incident Command System (ICS) is an excellent tool for controlling responses to emergency situations.

Case Study

The day was hot and muggy, like most in the dog days of summer. At a local health department, individuals were working at various tasks, from answering phone calls to performing Internet research. Other department personnel were out in the field conducting inspections and follow-up visits. Without warning, there were several loud cracks. The lights flickered, went out, came back for a moment, and then went out for a final time. Within a few minutes, emergency supervisors realized that most of the city, as well as the northeast section of the country, was without power. Employees as well as members of the general public were in the building, working or using the services of the health department. How should the department react to the power outage?

■ INTRODUCTION

Think about attempting to host a party for 300 guests without having some type of plan in place. Before deciding that such a task would be fun, remember that without a plan in place you would not have a guest list, you would not purchase food and beverages in advance of the event, and you would not have a space reserved for the event. Most people would consider a spontaneous gathering under such circumstances to be a disaster. The plans of many public health agencies for handling emergencies are uncomfortably close to the concept of an unplanned party. For the fortunate organizations that believe they are prepared, the question nags: Is the level of preparedness adequate? Many jurisdictions have prepared and practiced their plans. These jurisdictions ask: Was the plan OK? An affirmative response may provide some reassurance, but it raises another nagging question: Is OK good enough? Can the district afford to get by with a plan that is merely OK? Disaster preparedness plans should be as complete and workable as possible, yet retain flexibility and the ability to adapt to a variety of possible problems. Whether preparing for a party or a disaster, adequate planning cannot accurately forecast all contingencies. However, merely being OK is not likely to be sufficient.

This chapter provides insights into developing a disaster or response plan. It also offers some workable suggestions to include in an existing plan. Because of the extensive material needed to develop an adequate disaster plan, this chapter can only provide an overview. Public health and emergency response officials should review the extensive material on disaster preparedness planning available at the local, state, and national levels. Individual municipalities and departments should design plans that are best suited to their particular needs and vulnerabilities. Successful plans will include the needs, personnel, and specific disasters that could occur in their regions.

The text of this chapter provides a reasonable point from which to start. The resources at the conclusion of the chapter provide additional information and guidance. Taken together, the material provides a general idea of how to produce and implement preparedness policies for a community.

One preparedness expert summarized the process of emergency preparedness in a succinct manner: Failing to plan is the same as planning to fail. A well-developed and rehearsed emergency operations plan will enable a community to successfully respond to difficult situations with public health's limited resources.

PREPAREDNESS PLANNING

Public health practitioners are a vital component in the larger system of emergency providers who protect the health and safety of people and property during times of crisis. Responding to a major incident, whether caused by a terrorist action or a natural disaster, in a capable and timely manner is an important element in protecting the overall health and well-being of a given population. By applying the principles of assessment, policy development, and assurance, public health practitioners can ensure that their communities are prepared for terrorist attacks or natural disasters and also offer improved responses to everyday events.

Beginning to understand all of the available information on preparedness can be a daunting task. By utilizing a systematic approach, board members, health officers, and public health staff can be sure that they are making satisfactory progress with their efforts. Having well-defined goals enables agencies and individuals to work toward drafting a well-developed plan. It also minimizes the wasting of time and resources on nonpertinent items.

Plan Review

A successful frontiersman once remarked, "If I had six hours to chop down a tree, I'd spend the first four sharpening the axe." The initial step in creating a successful emergency protocol is to review the organization's existing plans and preparedness procedures. Such documents are frequently in plain sight on a slightly dusty bookshelf. There is no reason to totally abandon old plans. With some updating, these may be improved upon or adapted to address contemporary threats to public health. If the department currently does not have such plans, a clean slate provides an excellent opportunity to begin the most important aspect of disaster preparedness: developing and building relationships.

Developing Relationships

Identifying relevant stakeholders is a time-consuming but important task. Police, firefighters, hospital administrators, emergency medical responders, environmental officials, and local boards of health all have an interest in protecting the health of the communities and people that they serve. However, representatives from all of these groups rarely meet at the same table. Subgroup meetings are more common. Organizing a single meeting where the directors and staff of each department can meet each other is often difficult. Frequently, personal relationships must be established. Emergency responders use different words: "Three in the morning is not the time to exchange business cards." Trust must be built. Missing organizations must be identified. All of these processes require time.

Relevant organizations may be overlooked. Local examples include the Red Cross, the United Way, members of the clergy, service organizations (such as the Rotary, Lions, Boy Scouts, and Girl Scouts), and mental health professionals. Potentially interested state and federal agencies include emergency management agencies, National Guard units, the FBI, airport authorities, and environmental protection offices. Initial meetings may be required for attendees to simply get to know one another. Forging strong bonds and establishing mutual respect and trust are critical but time-consuming. Understanding the missions, objectives, resources, strengths, and weaknesses of each participating organization will be valuable when developing plans. More importantly, it will be known how each department will react during a crisis. Organizing and attending disaster committee meetings requires a commitment of time. Experts recommend meeting on a monthly basis. Integrating all individual organizational plans will provide the greatest protection for the entire community.

Integrating Plans

The activities of all interested local agencies must be melded. This may require surrendering some degree of organizational autonomy and independence for the overall success of a disaster plan. Lines of authority should be determined in advance. This can be accomplished using an Incident Management System or an Incident Command System. Developing contingency plans strengthens the overall emergency operations plan.

Communications and integration increase the probability that a plan will be successful in the event of a disaster.

Practicing Plans

Once plans are in place and personnel have had ample opportunity to review the plans, it is time to practice. Remember that practice doesn't make perfect. However, each drill improves individual skills and organizational readiness. Participants in training exercises will make mistakes. This merely serves as a reminder of how seriously such training should be taken. The manner in which the plan is practiced during a drill will be the way the plan is implemented during an actual operational response.

The All-Hazards Approach and Threat-Specific Planning

Developing an emergency operations plan can be accomplished in a timely fashion by utilizing a logical approach and considering issues that may have local importance. The master plan should reflect an *all-hazards* approach to emergency response, trying to identify all potential issues or situations that a local community might encounter. A universal plan should ensure that all agencies and community organizations know their roles and work together to mitigate any emergency, from a food-borne disease outbreak to an earthquake.

In addition to the all-hazard approach, local planning should also be threat specific, addressing potential problems that would only occur in a certain region. For example, International Falls, Minnesota, would not plan for a hurricane, and Tampa, Florida, would not plan for prolonged arctic conditions. The two approaches have obvious differences. All-hazard planning maximizes efforts and expenditures due to its extensive nature. Politicians can easily support threat-specific planning (Landesman, 2001).

Roles of the FBI and FEMA

Two important agencies related to disaster preparedness and response planning are the Federal Bureau of Investigation (FBI) and the Federal Emergency Management Agency (FEMA). The FBI is responsible for securing incident sites and conducting the criminal investigation during a known or suspected terrorist event. FEMA is the lead federal agency in the consequence-management period in any type of federally declared disaster. FEMA coordinates the recovery portion of the response effort for any disaster or incident. It is important to understand the relationship between crisis and consequence management when developing an emergency plan. The relationship between crisis management and consequence management is summarized in **Figure 26-1.**

The U.S. Policy on Counterterrorism is contained in Presidential Decision Directive 39. This presidential policy document delineates spe-

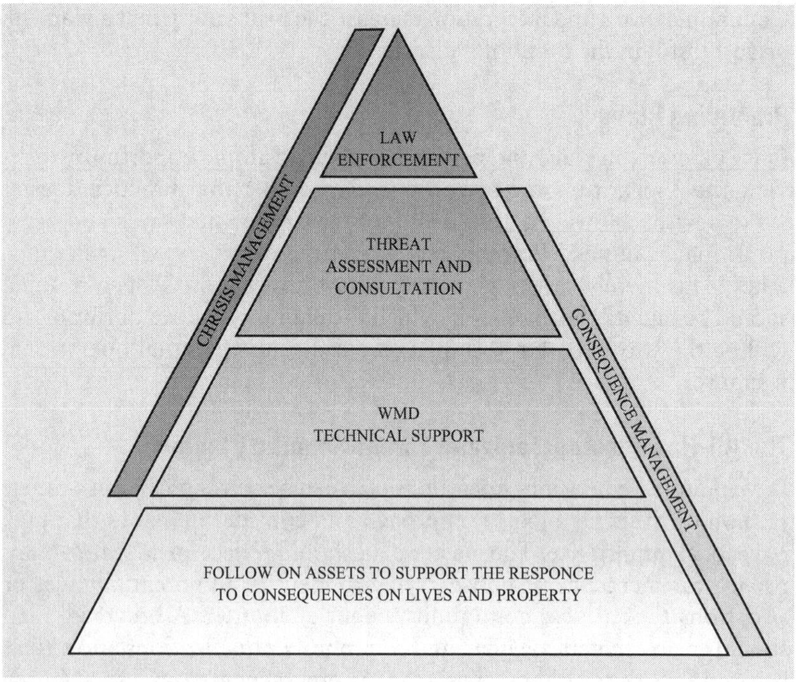

Figure 26-1 Crisis and Consequence Management
Source: Federal Emergency Management Agency (2004).

cific roles for both the FBI and FEMA in the event of a terrorist act. With the establishment of the Homeland Security Department, the activities of many different agencies are being coordinated.

Planning for Emergency Operations

Emergency operations plans should always be regarded as works in progress. Continuous quality-improvement activities should be undertaken to ensure that local plans work under a variety of circumstances or events.

Local public health agencies should ensure that they contribute to the all-hazards emergency operations plan of their local emergency management agency. This input should relate to health and medicine in general and the resources, such as epidemiology, that are specific to public health. Each public health agency should also have an internal emergency operations plan outlining the steps that will be taken in the event of an emergency. The details of an agency's plan should be coordinated with the master community plan. The designated public health emergency manager often has expertise that will be helpful in dealing with a biological event or disease outbreak. Details for such specific events are often contained in an appendix to an all-hazards plan. Infectious disease experts suggest that such an appendix be developed even if local emergency management personnel do not request a biological-event plan.

Potential collaborating organizations must conduct an assessment of potential threats and existing resources. The partners must pay particular attention to potential high-profile targets, such as electrical substations, pipelines, airports, and railroads. Stakeholders are excellent sources for accurate assessment information.

Based on the results of the inventory, workable plans of how to respond to these situations should be developed. Utilize services available from the stakeholders and formalize them through formal written memorandums of understanding. After the formal plan is written, have a formal review process with stakeholders. Establish deadlines for revisions to ensure that the plan will not be delayed. Conduct tabletop exercises with the completed plan. Apply the plan to several scenarios to validate its effectiveness.

After the plan is approved, train all response participants. These individuals don't necessarily need to know every portion of the plan, but they must understand how their agency fits into the plan and what their role will be in an emergency. Once plan participants have been trained and educated about the plan, begin staging drills with stakeholder support. Formally evaluate how the plan works in the field. Evaluate and document strengths and weaknesses and develop a corrective action plan to make any necessary adjustments.

REVIEWING AND ALLOCATING RESOURCES

A review of intra-agency resources is important when developing an emergency plan. All agencies involved in the development of the plan should make an assessment of the resources they have to offer. Such resources may include staff, equipment, and current emergency contact information for the agency. Agencies should also conduct an external resource inventory and determine what other individuals or groups in the community are able to offer. Personnel, equipment, and current emergency contact information are important pieces of information. Such information is important when developing emergency plans and incident action plans.

SAFETY

Staff members are public health's most important asset. When preparing for any crisis or adverse event, a well-trained and motivated staff is essential for success. Public health staff should be knowledgeable on a wide range of issues. Staff members should know the composition of biological agents, the proper use of personal protective equipment, and how to report to an emergency site. Training and discussion on these topics should be consistent and conducted prior to an event to reinforce concepts. During times of disaster, staff members will be called upon to perform their everyday duties and to assist with the disaster response. Generally, they will not be expected to perform duties outside of their normal duties. However, if they will be asked to perform tasks that are outside their job descriptions, staff will need to receive safety training in order to safely complete those tasks. Common concerns include proper procedures for traveling safely, working in unfamiliar areas, possible bodily injury from falls or other mechanical causes, and coping with biological, chemical, or nuclear contamination. Another training topic is how and when to use personal protective equipment.

Personal Protective Equipment

Personal protective equipment can be as simple as latex gloves or as complex as the use of an encapsulated suit. Training on how to properly and appropriately use personal protective equipment should be provided to all involved staff members. Specialized training and regulations exist for many personal protective items. These guidelines or requirements must be met. Certifications for use must be kept current. Developing and maintaining a training log is an excellent way to maintain appropriate certifications.

Public health departments should designate an emergency coordinator. This individual's duties include updating plans and specific contact information and serving as the liaison with other organizations in the emergency management community. An emergency coordinator often provides training for other health department personnel in the emergency operations center. The emergency coordinator often serves as the agency's public information officer.

THE PUBLIC INFORMATION OFFICER

A dedicated public information officer (PIO) is crucial when addressing an incident that has drawn or may draw media attention. A PIO often provides messages that are distributed to the general public through various information channels. The media appreciates having a single point of contact for information. This, too, is an appropriate role for the PIO. However, it is important to emphasize that the PIO does not have to be the designated spokesperson for an agency. In some cases, the PIO may only coordinate statements and spokespersons for the involved agencies. Make sure to review the amount of available time before designating the health officer or another high-ranking official as the PIO. During an emergency event, the health officer may not have the time or resources to lead the organization as well as provide a steady flow of information to the media. PIOs from organizations that comprise an emergency coalition should meet regularly to plan, prepare, and build relationships to properly communicate public health's message during a crisis. Additional information on communicating with the media can be found in Chapter 31.

Interacting with the Media

Many training courses that teach effective communications are available to PIOs. Dispensing information to the media at the proper time is an important skill. Training courses enable PIOs and other designated officials to perform their duties well. Members of the media will investigate to provide a story if one is not given to them.

Different elements of the media have the ability to reach large numbers of people quickly. These attributes are useful during a crisis. Members of the media are important allies during times of crisis as well as during normal periods. Where appropriate, members of the media should be included in training meetings and exercises. The goal is to embrace the media as stakeholders. If members of the media trust members of the crisis response team, they are more likely to be helpful and convey important information to members of the general public in a responsible and timely manner.

There are several important guidelines for working with the media. Major incidents may require joint press conferences with representatives from each of the agencies that are involved in the incident command system. This is especially true when joint decisions are being made under the unified command structure, a commonly used approach to managing emergencies. A joint information center may be designated as the central venue for ongoing information and risk communications. A PIO from the health department should be located at such a central facility. Whether the chief information officer is from the public health department will depend on the nature of the emergency and the structure of the unified command.

The Message

All requests from the media for information should be referred to the PIO. Once an official message has been formed by the unified command, no information should be conveyed to the media without the express permission of the PIO. Although conveying information to the public is a vital aspect of any emergency event, erroneous information can be disastrous. Radio and television reports help to spread information about topics such as evacuation, road conditions, and other relief efforts. This information must be disseminated in a responsible and accurate manner.

When a major incident occurs, people from media outlets from around the world may be present. It is important that media receive accurate and timely information from a source that can be controlled, such as the PIO. There may be a need to get written information to the public. This can be accomplished by distributing this material at public gathering places of such as shelters, town halls, schools, and disaster centers.

Relationships among public health, civic groups, and the media must be forged in advance (Levy and Sidel, 2002). All parties must expend care and effort. The PIO or his or her designee should monitor the media to ensure that the public is receiving correct messages. Trust established during training and preparation is an effective means to achieving this goal.

COLLABORATION AND COMMUNICATION

Collaboration and communication are complementary activities. Neither can be completed in an effective manner without the other. They are tools that facilitate the goals of building relationships and gathering resources.

Relationship Building

Developing relationships with other agencies is an important process that should occur before an incident takes place. By establishing both formal and informal relationships, the ability to provide and accept assistance during an incident is greatly simplified. Simply having coffee and speaking informally with other individuals from other agencies greatly moves the process forward. Writing a plan is important for a response during a disaster, but developing the plan enhances relationship building. The relationships will be invaluable during a crisis.

Resource Gathering

Simply knowing what resources are available from another agency is not sufficient. Other matters should be undertaken to ensure that those resources are available during a crisis. Only by inventorying the nature and availability of resources in a community will workers be able to determine what can be used during a particular incident. Once resources have been identified, it is wise to draft formal agreements regarding their use in an emergency. Two common vehicles for this purpose are a *memorandum of understanding* and a *mutual aid agreement*. By formalizing, in advance, contracts that ensure access to resources during an emergency, crisis workers will be in a good position to utilize these resources when the need arises.

Organizational leaders should always be looking for ways to offer or request resources. Active partners in planning, training, and drills are most likely to become responsible and prepared team members. Formal and informal interactions also provide alternative lines of communication that may be used during an actual incident. Clear, concise communications can only be expected when there is mutual respect and trust between organizations. By getting to know each other, the possibility of a jurisdictional dispute will be reduced. By knowing each other's terminology, codes, and procedures, all agencies stand to benefit. The most effective way to achieve this goal is to become a participant within the system.

THE PUBLIC HEALTH INCIDENT COMMAND SYSTEM

Not understanding policies and procedures during a crisis is a concern. A greater concern is when the organizations do not understand the flow of command and control during a crisis. This could have negative effects for public health during a disaster. The Incident Command System (ICS) system in use today provides coordination and control during public health emergencies. The ICS was developed as a consequence of fires that consumed large portions of wild land, including structures, in southern California in the 1970s. As a result of those fires, agencies saw the need to create a system that enabled them to work together toward a common goal in an effective and efficient manner. The ICS has undergone revisions over the years to improve efficiency. It is also referred to as the Incident Management System (IMS). Whether using the term ICS or IMS, the use of the system enables various types of incidents to be efficiently managed. The U.S. Department of Homeland Security is in the process of developing the National Incident Management System, or NIMS, to incorporate all levels of government response within the ICS.

The ICS/IMS is designed to initiate and maintain control of an incident from the time of onset until the incident is resolved. The *incident commander* or *incident manager* title can apply equally to a designated person or to the first person on the scene, depending upon the situation. The structure of the ICS/IMS can be established and expanded depending on the changing conditions of the incident. It is staffed and operated by qualified trained personnel from any designated department and may involve personnel from a variety of areas within the community.

The ICS/IMS is a comprehensive resource management system that ensures that resources are provided at the right time and at the right place. The ICS/IMS can be utilized for any type or size of emergency, ranging from a minor incident involving a single group of responders to a major emergency involving several agencies. The ICS/IMS ensures that systems and procedures are in place to rapidly obtain, stage, and utilize resources after an event has occurred. It enables agencies to communicate using common terminology and operating procedures. It also facilitates the timely combination of resources during an emergency. A similar system is used by the military (Maniscalco and Christen, 2002).

Common ICS Terminology

To function effectively, all personnel must use common terminology to communicate. This will ensure that all people from a variety of backgrounds will be saying and understanding the same concepts. For example, an agent is an employee in law enforcement while it transfers pathogens to a public health professional. Using simple and common terminology reduces confusion and the risk of mistakes. By having all parties involved in planning, the risk of communication mistakes will be greatly reduced.

Chain of Command

ICS/IMS is a top-down approach to management. If the incident commander or manager does not assign a duty to a subordinate, then the responsibility reverts to the commander. The system works best when the incident commander delegates responsibility and monitors progress. The individual serving as the incident commander (IC) must be a good leader and have a thorough knowledge of the incident as well as access to all needed resources.

Span of Control

It is important that there not be too many subordinates. In an emergency situation, a good rule of thumb is to have one person directly supervise three to seven individuals. When there are more or fewer subordinates, efficiency is greatly reduced and confusion can occur.

Division of Labor

It is unrealistic to expect one person to accomplish all of the tasks associated with an incident. Therefore, the work that must be accomplished should be divided up and delegated by the incident commander or manager. Not only is the responsibility delegated, but the authority to accomplish the required task is delegated as well. Delegating responsibility without providing resources is an invitation for failure.

The incident commander directs all aspects of the response and coordinates the efforts of subordinates. The commander must establish an Emergency Operations Center (EOC) or field Command Post (CP) and ensure that communications are established. Successful incident commanders quickly identify high-quality leaders and assign them to a section. Four section leaders are utilized in ICS: operations, logistics, planning, and finance. **Figure 26-2** depicts the ICS structure.

The *operations section leader* assumes control of actions directed toward directly resolving the situation. The operations leader often faces difficulties such as communication failures, personnel concerns, technical and infrastructure issues, and evaluation issues related to the incident (Levy and Sidel, 2002).

The *logistics section leader* ensures that supplies and personnel are available for the operations section. Without resources, the operations section is highly ineffective, and the incident will not be successfully mit-

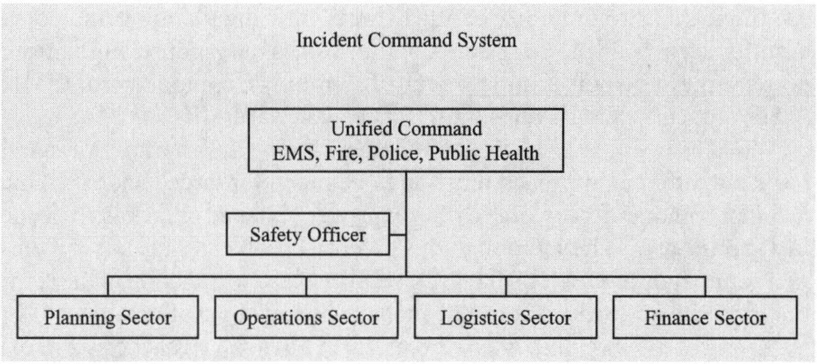

Figure 26-2 ICS Structure
Source: J. MacNeal (2003).

igated. An important issue facing logistics is long-term sustainability. The response to the World Trade Center attacks continued for months. Logistics may also have to provide for the emergency replacement of resources such as phone equipment. During the response to the September 11 attacks, the New York City Department of Health lost its phone service. The city's emergency response system had to relocate its operations to another building because it was located within four blocks of Ground Zero. This had been identified as an alternative in advance in the operations plan. Prudent planning includes continuity of operations and assuming that the primary facility may not be available.

The *planning section leader* develops a guide for the operations section to implement. This must be done in collaboration with other agencies and relevant experts. No single person can formulate a successful plan. The planning section leader may also use various computer resources.

The *finance section leader* should be proficient in fiscal principles. Even a small-scale response can be quite confusing when trying to establish the cost of resources from various agencies. The finance section leader is responsible for tracking personnel hours and supply expenses. This tracking is not only important for calculating overtime pay, but also for an occupational exposure assessments that may not be conducted for years after the event. Accurate record keeping is very important, because FEMA may reimburse many of the incident-related expenditures.

Command

The Integrated Emergency Management System (IEMS) is a conceptual framework that serves community-wide interests through an all-hazards approach. By using resources from federal, state, and local governments and private industry, IEMS works to maximize the allocation of resources. The goal of IEMS is to provide an overall system for agencies and individuals to render the highest possible level of service during times of crisis. IEMS seeks to minimize conflict by maximizing planning and coordination efforts. IEMS addresses the four stages of response: mitigation, preparedness, response, and recovery. ICS is only a component of IEMS. ICS is tactical while IEMS is more strategic in nature.

Whereas a single incident commander may be appropriate for small events, a different approach must often be taken for large incidents. One incident commander can quickly become overwhelmed or lack knowledge in a specific area. The solution to this potential problem is the use of a unified command structure. By having several key leaders function in the command role, a large incident can be managed in an efficient manner.

A *unified command structure* exists when all involved agencies and organizations are represented in the top tier of a local command structure. This is compatible with both ICS and NIMS. A unified command post will include the key leaders of emergency medical services, the fire department, law enforcement, and public health. With this type of structure, duplication of effort and opportunities for miscommunication are greatly reduced.

Consolidated incident action plans must use the objectives and working plans of all involved agencies. Integrating all organizations into the incident action plan and command structure ensures that all relevant issues are addressed. Often, this teamwork approach can safely mitigate incidents that would be impossible for a single agency to manage. A well-established communications infrastructure is critical to the success of a unified command structure. All agencies should be able to rapidly communicate with each other to report safety concerns or difficulties encountered when implementing tactics.

A functional unified command structure does not come into existence by accident. Deliberate actions are required to establish a working team that uses personnel from different agencies. Personal agendas must be set aside. Agencies must decide how the capabilities of various organizations will be coordinated and utilized. A successful unified command structure must be carefully planned and rehearsed before an incident. Begin by assessing what resources, personnel, and equipment each agency or organization can provide. Determine how normal agency activities will be conducted during an incident. Each agency will maintain its own identity, administration, and policies, but the agency must be able to coordinate within the overall command-and-control network.

Training is part of the process of development that advances and maintains individuals with an organization (Shafritz et al., 2001). To attain and maintain proficiency, regular practice sessions that utilize the incident command structure must be conducted. A local incident command structure may only be called upon once in the lifetime of public health professionals, but they must be ready. Training resources for ICS are widely available.

Historically, public health has accomplished much with limited resources. This record has been accomplished by using a systematic approach and relying on the relentless efforts of many public health practitioners. Public health practitioners must realize that a systematic approach to problem solving becomes even more important during nonroutine or emergency response operations. Some of these potential operations include county fair inspections, flu clinics, or presentations for the public.

COMMUNICATION DEVICES AND BACK-UP PLANS

Maintaining reliable and continuous communications during a crisis is a significant challenge. Planning for the use of several types of communication devices, establishing clear communication procedures in advance, and providing proper training to professionals and volunteers alike, also in advance, increases the potential for the effective transfer of vital information during an event. Each system or device has advantages and disadvantages that depend on the details of a particular incident.

Regular Telephone System (Landlines)

Traditionally, the regular telephone system has served as the main method of communication during small or medium incidents. To supplement the regular number of telephone lines, each city, town, or agency should have a bank of additional phone numbers established in advance and held in reserve for specific and immediate use during a crisis. Some numbers may be allocated to specific agencies or divisions in advance and prewired into emergency operations centers or into other facilities that are designated to become an emergency operation center in the event of an incident. The advantages of such an approach include ease of use and that the actual numbers can be published in crisis manuals in advance. Disadvantages include costs and the failure of the system due to power outages, destruction of the telephone line, or caller overload.

Cellular Telephones

With the prevalence of cellular telephones, cellular phone communications may serve well for an initial period. It may also fail partially or completely due to cell site failure or user overload. Cellular telephones are not completely separate from landlines. A portion of each cell phone connection is subject to transmission through landlines. Planners should discuss local network conditions with cellular service providers to see what safeguards can be included to assist in keeping emergency telephones in operation. Cellular telephone service is much less secure than landlines. During the response to the anthrax scare, members of the media eavesdropped on public health conversations that were conducted over cellular telephones.

Radio Communications

Government, business, military, utility, and public service agencies and ham radio operators have wireless communication capabilities on specific frequencies or bands (frequency ranges) of the radio wave spectrum.

Switching to radio for many communications during a disaster can free up telephone phone lines that can then be used by people in peril. However, scanners can be used to listen to radio transmissions. This is one disadvantage of radio. Another limitation is that communication operators must have radios appropriate for the particular band or frequency they are using as well as the authorization or a license to transmit. Ham radio operators are subject to these restrictions.

Computer-Based Communications

High-speed wireless radio communication capabilities are now available via computers during disasters. With the proliferation of personal computers, the use of e-mail and the Internet have become common, convenient, and effective means of communication. However, during a disaster, e-mail capabilities and Internet access may be seriously interrupted. Downed telephone, power, and cable lines or damage to central telephone facilities will eliminate access to e-mail and the Internet. However, provided with a portable generator, a radio communicator can utilize all modes of communication via computer, except voice. For this reason, some emergency operation centers have installed satellite-based Internet facilities backed up by generators for emergency power.

Automatic Packet-reporting System

Automatic packet reporting is a relatively new computer application that enables a radio to track events as they occur and graphically display information, such as object locations and their movements, on computer-generated maps. This information is used to locate or track police and fire vehicles and to monitor searchers. Data can be transmitted to all screens in a network, providing participants with continuously updated information. Many police and fire agencies are now installing such devices in their vehicles for ordinary and disaster situations.

Emergency Communications

Despite advances in radio communications via computer, voice communications via radio provide the fastest way to transmit and exchange critical information. Considering the vulnerability of landlines and cellular telephones, voice radio communications via ham radio continue to provide an established and reliable method for emergency communications. Since 1913, ham radio operators have provided emergency communications for large and small disasters until normal communications are restored. Ham radio operators who are members of local Amateur Radio Emergency Services and Radio Amateur Civil Emergency Services groups are trained emergency radio operators who can handle emergency communications. The operators can be coordinated in command posts, in emergency operations centers, or in the field. Ham radio operators can provide primary or backup communications. Emergency communications supersede all other radio communications and are prioritized to facilitate the proper passing of messages. Ham radio operators traditionally provide communications services for staff and displaced persons in emergency shelters set up during major incidents.

The Amateur Radio Emergency Service organization consists of licensed amateurs who have voluntarily registered their qualifications and equipment for communication duty when disasters arise and who have a sincere desire to serve. These volunteer communicators do not provide other services; they do not enforce laws or make major decisions. The Radio Amateur Civil Emergency Services organization also consists of licensed amateurs who have officially enrolled (with a background check) in a local organization to serve as radio communicators for civil-preparedness purposes during times of local, regional, or national civil emergencies, including war-related activities and natural disasters such as floods, fires, and earthquakes. All disaster responders maintain their gear and supplies in response-ready condition and are prepared to be self-sustaining for at least 72 hours.

Runners are an excellent use for official and spontaneous volunteers lacking specific expertise for the situation at hand. These people may assist experienced responders in a variety of capacities, from carrying physical messages to delivering equipment to assisting in the procurement of supplies, food, and water.

Local Emergency Radio

Many local fire districts, public safety organizations, and law enforcement agencies put out messages to the public. These communications pertain to emergencies, weather warnings, traffic conditions, and public safety. The most common location for such broadcasts is 530 on the AM radio band. The government supports the Emergency Alert System (EAS) and NOAA Weather Radio, which broadcast warnings and other information during emergencies.

Pocket Guides, Pamphlets, Emergency Resource Booklets

Many communities, local public health departments, and the Red Cross have published guides to help citizens be better prepared for and more self-sufficient during disasters. These excellent and convenient guides cover supplies, the amount and type of food and water to have on hand, first aid supplies and procedures, lists of medical centers, instructions on sheltering, and information on emergency radio stations and public and safety telephone numbers. They also provide specific instructions for major emergencies such as earthquakes, floods, and tornadoes and radiological, chemical, or biological occurrences. Terminology warning of impending weather conditions has been standardized. The term *watch* is used when a flood, fire, snowstorm, hurricane, or other adverse weather event is expected within 72 hours. The term *warning* denotes that adverse conditions are expected within 24 hours. *Alert* is used when conditions actually exist. Telephone books have emergency information, especially in areas surrounding nuclear power facilities and in areas of the country prone to earthquake and hurricanes.

CONCLUSION

The planning steps discussed in this chapter can be summarized. The initial step is to identify stakeholders in the community who can respond to an emergency. Stakeholders include traditional emergency service responders; health care providers; government agencies; support groups, such as the Red Cross; and community organizations, such as service and youth groups. By meeting with leaders of the stakeholder organizations well in advance, the various power bases and personalities that influence decision-making processes will be better understood. Schedule monthly disaster preparation meetings that include time for networking.

Conduct an assessment of community threats and existing resources. Evaluate the vulnerabilities a community may have, identify the threats that potentially exist, and inventory high-hazard facilities or populations. Gather input from all stakeholders whenever possible. Use information from the threat assessment to develop workable plans for responding to these situations. Note existing services that are available from the stakeholders and formalize access to them in writing. Once a formal plan is drafted, convene a formal review process with all stakeholders. Use of a formal system for reviewing and commenting on proposed plans will ease the revision process. Set deadlines for revisions to ensure that a plan is forthcoming. Conduct tabletop exercises with the completed plan. Practice using the plan with several different scenarios to validate the plan's effectiveness. Once the involved parties approve a plan, the process of educating the specific individuals who will respond should begin. These individuals don't necessarily need to know every portion of the plan, but they should know how their agency fits into the plan and what their role will be in an emergency. Once education about the plan has occurred, stage drills and evaluate how the plan works in the field.

The frontiersman quoted at the beginning of this chapter was Abraham Lincoln. He was an outstanding communicator who effectively managed the affairs of this country during a time of national crisis. Much can be gained from his type of thinking when considering disaster preparedness. Lincoln advocated spending far more time preparing rather than executing plans. Preparation also included considering unlikely as well as likely outcomes.

Returning to the unexpected loss of power, reaction plans were already in place. The building was secured to ensure the safety of both employees and members of the general public. Dedicated (with fully charged batteries) cellular telephones were used to share information with agency managers and staff as well as with outside contacts. The recipients of emergency information had been prearranged. Using these communication resources, officials were able to estimate the extent of the damage. Prearranged contacts with members of the media were included in the early information dissemination. The health department had a dedicated line to provide constant contact with representatives of the Metro Medical Response System and other local emergency officials.

Health department personnel were deployed based on the plan. Persons from the department went to the city's Emergency Operations Center to discuss developments and responses to the evolving situation. At the health department, stored vaccines were kept cold through the use of a portable generator. The generator at a secondary site had greater capacity. When officials realized that the outage would likely last for more than four hours, the vaccines were transported to the secondary site for storage. Other tasks began as a consequence of the expected duration of the outage. The emergency plan directed the health department to issue a press release on food safety and the well-being of the general public. Advice related to drinking water and sewage disposal was included to allay fears and enable members of the media to concentrate on other aspects of the emergency. The outage lasted for 17 hours. Because plans and procedures were in place and contacts had been arranged prior to the event, public health concerns were addressed with a minimum of disruption to the safety of the citizens. Adequate prior planning facilitated the rapid, timely, and coordinated responses of all emergency personnel.

References

Federal Emergency Management Agency. 2003. Available at www.fema.gov/pdf/rrr/frp/frp2003.pdf.

Landesman, L.Y. 2001. *Public Health Management of Disasters: The Practice Guide*. Washington, D.C.: American Public Health Association.

Levy, B.S., and Sidel V.W. 2002. *Terrorism and Public Health: A Balanced Approach to Strengthening Systems and Protecting People*. New York: Oxford.

Maniscalco, P., and Christen, H.T. 2002. *Understanding Terrorism and Managing the Consequences*. Upper Saddle River, NJ: Pearson Education.

Presidential Decision Directive 39, June 21, 1995. Available at www.fas.org/irp/offdocs/pdd39.htm.

Shafritz, J.M., Rosenbloom, D.H., Hyde, A.C., Riccucci, N.M., and Naff, K.C. 2001. *Personnel Management in Government: Politics and Process*, 5th ed. New York: Marcel Dekker.

Resources

Periodicals

Boscarino, J.A., Figley, C.R., and Adams, R.E. 2003. Fear of terrorism in New York after the September 11 terrorist attacks: Implications for emergency mental health and preparedness. *International Journal of Emergency Mental Health* 5(4):199–209.

Chi, C.H., Chao, W.H., Chuang, C.C., Tsai, M.C., and Tsai, L.M. 2001. Emergency medical technicians' disaster training by tabletop exercise. *American Journal of Emergency Medicine* 19(5):433–436.

Fong, T. 2003. Preparing for a disaster. Healthcare providers try to ready themselves for biological, chemical attacks without the benefit of government funding. *Modern Healthcare* 33(36):6–16.

Hodge, J.G. 2003. Protecting the public's health in an era of bioterrorism: The Model State Emergency Health Powers Act. *Accountability in Research* 10(2):91–107.

Jacobs, L.M., Burns, K.J., and Gross, R.I. 2003. Terrorism: A public health threat with a trauma system response. *Journal of Trauma* 55(6):1014–1021.

Knouss, R.F. 2001. National disaster medical system. *Public Health Reports* 116 (Suppl 2):49–52.

Levi, L., and Bregman, D. 2003. Simulation and management games for training command and control in emergencies. *Studies in Health Technology and Informatics* 95:783–787.

Olesker, S. 2002. Disaster preparedness: A multichannel platform is critical to a reliable emergency medical communication system. *Healthcare Informatics* 19(7):46–49.

Rollins, G. 2003. Preparedness: Disaster on-call. *Hospitals and Health Networks* 77(12):24–26.

Sharan, R.N. 2003. Preparedness to respond to possible acts of nuclear terrorism: Some strategies and recommendations. *International Journal of Radiation Biology* 79(3):217–219.

Turnock, B.J. 2003. Roadmap for public health workforce preparedness. *Journal of Public Health Management and Practice* 9(6):471–480.

Books

Amateur Radio Relay League. 2000. *ARES/RACES Emergency Communications Manual.* Newington, CT: Amateur Radio Relay League.

Byrnes, M.E., King, D.A., and Tierno, P.M. 2003. *Nuclear, Chemical, and Biological Terrorism: Emergency Response and Public Protection.* Boca Raton, FL: CRC Press.

Buck, G., Stilp, R., Bevelacqua, A., and Hawley, C. 2001. *Terrorism Handbook for Operational Responders.* Stamford, CT: Thomson Learning.

Haddow, G., and Bullock, J. 2003. *Introduction to Emergency Management.* Boston: Butterworth-Heinemann.

Henderson, D.A., Inglesby, T.V., and O'Toole, T. 2002. *Bioterrorism: Guidelines for Medical and Public Health Management.* Chicago: American Medical Association.

Novick, L.F., and Marr, J.S. 2003. *Public Health Issues Disaster Preparedness: Focus on Bioterrorism*. Sudbury, MA: Jones & Bartlett.

Web Sites

- Centers for Disease Control and Prevention (Training):
  www.cdc.gov/epo/training.htm
- Centers for Disease Control and Prevention Public Health Emergency Preparedness and Response Site:
  www.bt.cdc.gov
- Centers for Public Health Preparedness (Centers for Disease Control and Prevention):
  www.phppo.cdc.gov/owpp/CPHPLocations.asp
- Federal Emergency Management Agency:
  www.fema.gov/onp/ncb.shtm or training.fema.gov
- Homeland Security Presidential Decision Directive 5 (HSPD5):
  www.whitehouse.gov/news/releases/2003/02/20030228-9.html
- Incident Command System (Web-based training):
  www.wildlandfire.net
- National Response Plan:
  www.nemaweb.org/docs/national_response_plan.pdf
- Office of Justice Programs, Office of Domestic Preparedness:
  www.ojp.usdoj.gov/odp
- Oklahoma City National Memorial Institute for the Prevention of Terrorism:
  www.mipt.org
- Terrorism Aftermath Planning (United States Department of Justice):
  www.usdoj.gov/ag/terrorismaftermath.html
- U.S. Policy on Counterterrorism (Presidential Decision Directive 39):
  www.ojp.usdoj.gov/odp/docs/pdd39.htm

Organizations

Amateur Radio Relay League
225 Main Street
Newington, CT, 06111-1494
Phone: 860-594-0200
Fax: 860-594-0259
E-mail: hq@arrl.org
Web site: www.arrl.org

Centers for Disease Control and Prevention
1600 Clifton Road
Atlanta, GA 30333
Phone: 404-639-3311 or 404-639-3534 or 800-311-3435
E-mail: www.cdc.gov/netinfo.htm (Web form)
Web site: www.cdc.gov

Dekalb County Board of Health
Dekalb-Fulton Bioterrorism Response Plan
Center for Public Health Preparedness
445 Winn Way
Decatur, GA 30031
Phone: 404-294-3700
Web site: www.dekalbhealth.net

Federal Emergency Management Agency
500 C Street, SW
Washington, D.C. 20472
Phone: 202- 566-1600
Web site: www.fema.gov

CHAPTER

27

Integrated Crisis Preparedness

Ronald Burger
L. Fleming Fallon, Jr.
Jay MacNeal
Eric Zgodzinski

Chapter Objectives

After reading this chapter, readers will:

- Understand integrated crisis preparedness.
- Involve hospital personnel in crisis planning.
- Understand how to educate members of the general public on appropriate crisis responses.
- Appreciate the importance of handling mental health issues during a crisis.
- Know how to assemble immunization and drug prophylaxis programs.
- Know how to recruit and train volunteers.

Chapter Summary

Integrated crisis preparedness requires input and cooperation from a variety of personnel and stakeholders. Hospitals will be involved in most crisis responses, and demands for service will often exceed capacity in the event of a disaster. Alternative capacity must be secured, prepared, and staffed. Members of the general public must be educated on how to appropriately respond to an emergency. In the event of a threatened or actual bioterrorism attack, drug prophylaxis or immunizations may be required for large segments of the population. Mental health concerns and problems are likely to emerge during a crisis and remain after it has been resolved. Volunteers will be used to staff many health care positions. Recruiting, training, evaluating, and recognizing volunteers are important considerations.

Case Study

After a long flight from the Asia, passengers disembarked into a cool autumn afternoon in Midwestern America. Several of the passengers felt slightly tired, but all agreed that nothing would stop them from attending the local high school football games they had looked forward to all week during their conference overseas. As the evening approached, several of the passengers started to feel somewhat nauseous, but discounted the feelings as symptoms of jet lag. One by one, the passengers headed to their homes due to illness while others attended football games. By the next morning, several had been transported to local hospitals; others were severely sick and stayed in bed at home. Doctors at the various hospitals diagnosed many of the passengers as having influenza, whereas others were treated for possible food-borne illnesses. However, no tests were ordered, and there was no suspicion that the cases were related to a single source or exposure.

Two days later, several students and their family members had become ill. Some emergency response personnel also became sick. One physician with training in epidemiology questioned the apparent coincidence of three patients, two students who had been traveling abroad and an emergency room nurse, all having similar complaints. Suspecting a connection, the doctor made telephone calls to hospitals in the area. Other travelers and three hospital employees had the same constellation of symptoms. The physician notified the local health department.

Staff at the health department were briefed on the situation. They required several resources, but had trouble reaching the individuals who controlled supplies. The local health department wanted to implement its response plan, which required assistance from law enforcement and the state health department. No one could authorize the action. In addition, information was needed from each of the schools attended by the students.

Could any aspects of this scenario have benefited from an integrated approach to crisis preparedness? Can you identify any problems in the handling of the case?

INTRODUCTION

How and why disaster preparedness plans should be created was discussed in Chapter 26. The next task is to integrate planning and responses with agencies throughout the community. This enables organizations to know how they can assist each other and evaluate their joint plans and responses. Integrated crisis preparedness is the concept of building relationships and collaboration among multiple agencies before a crisis actually occurs.

HOSPITAL INVOLVEMENT

Information from hospitals can be extremely important during an incident. Information obtained from hospitals can dictate evacuation, containment, quarantine, treatment, and other response decisions for the community. Access to this information should be a formal part of any emergency plan. Informal and formal meetings with hospital staff can help to develop the relationships that are needed to collect and convey information. Hospitals are an integral part of the public health system in both times of crisis and when dealing with everyday concerns. Ongoing relationships between health department employees and leaders and hospital personnel will be very valuable during a disaster.

When disaster strikes, many people will go to a hospital because of the care it can provide and because it offers a feeling of safety. People assume that in any event, hospitals will have the antidote. Hospital may also be the conceptual ground zero of an outbreak. Individuals from the public will go there to seek treatment, accompanied by members of the media seeking stories. This provides a means to not only determine the cause of the health threat, but also a way to reach the masses through the media. Understanding the health threat may not always be as simple as asking questions or examining individuals. To improve their ability to define a possible threat to the health of the public, hospitals must share health information with their public health partners.

To protect the community and reduce the risk of further spread of disease, some type of early warning system should be developed that uses the information shared by hospitals and other venues. The area hospital should be part of any local surveillance system. The warning system should be established and tested prior to a disaster to determine the accuracy of data and the extent of injuries and illnesses that are used in the test situation. Surveillance systems are discussed in Chapter 29.

Just as an Incident Command System (ICS) is helpful when managing an incident, hospitals have their own type of management system. Public health planners and officials should understand the management system used by area hospitals. The most commonly used system is called the Hospital Emergency Incident Command System (San Mateo County, 2004). It was developed as a means for hospitals to respond to mass casualty incidents such as earthquakes. Much of the guidance for the Hospital Emergency Incident Command System comes from the California Earthquake Preparedness Guidelines (California Office of Emergency

Services, 1987). The basic principles of the Hospital Emergency Incident Command System are similar to those of the ICS system. Both are responsibility oriented, have common mission and terminology, are widely applicable, enable rapid resource transfer within and between facilities, have implementation flexibility for individual sections and branches, and impose minimal disruption to existing departments (Maniscalco, 2002). Using both the Hospital Emergency Incident Command System and the ICS facilitates information exchange and makes it easier for public health and hospitals to coordinate resources.

POPULATION EDUCATION

Education is a major component of the public health system. It must be included in integrated preparedness plans. Education for an incident caused by weapons of mass destruction should include basic definitions, precautions that should be taken, what to expect during an attack, and how to react after an attack. Preparedness education should be provided prior to a disaster.

Before an event, time and resources are available for education and preparation. Much of the groundwork for this type of education has already been established. The Centers for Disease Control and Prevention, the Red Cross, FEMA, and other agencies have developed fact sheets, procedures, and other information that can assist local health departments in delivering messages to the general public. Developing the message is difficult. Identifying delivery mechanisms and transmitting the message may be more problematic. Various methods, approaches, and information are needed for different communities or population subgroups. In the event of a radiation or chemical incident, the public may be advised to shelter in place.

For example, a rural department of health is unlikely to address the need for prophylaxis of 1 million individuals. Disaster preparations in Buffalo, New York, are unlikely to include hurricane preparedness. Conversely, similar preparations for Miami, Florida, do not include information on snow removal. Conduits for information exchange between a public health agency and the constituents it serves may include print, radio, television, billboards, Web sites, or town hall meetings. Any or all of these may be appropriate for a given agency and population. The utility of any specific method often changes as a disaster progresses. For example, billboards are inappropriate for providing immediate notification during a disaster. However, this is not the case before an event. A trained public information officer is a necessity. The role of a public information officer in organizing and transmitting messages was discussed in Chapter 26.

What is the message? When educating the public about a potential crisis event, simultaneous messages may be required. For example, during a crisis the message may be how to obtain safe water and food or how to properly board up a building. It may be that a current snowstorm is so severe as to limit travel on roadways to emergency vehicles. Responses to a biological agent may require informing the public how and where to report for vaccinations or immunizations or antibiotics to prevent or treat an infectious disease. A more challenging message to deliver is how to manage disaster-related fatalities.

Combating an infectious disease, such as smallpox, during a crisis event may include sheltering in place. This may be voluntary or through a quarantine or isolation function. Sheltering in place or quarantine was routinely practiced years ago in cities throughout the United States. It was used to control measles and other infectious diseases such as whooping cough (pertussis) and scarlet fever. Planning should include how, when, and where sheltering in place should occur. The use of this type of procedure may be required when hospitals or other places of care are filled to capacity. Under those conditions, the only way to control the spread of disease is to persuade individuals to stay at home or within designated shelters. This process will accomplish three objectives. (1) It will keep individuals who are contagious within a controlled area so the risk of infection to others is limited. (2) Uninfected individuals who are sheltered have a reduced probability of becoming infected. This protection is shared by others staying within their homes. (3) One of the main reasons for protecting a hospital is to prevent contamination of the facility.

To properly shelter in place, homes must be prepared. Food, water, and entertainment are needed to sustain the home's inhabitants for at least three days. A detailed list of supplies for preparing for a disaster can be found on the FEMA Web site (www.fema.gov/areyouready).

Successfully sending messages related to emergencies requires a team effort. Partnering prior to any event, practicing responses, and evaluating procedures are all extremely important when trying to protect the public's health as well as prevent panic and mental anguish.

■ MENTAL HEALTH

Mental health or stress management is important for both the public and staff who respond to a crisis. Local affiliates of national agencies for mental health are often available. Stress and mental health concerns accompany all disaster situations. Experienced planners remember that all members of a community, including rescue workers *and* members of the public, are affected.

Most local communities have boards of mental health that can take an active role in helping with education and responses to a crisis. In Toledo, Ohio, the Lucas County Board of Mental Health is currently planning for a variety of responses. The board has developed educational sessions on how local health department employees can handle stress during a time of crisis. In addition, they have contributed to pamphlets and protocols that can be utilized by both the general public and public health staff during a crisis. Finally, the group is developing extensive lists of mental health volunteers to respond during a crisis, such as the Red Cross Mental Health Disaster Action Teams.

SHELTER AND PROPHYLAXIS SITES

Staffing is a major concern for shelters that simply provide temporary housing for individuals and families. However, sites that will dispense antibiotics or immunizations are likely to require greater numbers of staff. The first site need is to provide shelter for the public. If in-place shelter is deemed necessary, it is fairly easy for members of the general public to house themselves in their own homes. However, this is only a viable option if the house is properly stocked with food and water and prepared prior to a disaster.

Local public health agencies often have concerns about sanitation, food safety, and the general well-being of shelter residents that must be addressed. Members of local government, not the American Red Cross, most often choose the locations for emergency shelters. However, the responsibility to manage and staff the shelter is often delegated to the Red Cross. The Red Cross may be the only provider of first aid in a particular neighborhood. Public health volunteers may be assigned to assist nurses and other personnel in the shelter.

Surveillance is an important aspect of shelters. Diseases and injuries that occur in shelters must be reported. Remember that under most circumstances, people with special needs cannot be easily accommodated or cared for in emergency shelters. Generally, local or state public health agencies have that responsibility. Pets are not accepted in shelters. Work with local animal control or humane society officials to arrange for the sheltering and care of family pets prior to any crisis.

Choosing the proper site for an emergency shelter is important. It should have ample space for sleeping, activities, food preparation, and, most importantly, adequate sanitary facilities. In many locations, local governmental planners have evaluated emergency shelters. Public health must ensure that the sites are environmentally safe. This includes properly disposing of all types of waste, maintaining cleanliness in the facility, and ensuring that safe food and water are provided for the occupants. Shelters must have the resources to continue operations for a sustained period of time.

Locations that will dispense drugs for treatment or prophylaxis or immunizations must also be designated. Dispensing sites must provide space for waiting, dispensing pharmaceuticals, and performing administrative duties. Such sites must have refrigeration facilities for pharmaceutical storage. A recognizable building such as a school, church, recreation center, or other public building is often a good location for a dispensing site.

Dispensing sites should have the capacity to store, prepare, and serve food for staff. It should have ample parking for the public entering the building, restrooms, and multiple rooms for educating the public on medications or procedures. Dispensing sites should be usable for both antibiotic dispensing as well as mass immunizations. Staff members must be flexible and trained to undertake both missions.

VOLUNTEERS

There are not sufficient numbers of professionals to adequately manage a crisis. Trained volunteer assistance is preferred rather than relying on random offers of help in times of crisis. Volunteers must be identified, organized, trained, credentialed, engaged, and evaluated.

Identifying Volunteers

Volunteers must be ready for a disaster or crisis. Volunteers should be identified, trained, and assigned in advance. Public health volunteers will have a range of skills, from individuals with little or no training to highly trained physicians and nurses with extensive experience. Medically trained professionals are relatively easy to identify. These will include physicians, nurses, veterinarians, and other medical professionals. However, these people will be in tight supply during a crisis. Other people, such as clerks, runners, and managers, will be needed to staff clinics and perform other support duties. One potential source for individuals with these skills is local government.

Developing, organizing, training, exercising, and evaluating a pool of volunteers from the community in advance of a disaster reduces confusion over and misuse of people's skills and decreases liability exposure during an event. Sources of potential volunteers include members of neighborhood emergency response teams, local emergency preparedness groups, ham radio operators, public service-oriented organizations, the Red Cross, the Salvation Army, Boy Scout and Girl Scout troops, high school students and teachers, employees from hospitals and medical centers, members of professional associations, paramedics, and personnel from search and rescue teams. Local government officials and employees should not be overlooked. In a crisis, many government departments will not be operational or will not be operating at full capacity. Many of these employees have valuable and useful skills. Community emergency response teams and the local branch of the Medical Response Corps should be included when planning for a disaster.

Organization

Public health professionals cannot complete the disaster preparedness process alone. The Red Cross is a particularly useful ally. One mission of the Red Cross is to train volunteers, equipping them with emergency survival skills. A local Red Cross chapter may have teachers who can assist in training volunteers. Because of liability issues, the Red Cross cannot provide supervision during an emergency.

Documentation and verification of volunteer and professional training is essential. Personal information, skills, and experience should be included in a database. Maintaining the confidentiality of a volunteer database and deciding who will have access to the information are serious issues. Appropriate volunteer coordinators must be identified and cleared in advance.

Implementation

Implementation of a disaster preparedness plan can be daunting and time-consuming. Full preparation includes selection, training, evaluation, and assignment of volunteers to staff clinics or medical responses associated with the Strategic National Stockpile.

Emergency preparedness plans should include at least two methods of calling or notifying previously identified volunteers for duty. It is important that this list be shared with emergency medical assistance and other agencies that may need to call upon individuals if the main organizing agency is overwhelmed or unable to respond.

Some communities have created a computerized mobilization system. When agencies are activated and their staffing needs are known, volunteers should be put on standby or told to report for duty. Scheduling and assigning primary, secondary, and tertiary responders should proceed according to a prearranged plan. This ensures the effective use of volunteer skills and expertise and provides a steady supply of well-qualified volunteers throughout the duration of the event. It is essential to rotate volunteer responders during the event to avoid physical and mental fatigue. Remember that volunteers must be fed and housed during practice drills and emergency events.

Credentialing

One of the most difficult aspects of using volunteers is the initial credentialing and continuing education. For many positions that must be staffed during a crisis, simple questions and basic background checks are sufficient. Professionals are credentialed as a condition of continued employment. Emergency agencies should keep copies of annual registrations or licenses. Data may be required from multiple agencies and organizations.

Volunteers should be issued special identification cards to be used during emergency drills or operations. Several examples of such cards are currently available. Some cards are quite simple; such cards have a photograph and the person's name and other pertinent information. Some identification cards have a bar code. Others features a magnetic strip that contains encoded information. Cards can also have computer chips on them to store data. Cards having magnetic strips or computer chips are easy to use and can contain much information. However, the electromagnetic pulse of a nuclear explosion may alter the encoded data, a possible limitation on the utility of those identification cards containing magnetic strips or computer chips.

Maintaining Interest

An ongoing concern of any program that relies on volunteers for assistance is sustaining their interest over relatively long periods of time. Periodic practice sessions or simulations can help to dispel complacency and maintain interest in the goals, objectives, and operations of a program. Tabletop exercises provide excellent training opportunities and incentives for volunteers to learn more and better develop their skills. They also enable volunteers to interact with the people with whom they will be working during disasters. Allowed to practice their skills, volunteers will be more likely to continue their service to a program. The cost of tabletop and other exercises includes direct expenditures for supplies, but it reduces recruitment expenses for replacement volunteers.

Newsletters can be used to help maintain interest. Successful newsletters include information about current events and program updates. Providing regularly scheduled forums for speakers and management reviews of past training exercises and lessons learned from them are useful ways to maintain volunteer interest.

Evaluation

Integration of volunteer teams means that volunteers must be properly educated about performing their jobs as well as learning to work with other emergency workers. To accomplish this goal, volunteers must have joint training sessions. Their exercises must be evaluated based on response time, performance, and overall execution of the exercises as individuals and as teams. The performance of the health department and its activities must also be evaluated. Exercise and evaluation protocols are available from a number of sources, such as federal and state emergency management agencies.

All volunteers should be categorized in advance based on their areas of expertise, personal and professional interests, training status, certifications, and experience level. Each volunteer's skills and experience should be periodically reviewed. Every volunteer should have a working knowledge of the Incident Command System. All must be thoroughly familiar with the terminology used. Procedures for processing and using spontaneous volunteers must be in place. Unexpected volunteers must be evaluated on the spot and quickly utilized. Integrating all agencies and volunteers in an exercise will test the overall ability to react, mobilize, use and coordinate volunteers. It also ensures that volunteer participation will be successfully managed.

FEDERAL THREAT LEVELS

Federal directives and agencies may guide local disaster response efforts. The Department of Homeland Security (DHS) has developed a color-coded system to inform the public of current relative risk levels for terrorist attacks. The colors have actions associated with them. Additional details can be found at the DHS Web site at www.dhs.gov/dhspublic/index.jsp (Department of Homeland Security, 2004). The color-coded system is shown in **Figure 27-1**. Each condition is described in the following list:

- **Low Condition (Green)**. This condition is declared when there is a low risk of terrorist attacks.
- **Guarded Condition (Blue)**. This condition is declared when there is a general risk of terrorist attacks.
- **Elevated Condition (Yellow)**. This condition is declared when there is a significant risk of terrorist attacks.
- **High Condition (Orange)**. This condition is declared when there is a high risk of terrorist attacks.
- **Severe Condition (Red)**. This condition reflects a severe risk of terrorist attacks.

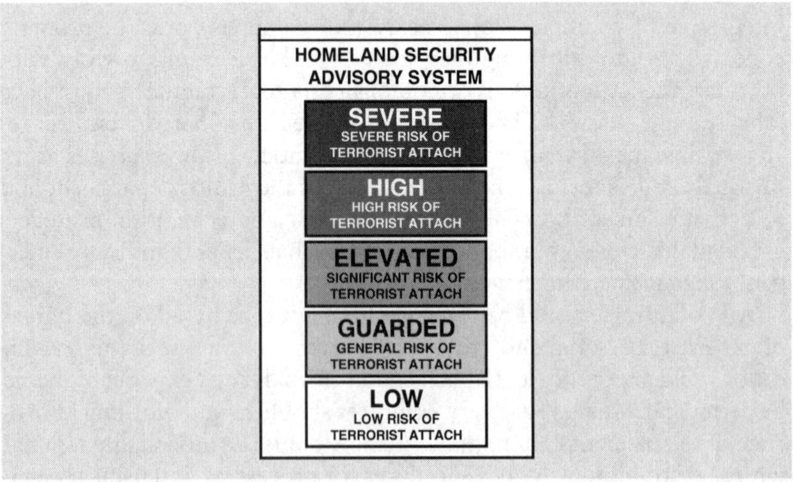

Figure 27-1 Federal Threat Levels

Source: U.S. Department of Homeland Security.

Local agencies and organizations should determine what these threat levels mean for them. Their emergency plans should delineate measures to be taken when specific threat levels are issued by the DHS. The American Red Cross provides recommendations for appropriate individual reactions in homes, schools, and workplaces based on each threat level (American Red Cross, 2004).

Soft targets include large groups of people, such as those attending a sporting event or concert. *Hard targets* include buildings, infrastructure components, and other objects or structures. An inventory of soft and hard targets in a locality should be created during initial planning meetings. The inventory should be periodically reviewed and amended. Planners must communicate with local officials and leaders to determine how their communities will react to the threat levels established by the federal government.

GEOGRAPHIC INFORMATION SYSTEMS

A Geographic Information System (GIS) is a computer-based system that combines layers of information about specific locations, thus enhancing understanding of a particular site. Specifically, GIS uses computer software, hardware, information, and personnel to manipulate, analyze, and present data that are linked to a spatial location.

GIS is a useful tool for preplanning as well as evaluating a disaster as it progresses. For example, GIS enables incident commanders to track the spread of an infectious disease through a community. Disaster preparedness should include identifying information sources that are available in a community. Planning and development offices are often useful resources. State and federal governments are potential resources. Federal agencies having GIS-ready data include the U.S. Geological Survey and the Agency for Toxic Substances and Disease Registry. During a crisis, the ability to use GIS-ready data is invaluable in assessing an emergency situation.

AFTER-ACTION REPORTS

After-action reports are essential. Such reports enable agencies to identify and improve their deficiencies. By being honest with themselves, agencies are able to critically evaluate and respond to poor performance areas. After-action reports should discuss aspects of operation that are performed well and underscore staff competencies. Integration of after-action reports enables multiple agencies to review organizational performance. Allowing other agencies to review activities increases understanding of deficiencies. More importantly, it contributes to correcting deficiencies.

CONCLUSION

The people and organizations in the chapter-opening case could benefit from an integrated approach to crisis preparation. Having a plan that had been tested and evaluated is the first requirement. An active surveillance program is the second requirement. These alone could have alerted authorities of the emerging problem. Data from hospitals should have triggered a response if early surveillance systems missed the illness reports from the report normally filed by members of the crew of the airplane on which the affected persons entered the country.

Emergency room physicians in hospitals close to international airports must routinely collect recent travel data. They must be familiar with uncommon diseases or have access to such expertise. Consultants must be called in cases of unusual illnesses. Access to supplies must be arranged in advance. The local health department and law enforcement agencies should use the Incident Command System. Mutual assistance compacts should be written and accepted by the political leaders of all involved organizations.

In a disaster situation, time will be in short supply. Being prepared, trained, and ready will increase the probability of minimizing injuries and losses. Lack of preparation and confusion during a disaster are likely to be paid for with lost lives and increased suffering.

References

American Red Cross. 2004. Homeland security advisory system recommendations. Available at www.redcross.org/services/disaster/beprepared/hsas.html.

California Office of Emergency Services. 1987. *Earthquake Preparedness Guidelines for Hospitals*. Sacramento, CA: California Office of Emergency Services.

Maniscalco, P. 2002. *Understanding Terrorism and Managing the Consequences*. Upper Saddle River, NJ: Prentice Hall.

San Mateo County, California. 2004. Hospital Emergency Incident Command System. Available at www.emsa.cahwnet.gov/dms2/heics3.htm.

U.S. Department of Homeland Security. 2004. Homeland security advisory system. Available at www.dhs.gov/dhspublic/display?theme=29.

Resources

Periodicals

Benedek, D.M., Holloway, H.C., and Becker, S.M. 2002. Emergency mental health management in bioterrorism events. *Emergency Medical Clinics of North America* 20(2):393–407.

Bledsoe, B.E., and Barnes, D.2003. Beyond the debriefing debate: What should we be doing? *Emergency Medical Services* 32(12):60–68.

Chandley, M. 2001. Before the experts arrive. *Journal of Psychosocial Nursing and Mental Health Services* 39(6):12–20.

Eyre, A., Fertel, N., Fisher, J.M., Gunn, S.W., Hampton, D., Lederman, B., Posner, Z., Preobrajensky, V.N., Rebonato, M., Riboni, V., Rodriguez, D., Shih, C.L., and Yamamoto, Y. 2001. Disaster coordination and management: Summary and action plans. *Prehospital and Disaster Medicine* 16(1):22–25.

Simon, J.D. 1999. Nuclear, biological, and chemical terrorism: understanding the threat and designing responses. *International Journal of Emergency Mental Health* 1(2):81–89.

Simon, R., and Teperman, S. 2001. The World Trade Center attack. Lessons for disaster management. *Critical Care* 5(6):318–320.

U.S. Department of Health and Human Services. 2004. Communicating in a Crisis: Risk Communication Guidelines for Public Officials. Document SMA 02-3641. Available from 800-789-2647 or www.mentalhealth.org.

Books

Bevelacqua, A.S., and Stilp, R.H. 2004. *Terrorism Handbook for Operational Responders.* Albany, NY: Delmar.

Kirschenbaum, A. 2003. *Chaos Organization and Disaster Management.* New York: Marcel Dekker.

Spigarelli, J.A. 2002. *Crisis Preparedness Handbook: A Comprehensive Guide to Home Storage and Physical Survival.* Alpine, UT: Cross-Current Publishing.

Ursano, R.J., Fullerton, C.S., and Norwood, A.E. 2003. *Terrorism and Disaster: Individual and Community Mental Health Interventions.* New York: Cambridge University Press.

Webb, N.B. 2003. *Mass Trauma and Violence: Helping Families and Children Cope.* New York: Guilford Publications.

Web Sites

- Agency for Toxic Substances and Disease Registry:
  www.atsdr.cdc.gov
- American Red Cross:
  www.redcross.org
- Center for Risk Communications:
  www.riskcommunication.org
- Community Emergency Response Teams:
  www.usafreedomcorps.gov
- Geographic Information Systems:
  www.gis.com
- Medical Response Corps:
  www.medicalreservecorps.gov
- National Partnership for Workplace Mental Health:
  www.workplacementalhealth.org
- U.S. Geological Survey:
  www.usgs.gov

Organizations

American Red Cross National Headquarters
2025 E Street, NW
Washington, D.C. 20006

Phone: 202-303-4498
Web site: www.redcross.org

Centers for Disease Control and Prevention
1600 Clifton Road
Atlanta, GA 30333
Phone: 404-639-3311, 404-639-3534, or 800-311-3435
E-mail: www.cdc.gov/netinfo.htm (Web form)
Web site: www.cdc.gov

Federal Emergency Management Agency
500 C Street, SW
Washington, D.C. 20472
Phone: 202-566-1600
Web site: www.fema.gov

U.S. Department of Health & Human Services
200 Independence Avenue, SW
Washington, D.C. 20201
Phone: 202-619-0257 or 877-696-6775 (toll free)
Web site: www.hhs.gov

U.S. Department of Homeland Security
Washington, D.C. 20528
Web page: www.dhs.gov/dhspublic/index.jsp

CHAPTER

28

Crisis Management

Ronald Burger
L. Fleming Fallon, Jr.
Jay MacNeal
Diana Wilde
Eric Zgodzinski

Chapter Objectives

After reading this chapter, readers will:

- Understand the Incident Command System.
- Appreciate the value of communications and the need to develop trust and credibility before an emergency occurs.
- Understand that unpredictable mental reactions may surface in response to emergency situations.
- Know how to staff and operate an emergency operations center.
- Know how to manage human and material resources during a crisis.
- Understand the role and importance of technology in managing crisis situations.
- Delineate state and federal sources of assistance.
- Know how to conduct an after-event debriefing.

Chapter Summary

Successful crisis management requires adequate planning, preparation, and practice. Roles must be learned, and trust must be developed among key crisis leaders. Emergency team members will react to crisis situations in different ways. All persons involved in an emergency are at risk of developing a post-traumatic stress disorder. Incident commanders must be able to successfully manage human and material resources. They must also appreciate the role of technology in crisis management and be able to use technology-based resources in an appropriate manner. Assistance is available from state and federal agencies. After-event briefings provide critical information and guidance for future crisis events.

Case Study

On October 19, 1991, a fire burned three acres in a valley in Oakland and Berkeley Hills, California. The area is across the bay from San Francisco. Local firefighters put out the blaze and went home to dinner.

The next morning, a spark from the previous day's fire was picked up and blown into a fuel-rich wooded area by fierce northeast winds. Influenced by the winds in the canyon, the spark erupted into a new fire, gained momentum, and moved directly from tree cover to houses. The fire intensified so quickly that within 15 minutes it had developed into a major firestorm with a thermal column that looked and acted like a tornado. This new fire blackened the sky for miles, raged through prime hill areas for 10 hours, jumped an 8-lane freeway with its airborne flaming material, and torched homes at the rate of one every 11 seconds.

The fire defied every effort to stop its progress until thousands of residents, volunteers, and professional firefighters pulled together hundreds of pieces of fire-fighting equipment and attacked the fire on several fronts. The battle continued well into the night until the gale-force winds started to subside. By the time the fire was declared contained two days later, it had burned more than 1,600 acres, destroyed 3,354 residences and 456 apartments, killed 25 people, injured 150, caused an estimated $1.5 billion in damage, and displaced over 5,000 people.

What public health plans and services should have been available and implemented during and following this conflagration?

INTRODUCTION

Chapter 26 discussed various aspects of disaster planning. In Chapter 27, integrated crisis preparation was reviewed. The present chapter extends these concepts to managing a crisis during an actual event. Chapter 29 will focus on bioterrorism.

Terrorism

On September 11, 2001, many people were violently introduced to terrorism. However, terrorism is not a new phenomenon. Even in the realm of public health, forms of terror were practiced throughout the twentieth century. From the perspective of crisis management, terrorism is similar to other natural disasters. Natural disasters, like terrorist incidents, cause confusion and problems with communication. Unlike natural disasters, terrorist events add a mental dimension that is linked with unremitting fear. The mental images impair the ability to adequately assess information and make appropriate responses. However, if emergency planners and incident commanders remain calm, plan adequately and prepare with diligence, the challenges of terrorist incidents can be successfully managed by trained crisis managers. Terrorism is discussed in greater detail in Chapter 29.

UTILIZATION OF THE INCIDENT COMMAND SYSTEM

When an incident occurs, immediate activation of the Incident Command System is necessary to limit the impact of the event. The leader or incident commander for a public health event may initially be a sanitarian or public health nurse who happens to be the first responder to an incident. The incident commander must accomplish many tasks to ensure a safe and efficient operation while developing an appropriate approach to the incident. Constant evaluation of response objectives and tactics is crucial as the incident progresses. The incident commander must immediately focus on three priorities. The highest priority is to save and preserve life. The next priority is to stabilize the scene of the event. This also means taking steps to prevent the crisis from escalating. The lowest priority is to protect property, conserving and preserving it as possible and appropriate.

The incident commander must use these priorities to survey the scene and develop an immediate plan for action. The incident commander initially has a very important role and must begin to coordinate the response efforts of all of the people and resources at the scene. This must be undertaken with a high regard for responder safety. For example, the incident commander must assess the situation and decide what types of personal protective equipment may be needed or how individuals will be rotated to decrease risks associated with physical and mental exertion. Safety of personnel must be a constant priority for an incident commander.

While the immediate safety of emergency responders is being ensured, the incident commander next creates and activates a command post. The incident commander then appoints a safety officer or assumes the responsibility. Next, the incident commander must appoint four main section leaders to handle differing duties. This management team will provide information to the emergency operations center if and when it is activated. The initial incident commander may serve the best interests of the response team if the group is located in the emergency operations center. Other personnel in the field or at the site of an emergency may be more effective in coordinating response efforts. In such a situation, overall command should be transferred to a replacement incident commander. Using the incident command system, smooth transfers of command can be easily accomplished.

It is important for the incident commander to begin thinking about ways to formulate response objectives and to develop an incident action plan. The incident commander should consult with the command staff to determine the best approach to the incident. The approach may be defensive, such as sheltering in place. It may be offensive, such as a mass prophylaxis antibiotic or immunization campaign. The best action may be nonintervention. Regardless of the approach selected, an effective communication effort will usually alleviate fears among members of the public. Any selected action must be well thought out, documented, and evaluated. After the incident, it will most likely have to be justified to the general public.

Any plan of action must include safety considerations and be consistent with existing emergency plans. Capabilities and standard operating guidelines of response organizations must also be considered.

Decision making is a critical skill for incident commanders. Making timely decisions is important. Frequently, an incident commander must make decisions based on limited information. Because many of these decisions may have serious consequences, a systems-based approach should be undertaken. One such system is the DECIDE method that is taught to hazardous materials responders (**Figure 28-1**).

The occupational health principles of anticipate, recognize, evaluate, and control provide an alternative method that can be used when making decisions during an incident. By anticipating and preparing, potential incident commanders will be ready to respond when the need arises. Rapid recognition will enable them to limit casualties and ill effects on the community. Risk evaluation guides decision-making efforts and is useful when evaluating or revising action plans. Controlling risk eventually enables citizens to return to their communities and resume pre-event activities.

By implementing the Incident Command System under the control of a unified command structure, emergency response leaders can use the resources of agencies and organizations in an effective manner. An intra-

Detect the presence of hazard

Estimate likely harm without intervention

Choose the response objectives

Identify action options

Do the best option

Evaluate Progress

Figure 28-1 The DECIDE method

agency approach to response is necessary because no single agency or organization can effectively respond to all types of incidents. By working together as a team, great goals can be accomplished and the health of the public can be protected during threatening times.

■ COMMUNICATIONS

During any incident, reliable communications are critical. As the scale of an incident grows, the importance of communications becomes even more critical. The Health Alert Network is an important set of procedures that are used to contact and inform individuals of a crisis. The network involves telephone trees, e-mail chains, radio networks, and facsimile transmission lists. These components are purposefully redundant to maintain communications under a variety of emergency conditions and when some elements may be unavailable. It is important that the emergency operations center, the people in a command post, all sector leaders, and any on-site workers be able to communicate with each other. The ability to communicate enables constant evaluation and continuous adaptation. During a response to an incident, the needs of responders can rapidly change.

Approximately 70 percent of communications are nonverbal. Personal and informal communications are both reliable and desirable. However, although informal communications are useful during an emergency, they are limited. Public health managers must learn to utilize all available methods and channels of communication and use the incident command center as an information and resource exchange mechanism. One example of the importance of communications and building relationships in advance of an incident is the following comment. At the time of the comment, one of the authors (G.B.) was the Commissioner of Health for the State of Maryland.

> We spoke to people we knew as trusted colleagues in channels that were well rehearsed to get the information and get it quickly. This is not to say, however, that these informal relationships should usurp formal hierarchy but should be integrated into a command and control structure that relies on established lines of authority with well-defined roles and responsibilities at all levels. The exercise and use of this command structure by all levels will minimize the need to rely on informal communication structures. (Casani et al., 2003)

Communication Methods

Telephones and fax machines are two available communication options. However, during major emergencies, telephone lines may become overburdened and thus become unreliable for conveying critical information. For example, during the New York City response to the September 11 terrorist attack on the World Trade Center, important communication links could not be made due to overuse (Levy, 2003). During emergencies related to natural disasters such as hurricanes or earthquakes, normal communication lines may be disrupted.

Methods and systems are available that will allow provide a high priority to emergency personnel so that they will have increased access to telephone company trunks. Such systems must be arranged and approved in advance. Radio communication needs must be addressed prior to a crisis. Portable radios have limited range and may require the use of a repeater system. In addition, towers that provide repeater service may be destroyed during a crisis.

Computer-based messaging such as e-mail is useful, but it may be dependent on the public telephone system, and thus may be disrupted during a crisis. Organizations may decide to have an alternative Internet service provider that is located in another state or region. Management during a crisis would most likely require e-mail usage or Internet access. Another alternative to both cellular and landline telephones is a satellite telephone. Remember that cellular telephones require both towers and land lines for normal function. Many emergency situations may interrupt one or both of these components.

Amateur radio operators can be of assistance when normal communication systems fail. Local emergency radio systems can rapidly provide information to large groups of citizens. The Emergency Broadcast System, now enhanced by the Emergency Alert System, is a way to rapidly communicate with citizens via a one-way broadcast method. Use of these systems should be written into emergency plans and tested on a regular basis.

Runners are actual people who are used to convey messages when all other means have failed. The use of runners is slow and less desirable. However, runners may be the only means of communication available in some emergency situations.

Most likely, more than one type of communication modality, device, or pathway will be needed to effectively manage and respond in a crisis situation. Using different modes of communication and understanding how they work prior to a crisis will improve responses during an emergency.

Support Staff

During a crisis, it is important to clearly communicate with all staff members and provide them with all pertinent, nonclassified information. This information will enable staff to perform their duties in a more efficient and informed manner.

Providing staff with updated information also greatly improves their physical safety. Working with outdated information does not lend itself to accomplishing difficult objectives in a safe manner. In post-event debriefings, experienced incident commanders have reported that information often becomes obsolete in a matter of minutes.

Staff accountability is also important. Knowing the locations of staff members and when and to whom they should report during a crisis is an important responsibility of crisis management team leaders. The specifics of a given emergency event will determine how, when, and where staff will be dispatched. The same crisis specifics will also determine their immediate goals. A crisis leader's main responsibility is ensuring the safety of emergency response personnel.

Communicating with the Media and the Public

A public information officer should be an integral member of any crisis management effort from the beginning of the response. The public information officer should attend all internal briefings so that he or she understands what is going on. Public information officers should understand the limits and responsibilities of their positions. In addition to developing messages with other agencies, they should understand the limits of what they are permitted to say. This responsibility calls for judgment and maturity. All collaborating agencies must issue communiqués that are in agreement. During an emergency, issuing different messages can cause panic and decrease credibility. Messages must issue needed information. First and foremost, they must instill calmness and vigilance.

Emergency Alerts

Various elements of the media have important roles and responsibilities during a crisis. Arrangements and contacts with persons in the media must be established before a crisis actually occurs. Time is required to establish trust. The Emergency Alert System has been in place for years. This system can be activated by a local emergency management agency. It provides a useful way to warn people of impending natural disasters such as hurricanes or floods. It can also be used in the event of a biological, chemical, or terrorist attack. Public messages must be precise and clear as to what actions are expected and must be broadcast in a timely manner.

During and After an Event

The type of disaster and its expected duration largely dictates the procedures that will be employed and the actual messages that will be broadcast. Will the crisis require portions of a population to be evacuated or relocated? How long will disruptions of normal routines last?

What is the most efficient venue for communicating with members of the general public? Efficiency must be assessed from several directions. From the perspective of an incident commander, the easiest medium to contact may be the most efficient. From the perspective of a public information officer, the medium that will broadcast to the greatest potential number of people may be the most efficient. From the perspective of the public, the medium to which they have access may be the most efficient. In the final analysis, using all available media may prove to be the best choice.

The presented message must convey the severity of the situation, but it must be presented in a way that does not panic the public. Preparing messages in advance is an appealing possibility. However, the opportunities for phoniness and generalities usually reduce the utility of such efforts. When a public information officer is asked to present information to the public in person, such as during a news spot or a special report, the best advice is be truthful.

After a crisis has been resolved, questions will be raised. Media releases can be used to transmit important information in the immediate wake of an event. After normal routines have been reestablished, more probing and critical questions are likely to be raised. Three prior points have relevance. First, all members of the crisis team who have been authorized to speak to the public should understand and respect any information boundaries that may be required. Second, all team members should deliver a consistent message. Third, all spokespeople should be truthful.

Evacuations

This is an important action that is often resisted by persons in potential peril. Many agencies must cooperate closely to coordinate and communicate an evacuation in an orderly and timely manner. Evacuations may be required by impending natural disasters, such as hurricanes, or environmental accidents, such as chemical spills or gas leaks. Public health personnel must be ready to assist even though they are unlikely to request an evacuation. Prearranged plans should describe expected roles and actions in the event of an evacuation. Public health may be called upon to provide technical assistance to the incident command with reference to evacuation. Part of an effective evacuation plan is preparing shelters and other venues to house people who are displaced. The public information officer has an important role in an evacuation. Media releases are often jointly drafted and released. Well-planned and coordinated evacuations minimize injuries. They also minimize loss of life during the event for which the evacuation was ordered.

EMERGENCY OPERATIONS CENTERS

To properly manage a crisis, an emergency operations center facility should be secured. Ideally, this should have been arranged during the planning phase and before the fact. During a crisis or a practice drill, only authorized personnel should be admitted to the facility. The facility should be free-standing, meaning that it can be self-sufficient for prolonged periods of time. To maintain self-sufficiency, the facility should have a dedicated power source, communications capabilities, sufficient food and water, and sleeping facilities for both staff and an unanticipated number of additional officials or other people who might gain entrance.

During times of activation, staff members should rely on the training they have received concerning the emergency operations center. Staff should be preassigned to all affiliated command facilities, including the local emergency operations center as well as state and federal emergency operations centers. Such assignments will be determined by the nature of the crisis. Initially, plans should prepare for the emergency center to operate continuously (over 24 hours) for the first several days of a crisis. This requires staffing preparations. Public health personnel should be included in the staffing roster. Shift leaders should plan on periodically briefing staff throughout the crisis so that everyone remains informed.

By having agency heads working under a unified command in an emergency operations center, operational organization and proper resource allocation become easier. Local resources may require supplemental support by state or federal personnel and assets. Agreements to provide or share such resources should be made in advance. The emergency operations center should have the ability to request or allocate resources from or to appropriate agencies.

Another communication requirement is to prepare call lists for employees along with any other needed contacts. Alternative or back-up contact numbers provide additional assurance that people will be located and contacts will be established during an emergency. These tasks, too, must be completed in advance. If the crisis is biological in nature, a public health professional may be called upon to lead the response effort. This may change as other information or personnel become available. Other crises will have different levels of need for responses from public health personnel.

MENTAL HEALTH

Mental health is often relegated to a secondary position within many public health activities. Mental health is an important aspect of any emergency situation. This is true for emergency response workers as well as victims of the incident. An important aspect of crisis preparation is establishing communication pathways and resource personnel for all concerned. When responding to a crisis, mental health leaders should be familiar with all emergency plans and decision protocols.

Mental health personnel responding to a crisis must provide quick and accurate information to the general public. The message of keeping calm and in control of oneself must be conveyed to the general public by elements of the media or any other means. Two central mental health messages include coping with stress and processing catastrophic upheaval and loss.

Mental health professionals must continually adjust their messages as the nature of a crisis changes. Different forms of support are required for victims and response personnel. Different degrees of support are needed as a crisis evolves and ultimately resolves itself. Mental health services are frequently required for a long time after an incident has been concluded. Post-traumatic stress disorder is well documented (First and Tasman, 2004; Horowitz, 2002; Levin et al., 2004). The implication is that mental health services must be as readily available as other emergency services.

Several issues related to mental health must be addressed in planning and implementing a crisis management plan. The services of appropriately qualified mental health professionals must be secured in advance. Messages must be constructed for release to the public. These must be sensitive to the specifics and gravity of any crisis. Support must be available and provided to emergency personnel during and after an event. Mental health professionals must be sensitive to their role in responding to crisis situations. The specifics of all mental health responses during any crisis differ and depend on the nature, severity, and duration of an emergency.

RESOURCE MANAGEMENT

Once internal and local resources already on scene have been expended or used up, additional resources may be needed. Assistance from neighboring regions or the state and federal reserves may be requested. Local requirements are discussed among incident command leaders in the emergency operations center. Requests for assistance should be made in a timely fashion. Logistic factors such as existing supply levels and the time required for procurement, loading, and transportation of replacement supplies must be factored into the timing of requests for assistance. Other demands on sources of replacement supplies must also be considered.

TECHNOLOGY

A number of technologies may be useful to public health professionals both during and after a crisis.

Surveillance and Tracking

Most of the usual activities of a public health department must continue during a crisis. However, some modifications of standard operating procedures may be in order. Disease surveillance provides a convenient example. Under normal conditions, persons with reportable diseases may be actively sought out, personally interviewed, or medically reviewed. During an emergency, some or all of these activities may be replaced by simply making an entry into a computer database. Such modifications of normal procedures should be considered and planned for in advance.

Disease tracking during an emergency may require alternative techniques and organizational strategies. Interviews still have relevance, although available personnel resources may be depleted. A form of organizational triage is useful in such situations. Interviews should be reserved for individuals who have diseases that may impact the emergency. If isolation or quarantine is required, appropriate processing is needed to properly carry out activities to protect the general public. The triage and processing system can be computerized. Handheld devices or field laptop computers can be utilized to expedite initial processing, appropriate or legally required notification, and transfer of data into permanent records. These changes in normal routine should be included in the emergency planning process.

Analysis

Computer programs are available to analyze data and generate statistics. Program operators must be thoroughly familiar with the operation of all software programs that will be used during an emergency situation. Information processors should have basic knowledge of computer hardware, because support personnel may not be readily available during an emergency. Prudent planners provide for backup computers that have needed software programs loaded in advance. During a crisis, information feeds should provide raw data to both primary and backup computers. This will reduce downtime if the primary computer malfunctions. If possible, data coming into computers should be linked with GIS coordinates. Such data can be displayed in a pictorial manner. This is potentially far more useful than tabular arrays of the same information.

Output from data received during a crisis must be generated quickly and be accurate. Although both are desirable, accuracy is generally more important. Incident commanders may use the output to make decisions affecting lives. It will also be used for media updates. Finally, documentation will ultimately be required. After the event, questions will be asked concerning activities, decisions, and outcomes. Analyzing why particular procedures were used is an excellent topic for pre-event drills.

STATE AND FEDERAL ASSISTANCE

A declaration or state of emergency is made by an elected official of a city, county, state, or federal government. Local regulations determine the level at which such a declaration may be made. The level at which a declaration is made also determines the resources that can be requested. The usual rationale for a declaration of emergency is that the lives or property of a large number of people are at risk or that an event has overwhelmed the available resources in an area. **Figure 28-2** outlines the system used by a local health department to request outside assistance from an emergency management agency in adjacent jurisdictions, the state government, or the federal government.

State Assistance

The states have recently developed a system of mutual aid to provide assistance to each other in times of disasters. An *emergency management assistance compact* is a mutual aid agreement and partnership between states. Such compacts were developed to address natural disasters, such as hurricanes, earthquakes, and tornadoes, and environmental disasters, such as wildfires, toxic waste spills, and explosions. Terrorism has been added to the list of disaster situations. An emergency management assistance compact offers a rapid way for states to provide personnel and equipment to help disaster relief efforts in other states.

Emergency management assistance compacts provide aid when state and local resources are overwhelmed and federal assistance is inadequate or unavailable. Requests for emergency management assistance compact assistance are legally binding. States and jurisdictions that request help are responsible for reimbursing all out-of-state costs and are liable for out-of-state personnel. Providers of aid will not incur a financial or legal burden for their help. Generally the Federal Emergency Management Agency will assist with financing such efforts.

Receipt of a request does not obligate a state to provide assistance. In practice, a request would be refused only if the requested resources were already in use and thus unavailable. The simplicity of an emergency management assistance compact request eliminates bureaucratic wrangling. States are now helping one another due, in large measure, to the protocols of emergency management assistance compacts.

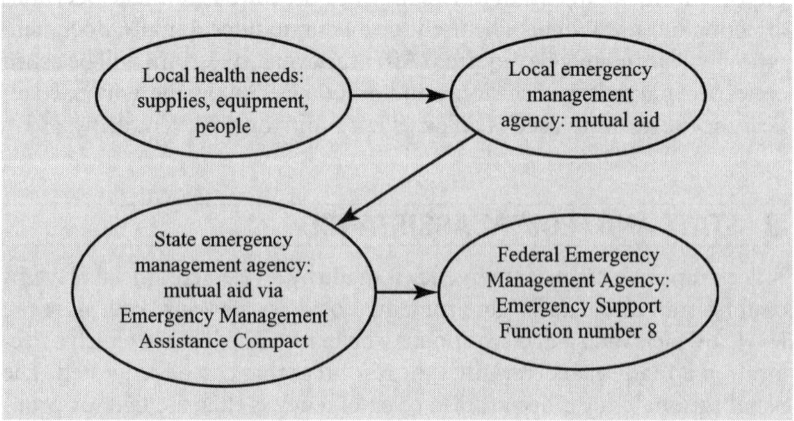

Figure 28-2 Requests for Outside Assistance

Federal Assistance

The Robert T. Stafford Disaster Relief and Emergency Assistance Act, as amended, delineates resources and response options that can be provided by the federal government. Specific details are contained in the Federal Response Plan. The Stafford Act provides for assistance to state and local governments when a major disaster or emergency overwhelms their ability to respond effectively to save lives; to protect public health, safety and property; and to restore their communities.

The Federal Response Plan is an all-hazards approach to disasters. It describes the policies, planning assumptions, concept of operations, response and recovery actions, and responsibilities of 25 federal departments and agencies and the American Red Cross. These resources become available after the president declares a major disaster or emergency. The Federal Response Plan has proven to be an effective framework for coordinating delivery of federal disaster assistance to state and local governments. Since the Stafford Act was signed in 1992, federal agencies have demonstrated that they can work together to achieve the common goal of efficient, timely, and consistent responses and facilitate economic and social recovery in affected areas.

The Federal Response Plan employs a functional approach that groups the types of assistance that are most likely to be needed into 12 Emergency Support Functions (ESFs). These functions include immediate assistance, such as mass health care and medical services, and help to sustain recovery efforts. Support capabilities, such as transportation and communications, also are included. Agencies are expected to provide mutual assistance when participating in a crisis response. Based on their resources and capability to support one or more functional areas, other agencies have been designated to provide assistance to one or more of the primary agencies. The complete list of primary functions and the agencies responsible for coordinating them are listed in **Figure 28-3**.

ESF 8 is of particular interest. The primary federal agency to coordinate health and medical care is the Department of Health and Human Services. States receive help in assessing health and medical needs and in providing health surveillance, medical personnel, and supporting equipment and supplies. Resources are provided to evacuate injured or threatened persons, provide hospital care, and support recovery workers with food, shelter, and other personal care as needed. Consultation resources are provided for mental health and problems associated with radiological, biological, and chemical contamination. Specialized personnel and equipment are available to provide potable water, sanitation, and solid waste disposal. Veterinary and vector control services are available. If needed, victim identification and mortuary services can be provided.

Three other forms of response to specific events are coordinated by the federal government. The Federal Radiological Emergency Response

Resources provided by the federal government are grouped into 12 Emergency Support Functions (ESFs):

- ESF 1: Transportation. Providing civilian and military transportation.
  Lead agency: Department of Transportation
- ESF 2: Communications. Providing telecommunications support.
  Lead agency: National Communications System
- ESF 3: Public Works and Engineering. Restoring essential public services and facilities.
  Lead agency: U.S. Army Corps of Engineers, Department of Defense
- ESF 4: Fire Fighting. Detecting and suppressing wild land, rural, and urban fires.
  Lead agency: U.S. Forest Service, Department of Agriculture
- ESF 5: Information and Planning. Collecting, analyzing, and disseminating critical information to facilitate the overall federal response and recovery operations.
  Lead agency: Federal Emergency Management Agency
- ESF 6: Mass Care. Managing and coordinating food, shelter, and first aid for victims; providing bulk distribution of relief supplies; operating a system to assist family reunification.
  Lead agency: American Red Cross
- ESF 7: Resource Support. Providing equipment, materials, supplies, and personnel to federal entities during response operations.
  Lead agency: General Services Administration
- ESF 8: Health and Medical Services. Providing assistance for public health and medical care needs.
  Lead agency: U.S. Public Health Service, Department of Health and Human Services
- ESF 9: Urban Search and Rescue. Locating, extricating, and providing initial medical treatment to victims trapped in collapsed structures.
  Lead agency: Federal Emergency Management Agency
- ESF 10: Hazardous Materials. Supporting federal response to actual or potential releases of oil and hazardous materials.
  Lead agency: Environmental Protection Agency
- ESF 11: Food. Identifying food needs; ensuring that food gets to areas affected by disaster.
  Lead agency: Food and Nutrition Service, Department of Agriculture
- ESF 12: Energy. Restoring power systems and fuel supplies.
  Lead agency: Department of Energy

Figure 28-3 Emergency Support Functions
Source: Federal Emergency Management Agency (2004).

Plan covers nuclear or other radiological emergencies. The National Contingency Plan provides assistance for incidents involving hazardous materials. The Terrorism Plan was created to coordinate responses to terrorist attacks. These preparations, in combination with the Federal Response Plan, are being combined into a single, all-hazards plan for federal response to assist states. The proposed single protocol is known as the National Response Plan.

POST-EVENT ACTIVITIES

Ending a disaster response or emergency operation is almost as important as beginning it. Pre-incident planning should include objective criteria for concluding an operation. Agreement on how to end an operation can help to avoid problems in the future. After the incident response has concluded, the response to the event should be evaluated. Documentation generated by the event should be collected and filed.

Demobilization

Demobilization is the removal of a portion or all of the response personnel or organizations. Fatigue may precipitate withdrawal of persons. Lack of resources may limit the usefulness of response workers. Personnel may be withdrawn because operational goals have been met. Personnel and resources may have been provided by cooperating agencies; any restrictions on their time must be respected. Demobilization should be practiced in drills. Demobilization procedures must be documented before an event and used when needed. Demobilization is a necessary part of any disaster response.

Emergency workers may not want to be dismissed. This phenomenon grows as the duration of a response increases. It is also influenced by emotional factors. Some responders may be personally involved, surviving when friends or loved ones have not. They often experience a mixture of responsibility and guilt. Some emergency personnel face the return to a relatively bland job. When emergency response duties are perceived as being exciting, returning to regular work is often avoided. These issues should be discussed in advance by event planners. Appropriately trained counseling resources should be provided if such issues arise.

Event Evaluation

Self-evaluation is often an unpleasant task. However, it is a necessity. Occupational Safety and Health Act regulations require that a proper debriefing be conducted after an event response has concluded. Three components that should be included in a proper termination evaluation are debriefing, post-incident analysis, and critique.

A *debriefing* should be conducted immediately after an incident response is concluded. In the event of a long-term response, incident commanders or senior assistants should attempt to debrief workers at the conclusion of their shift or rotation. The debriefing is used to determine what objectives were completed and provides an ongoing progress evaluation of the incident action plan. During the debriefing, emergency workers should be advised of potential environmental exposures and their consequences. This is especially important when responding to events involving biological or chemical agents such as phosgene or asbestos, which may involve significant delays between exposure and the onset of symptoms. Workers should be advised as to what signs or symptoms to watch for and how they should respond if health changes are observed. Emergency responders should be reminded of the possibility of post-traumatic stress disorder.

During a *post-incident analysis,* data from debriefing sessions are reviewed. Evaluating progress is a primary goal of analysis. Incident commanders use the results of analysis to determine their next objectives. After the response phase of an event is concluded, planners should review the entire emergency plan. Revising plans using actual experience is a positive step that improves future responses.

The *critique* provides an opportunity to critically evaluate response efforts. What actions and operations were undertaken and concluded in a satisfactory manner? What was handled in a less-than-satisfactory manner? Were the lives of responders put at risk? What aspects of the operation could be improved in the future? What approaches could be modified? Were commands given and carried out in a timely manner? Individuals conducting a critique must be honest with each other. The goal is improving both the process and the team.

Documentation

Gathering records from the incident is important. This should be an ongoing task. Some incident commanders assign this task to a single individual. If data collection is not ongoing during the incident, the task should be addressed as soon as possible and practical after demobilization. This should minimize the chance that relevant data will be overlooked. Recall accuracy tends to decline as time passes. Waiting to collect data potentially degrades learning from the incident and may limit future preparations. Interview data also contributes to a paper record of the event. From a legal perspective, proper documentation is important and can influence rights to compensation for exposure to environmental agents during the event for workers and members of the public.

■ CONCLUSION

This chapter has discussed issues related to crisis management. Adequate planning, appropriate training, and sufficient resource allocation should enable incident commanders to successfully manage a crisis. Crisis management is a process that begins with planning and preparation. The crisis management plan is then put into practice and evaluated at the conclusion of the crisis. The process of evaluation initiates the next cycle. Professionalism, preparation, and communication are the keys to managing a crisis response in a timely and competent manner.

The major and unprecedented Oakland and Berkeley Hills firestorm exposed many weaknesses in the crisis responses of local, county, and state agencies. It also raised unplanned operational issues among firefighters. Little, if any, time had been spent in creating a plan for fighting fires in local urban and wild areas. In particular, the fire involved two adjacent city and county jurisdictions as well as an expanse of regional parkland.

During the conflagration, police and fire personnel experienced great difficulty warning residents to leave the area ahead of the fast advancing inferno due to narrow roads, poor interagency communications, and minimal coordination between bordering agencies. One city had its own emergency radio communication frequencies that were not accessible on standard radios and that differed from those used by all other agencies throughout the state. The city's fire hydrants had 3-inch valves that were incompatible with standard 4-inch hose connectors. This necessitated trucking in hose adapters to the scene, causing a critical delay in early efforts to fight a huge, fast-spreading fire.

Many neighborhoods were destroyed on the first day of the fire. Late on that day, a significant number of residents required immediate assistance with food, water, shelter, first aid or hospitalization, clothing, and other necessities. They also wanted to contact concerned family and friends and needed help in finding lost pets or housing their pets somewhere other than in the temporary shelters. Red Cross regulations prohibit people from bringing pets into its emergency shelters.

Later that night a welcome rainfall aided firefighters. However, this quickly contributed to a major public health issue. Raw sewage from overflowing septic tanks ran down the steep, newly deforested terrain.

Mail delivery became an enormous problem during the first few days after the fire was controlled. This was quickly followed by frustration among insurance adjusters. Many companies flew in personnel. The out-of-state adjusters were unfamiliar with California's high-priced real estate, furnishings, and belongings. They could not communicate with home offices or claimants. Not understating local values, they made inequitable adjustments. They were overwhelmed and under prepared for the task they were asked to perform.

As a result of lessons learned from this fire, several changes were made. The local public water department has a better understanding of water supply needs in the event of a major fire. Plans now call for shutting off water in neighboring areas to increase the flow of water to fire areas. Standard radio frequencies have been assigned to all local, county, and state agencies. All fire hydrants throughout the state have been fitted with standard-size valves. Power companies are now prepared to shut off gas and electricity at critical locations so that broken utilities do not continue to feed fires. City, county, and state agencies have established guidelines for the immediate designation of a public relations person or team to provide a single, central source of reliable information during any major crisis. This person will aid emergency workers and inform and direct the public. Centralized communication centers have been identified. They are ready to serve as sources of information regarding various relief agencies available to victims of any type of catastrophe.

As an additional result of this fire, an Incident Command System model was developed. This model created a known chain of command and prescribed a set of actions and responsibilities that go into effect whenever local, county, or state emergency personnel respond to a critical incident. Both police and fire departments use this system on a daily basis. Additionally, all counties in California must now have well-equipped, stand-by emergency operating centers ready for immediate use should an area-wide or severe emergency arise.

As for Oakland and Berkeley, the Hills Emergency Forum was established with the goal of coordinating the services of the local cities, counties, and parks; the power, water, and sewer companies; the watershed management department; and the public health agencies. Much has been accomplished, and many positive changes have occurred since October 1991. These have only come about by the collaborative efforts of these agencies. Determined citizens have been at the heart of the effort, volunteering their time so that this region will never again be susceptible to or sustain such a massive and devastating firestorm.

References

Casani, J., Matuszak, D., and Benjamin, G. 2003. Under siege: One state's perspectives of the anthrax events of October and November 2001. *Biosecurity and Bioterrorism: Biodefense Strategy, Practice, and Science* 1(1):43–45.

Federal Emergency Management Agency. 2004. Available at www.fema.gov/about/esf.shtm

First, M.B., and Tasman, A. 2004. *DSM-IV-TR Mental Disorders: Diagnosis, Etiology, and Treatment.* New York: Wiley.

Horowitz, M.J. 2002. *Treatment of Stress Response Syndromes.* Arlington, VA: American Psychiatric Publishing.

Levin, B.L., Hennessey, K., and Petrila, J. 2004. *Mental Health Services: A Public Health Perspective*, 2d ed. New York: Oxford University Press.

Levy, B. 2003. *Terrorism and Public Health.* New York: Oxford University Press.

Resources

Periodicals

Bledsoe, B.E., and Barnes, D. 2003. Beyond the debriefing debate: What should we be doing? *Emergency Medical Services* 32(12):60–68.

Castellano, C. 2003. Large group crisis intervention for law enforcement in response to the September 11 World Trade Center mass disaster. *International Journal of Emergency Mental Health* 5(4):211–215.

Covello, V.T. 2003. Best practices in public health risk and crisis communication. *Journal of Health Communication* 8(Supplement 1):5–8.

Domino, M.E., Fried, B., Moon, Y., Olinick, J., and Yoon, J. 2003. Disasters and the public health safety net: Hurricane Floyd hits the North Carolina Medicaid program. *American Journal of Public Health* 93(7):1122–1127.

Garcia, E., and Horton, D.A. 2003. Supporting the Federal Emergency Management Agency rescuers: A variation of critical incident stress management. *Military Medicine* 168(2):87–90.

Garrett, N.Y., Yasnoff, W.A., and Kumar, V. 2003. Emergency implementation of knowledge management system to support a bioterrorism response. *Proceedings of the American Medical Informatics Association Symposium* 849–853.

MacVaugh, T.W. 2003. Planner must be good at crisis management. *Hospital Material Management* 28(7):14–16.

Mitchell, A.M., Sakraida, T.J., and Kameg, K. 2003. Critical incident stress debriefing: Implications for best practice. *Disaster Management and Response* 1(2):46–51.

Mitchell, J.T. 2003. Major misconceptions in crisis intervention. *International Journal of Emergency Mental Health* 5(4):185–197.

Peek, L.A., and Sutton, J.N. 2003. An exploratory comparison of disasters, riots and terrorist acts. *Disasters* 27(4):319–335.

Books

Brown, L. 2004. *Media Relations for Public Safety Professionals.* Sudbury, MA: Jones & Bartlett.

Bullock, J., and Haddow, G. 2003. *Introduction to Emergency Management.* New York: Butterworth-Heinemann.

Dunn, V. 1999. *Command and Control of Fires and Emergencies.* Tulsa, OK: PennWell Corporation.

Hillard, R., Zitek, B., and Gebler, B. 2003. *Emergency Psychiatry.* New York: McGraw-Hill.

Latourrette, T., Bartis, J., Peterson, D.J. 2004. *Protecting Emergency Responders: Community Views of Health and Safety Risks and Personal Protection Needs.* Royal Oak, MI: Rand Publishing.

Schoenfeld, D.J. 2002. *How to Prepare for and Respond to a Crisis.* Alexandria, VA: Association for Supervision and Curriculum Development.

Web Sites

- Centers for Disease Control and Prevention Health Alert Network: www.phppo.cdc.gov/han
- Department of Health and Human Services: www.dhs.gov/dhspublic/index.jsp
- Department of Homeland Security: www.dhs.gov/dhspublic/index.jsp
- National Center for Post-Traumatic Stress Disorder: www.ncptsd.org
- National Institute of Mental Health—Post-Traumatic Stress Disorder: www.nimh.nih.gov/anxiety/ptsdri1.cfm
- Veterans Administration: www1.va.gov/pubaff/ptsdprtr.htm

- U.S. Public Health Service:
  www.usphs.gov

Organizations

Centers for Disease Control and Prevention
1600 Clifton Road
Atlanta, GA 30333
Phone: 404-639-3311, 404-639-3534, or 800-311-3435
E-mail: www.cdc.gov/netinfo.htm (Web form)
Web site: www.cdc.gov

Crisis Management Institute
P.O. Box 331
Salem, OR 97308
Phone: 503-585-3484
Fax: 503-364-0403
E-mail: info@cmionline.org
Web site: www.cmionline.org

Federal Emergency Management Agency
500 C Street, SW
Washington, D.C. 20472
Phone: 202-566-1600
Web site: www.fema.gov

U.S. Environmental Protection Agency
1200 Pennsylvania Ave., NW
Washington, D.C. 20460-0001
Phone: 202-272-0167
Web site: www.epa.gov

CHAPTER

29

Bioterrorism

Ronald Burger
L. Fleming Fallon, Jr.
Eric Zgodzinski

Chapter Objectives

After reading this chapter, readers will:

- Know the history of bioterrorism.
- Understand how to plan for a bioterrorism event.
- Know various methods of bioterrorism surveillance.
- Appreciate the implications of bioterrorism on community health.
- Recognize problems associated with imposing a quarantine.
- Understand issues related to a mass prophylaxis campaign.
- Know how to plan and coordinate a mass treatment program.
- Appreciate bioterrorism-related issues.

Chapter Summary

Bioterrorism has become a major concern in the opening years of the twenty-first century. Prior to 2001, anthrax was present but declining as a global health threat. However, in 2001, it became a weapon. The World Health Organization declared the eradication of smallpox in 1978. The specter of its return as a weapon has generated much activity as governments prepare for a smallpox attack by bioterrorists. Sarin, a nerve agent, has been used to attack subway riders in Tokyo.

This chapter introduces concepts related to preparing for a bioterrorism attack. Planning and preparation are crucial to a successful response to a bioterrorism event. Surveillance is an important aspect of preparation. Most health care facilities will be unable to cope with the demands for treatment in the event of a bioterrorism incident. Alternatives must be established and protocols developed for processing persons seeking treatment. The possibility of quarantine will be examined. Resources and plans for mass prophylaxis or treatment will also be explored.

Case Study

A class of tenth graders was studying recent events. One of the students asked the instructor if the virus that causes Bolivian hemorrhagic fever could be used as a weapon. The teacher had no cogent reply. He had never heard of the disease and had no knowledge of local preparations for a bioterrorism attack. He decided to use the question as the basis for a class project. What aspects of bioterrorism should the class explore? What groups or individuals should be interviewed by members of the class? Why?

INTRODUCTION

Contemporary news is rife with reports of terrorism. Acts of terrorism have been reported for decades. It became more commonplace during the closing years of the twentieth century and the start of the twenty-first. The events of September 11, 2001, brought terrorism to the United States and imprinted terrorism in the minds of many Americans. Public health professionals made significant leadership contributions during the response to the terrorist attacks of late 2001. Planning efforts have begun to minimize the damage and societal interruption of future attacks. Nuclear and chemical terrorism are frightening and complex. Specific agencies have been assigned to make preparations and oversee future responses to both of these forms of terrorism. Members of the public health community will be asked to assume major responsibilities in responses to intentional or unintentional releases of chemical or radioactive materials. Public health officials may be asked to assist with evacuation decisions, provide health and medical care, coordinate counseling, provide advice and guidance related to the health effects of released substances, identify appropriate protective substances or gear, control diseases, and monitor the progression and status of diseases. The environment is within the professional purview of public health. As such, public health will be asked about issues affecting air, food, water, soil, and shelter. Nuclear and chemical agents usually can be quickly detected and accurately identified. However, biological agents often do not have characteristics that allow for rapid detection and identification. This slows the delivery of treatments and antidotes.

It is tempting to assume that the federal government will protect local communities from acts of biological terrorism acts through intelligence and other defensive activities. This is unrealistic given the size and open characteristics of American society. Local governments must participate in keeping their communities as safe as possible. Biological agents can infect an entire population through contamination of the water supply, food, or open air. Although such large-scale attacks should be considered, experts think that the release of biological agents in a smaller area, such as building ventilation or water systems; areas in which the public is gathered, such as sporting, cultural, or other public events; or shopping centers or schools, is more likely (Purver, 1995).

Biological agents have many associated variables and patterns that must be understood before any specific treatment can be offered. The source and methods of delivery and release of the agent must be identified. For these reasons, it is imperative to prepare for all facets of biological terrorism.

HISTORY

Many of the earliest contributions from the discipline of public health involved biological agents and the diseases that they caused. Public health professionals have made significant contributions to society by educating members of the general public about diseases and disease avoidance. These contributions were discussed in greater detail in Chapter 2.

On September 11, 2001, many people were violently introduced to terrorism. Bioterrorism involves the use of a biological agent. Terrorist events add a mental dimension that is linked with extreme fear. The mental images impair the ability to adequately assess information and make appropriate responses. Terrorist events are usually intended to inflict both mental and physical damage. Biological agents have been used as weapons for centuries. Most historians agree that the use of such weapons did not constitute terrorism due to the absence of a mental component. The distinction may be moot.

Biological agents, notably smallpox and measles, have been used as weapons by Europeans who sought to conquer native peoples in the Western hemisphere. Chemicals that exerted toxic effects on biological systems were used in the First World War. More recently, the chemical agent Sarin was used as a terrorist weapon by a Japanese group. Other groups have employed chemical agents to inflict biological harm in the Middle East.

In more recent times, public health workers have helped to track and detect biological agents that have been used as weapons by terrorists. Current education efforts about biological threats and agents have been targeted at police officers, firefighters, and safety personnel from other related agencies. This integration has been useful in preparing personnel to react appropriately in the event of the use of biological agents.

PREPARATION

When preparing for a biological incident, it is imperative that public health personnel integrate and communicate effectively with a variety of community and regional partners. If a major biological release occurs, no single agency, including public health, could effectively sustain a response. Standard emergency responders, hospitals, health care providers, the media, and academia should all be included in a response. Do not overlook representatives from state and federal agencies such as the military and the FBI.

During a biological crisis, the most important resource is staff members. Environmental specialists or sanitarians have the training to conduct investigations. Epidemiologists can collect data and assist in data analysis. Clinic staff can be reassigned to duties that utilize their special skills. During a crisis, clerical staff can assume the duties of other staff and conduct normal departmental operations. The key to ensuring this capability is providing supplementary training in advance. Mental health specialists will have major responsibilities related to the stress and fear caused by a crisis event. Both employees and members of the public will require mental health services.

The Centers for Disease Control and Prevention (2004a) has issued guidelines for local health departments in the event of a probable or confirmed bioterrorist incident or threat. Health commissioners or local health officers who are notified or otherwise become aware of a bioterrorist incident or threat should immediately contact the nearest FBI field office. Local law enforcement officials also should be notified. The FBI has been designated as the agency that will manage the response to a bioterrorism threat. The public health response will be most effective if the FBI supports the overall response. Incidents that require notification are listed in **Figure 29-1**. After ensuring that federal law enforcement officials have been notified of a potential incident, officials from the state health department should be notified. Coordination between public health professionals at all levels will be necessary in the event of an actual attack.

a. One or more cases, definitively diagnosed with one or more of the following:
   - Any case of smallpox or pulmonary anthrax (such a disease in even one case would strongly indicate the likelihood of bioterrorism).
   - Uncommon agent or disease (e.g., *Burkholderia mallei* or *pseudomallei*, smallpox, pulmonary anthrax) occurring in a person with no other explanation.
   - An illness caused by a microorganism with markedly atypical features (e.g., features suggesting that the microorganism was genetically altered)
   - An illness due to aerosol or food or water sabotage, as opposed to a usual transmission route.

b. One or more clusters of illnesses that remain unexplained after a preliminary investigation.

c. Deliberate chemical, industrial, radiation or nuclear release.

Figure 29-1 Notification Criteria for the FBI

Source: Centers for Disease Control and Prevention (2004a).

If an attack occurs, three factors must be considered: detection, containment, and treatment. *Detection* simply means confirming that a bioterrorist event has occurred and identifying the involved agents. *Containment* means isolating infected persons to minimize the spread of the disease and isolating the agents adhering to contaminated items. *Treatment* means intervening with appropriate medical or psychological modalities to cure infections or alleviate suffering. Various agencies within the federal government are developing protocols to detect biological contamination of humans. As these protocols are developed, relevant personnel in local health departments must be trained in their use.

As soon as an attack has been verified, the disease must be contained and its spread minimized. Containing the spread of an infectious disease involves intrusive measures such as a isolation with quarantine that limit personal and civil liberties. Working with relevant government agencies, local health department personnel should develop and implement a standardized approach to isolating and treating infected individuals. Protocols must include isolation and treatment of exposed persons as well as isolating and decontaminating or destroying clothing and other exposed items in a manner that does not also contaminate the environment. Plans must ensure that health care facilities such as emergency departments, hospital inpatient areas, and physicians' offices are protected from contamination. Health care personnel must be trained and practice performing their assigned duties while wearing personal protective equipment such as exposure suits and respirators.

Treatment of persons exposed to biological agents will depend on the agent used and the availability of appropriate resources. Effective treatment includes isolating the attack so that the routine needs of people living or working in the area of the attack can be served. Secure methods of communication must be established to enable communication among personnel at local, regional, and national levels to alert health departments of suspected or confirmed bioterrorist threats or events. Communication plans for informing the public about bioterrorist incidents must be developed in advance.

Planning efforts must assess the capacity of the health care delivery system. Providers of care will require psychological and physical support. Alternatives to hospitals must be identified and prepared. Home health agencies and hospices may be utilized to expand treatment capacity by confining infected persons to their homes. Portions of telephone and other communication systems must be protected from the inevitable flood of calls that will accompany a bioterrorist attack.

■ SURVEILLANCE

In addition to specific intelligence developed by the federal government, public health surveillance is an important element in the warning system for a bioterrorist attack. Vulnerable populations and targets should be identified during the planning process. Once a surveillance system is in place, it should be tested prior to an event.

Surveillance systems can be extremely complex. Identification of a possible attack is only the beginning of the process. Presumptive identifications must be confirmed. Means must be available to relay pertinent information to appropriate personnel throughout the community. Telephones and facsimile systems are logical routes for notification. However, their successful use assumes that the telephone system is available. Reserving capacity in advance or installing dedicated lines to connect important organizations and response elements can ensure this capability. Protocols should be established for accessing data, and specific times for sending reports should be set. The fundamental goal of an effective surveillance system is to obtain data on the types of diseases that are being observed or reported and knowing the number of sick or symptomatic individuals.

Surveillance activities during and after an event are similar to those during pre-event surveillance. Data are needed on the number of affected individuals and the types of diseases. Data on the size and extent of contaminated areas also are needed. This is required for decontamination and possible quarantine activities. After an initial exposure has occurred and those first affected have been treated, concern shifts to controlling the spread of the disease as well as struggling with possible hostile working conditions. Post-event surveillance requires that redundancies be built into the system for gathering and reporting information. Depending on the number of affected individuals, non-public-health personnel may be required to conduct interviews and follow up with affected people. These people must be identified and adequately trained in advance.

Syndromic data collection is a currently used method of surveillance. Hospitals, labs, and other entities use specific codes for different symptoms. Computers are used to detect patterns and tentatively identify particular diseases. Syndromic surveillance requires that data are entered in a timely manner using appropriate codes. All elements of a surveillance system in a particular region must supply data. All must use the same computer software. Staff must be assigned to perform this work. Lapses in the system potentially jeopardize the safety of all persons in a particular region.

Sentinel site is another useful form of surveillance. Routine reporting data for health care facilities are automatically compared with a program that has pre-set thresholds for diseases of interest. When thresholds are exceeded, personnel are notified to investigate the situation. This system has the advantage of being relatively inexpensive and easy to operate. However, it may not provide early warnings because it depends on timely and accurate data input. It is most useful for analyzing data from a relatively large region.

Informal systems also are in use. The essence of such a system is a conversation among colleagues. One relays details about an unusual case. After the casual conversation, a report may be made. This is the least-expensive system to operate. It is also useful for building interpersonal relationships. However, it assumes that persons will recognize an unusual constellation of symptoms and report them to an appropriate person. It also assumes that a mechanism is in place to report unusual findings to a local collecting point and that someone is available and trained to act on the information. Most authorities would agree that such a system is better than having no system, but that it has great potential for failure. It is also the most common system currently in place in the United States.

Communication of surveillance information can be as simple as using a telephone or as complex as using a networked computer system. Advanced technology is generally preferable, but costly. Whatever system is used locally should have redundancies for collecting and distributing information to key individuals and organizations in the area.

■ COMMUNITY HEALTH

The ability to respond to a bioterrorist attack in a timely and adequate manner will improve overall community health and provide for a stronger public health infrastructure. Monitoring and testing of biological agents can be time consuming. If improper procedures are used, it can also be dangerous. For example, material from a suspected smallpox lesion must be processed in a Bio-Safety Level 4 (BSL-4) facility. Obviously, it cannot simply be sent to a regular hospital facility.

When responding to an infectious agent that is presumed to be biological, the public health department may not always send the sample to a federal or military laboratory for testing. Federal or military laboratory facilities are used to identify extremely hazardous pathogens or unusual bacteria or viruses. Examples of non-biological agents include chemicals in gas or solid form that can cause nerve damage or other toxic effects. The local hospital lab may initially identify a suspected biological agent as pneumonic plague or tularemia. Identification by a local laboratory can save time. Biological agents may be common bacteria. Well-placed salmonella typhoid in multiple salad bars can be as deadly as many more exotic agents. Public health or local hospital laboratories are essential for detection and surveillance of common as well as exotic biological agents. It is important to ensure that sufficient resources are available to respond to a biological crisis. The Laboratory Response Network was established using Centers for Disease Control and Prevention bioterrorism funds. Each state has designated laboratories that have been set up to test for certain agents.

After a biological event has been identified, monitoring and epidemiological surveillance are needed. Identifying an index (first) case of a disease begins the reaction process. Later cases must be monitored for disease status. The environment in which the affected person lives or works also must be investigated. Any residual biological agent may pose an environmental health risk within the affected area. Decontamination or quarantine may be appropriate. Post-event testing includes analysis of environmental elements associated with the event. These include water, air, radiation, or food.

QUARANTINE AND ISOLATION

Quarantine and isolation are words that conger up bleak and dark thoughts. For many, the idea of quarantine and isolation invokes the breakdown of all civic and Constitutional norms. For others, it provides a sense of comfort and protection. In public health, it is the last resort for containment and control of a situation that could extract a great price from the population. The price can be economic through lost production due to an infectious agent that prevents people from working or restricts individuals from traveling into an affected area. More important is the potential loss of life or long-term morbidity within a community that may be caused by an infectious agent if quarantine is not imposed.

Quarantine and isolation evokes images of the Middle Ages and people dying of bubonic plague. The practice of quarantine originated when cities unaffected by the plague prohibited potentially infected ships from docking in their harbors. In the United States, the right of public health agencies to impose a quarantine is derived from the U.S. Constitution's allocation of police powers.

Contemporary definitions of quarantine and isolation involve restricting the movement of sick persons or those presumed to be infected with a contagious disease. This is most often imposed in a hospital, but it can be undertaken at home or in a dedicated isolation facility. Quarantine and isolation can also restrict the movements of well persons who have been presumed to be exposed to a contagious disease. Such an action can be taken within a single home, a dedicated facility, or an entire community. Quarantine and isolation are usually requested with voluntary compliance. However, they can be legally imposed.

The processes for declaring quarantine and isolation vary from community to community. For most, the declaration of quarantine and isolation must be made by a designated public health official at the local, state, or federal level. The declaration and process for quarantine and isolation are governed by regulations.

Of major concern is how public health and local police will enforce a large-scale quarantine and isolation. Few, if any, cities have sufficient security forces to fully enact and protect the integrity of a large-scale quarantine. Even with the addition of resources such as the National Guard, major questions still exist. How will individuals be prevented from leaving an area or kept within their homes or public shelters? Are security personnel empowered to use force to maintain a quarantine and isolation? If so, how much and under what conditions? Infected individuals leaving a contaminated area have the potential to spread a lethal disease. Such questions do not have easy or clear-cut answers. The optimal resolution may be education of the general public prior to the issuance of a quarantine and isolation order.

As part of any preparation for a bioterrorist event, the general public should be told that quarantine and isolation are essential for their well-being. The success or failure of the quarantine and isolation, and subsequent life or death of many people, depends on everyone obeying a quarantine and isolation order. People should be told to seek shelter in place, which means that they should simply stop traveling and stay put. Sheltering in place minimizes the possibility of contaminating others while simultaneously protecting them. Remaining within the quarantine and isolation area increases the chances of receiving needed treatment or prophylaxis.

MASS PROPHYLAXIS

After calming the public's fears about a biological agent, an important role for public health is treating the general public. Most biological agents require prophylaxis within a day of exposure. Response times vary depending on the agent involved. The Centers for Disease Control and Prevention has produced guidance documents for administering prophylaxis to entire populations within a 10-day period (Centers for Disease Control and Prevention, 2004b). Some cities have reduced this period to five days or fewer. Every community and region should develop plans to ensure that all people can receive appropriate treatment in a timely manner.

Specific treatment depends on the agent that has been released. Antibiotics will be necessary if the agent is anthrax. If the agent is smallpox, vaccinations will be required. The federal government has developed a system to stockpile and move large amounts of drugs and other materials that may be needed during a biological attack or incident where pharmaceuticals and other medical supplies and equipment might be requested by state and local health authorities.

The program is known as the Strategic National Stockpile (Centers for Disease Control and Prevention, 2004c). The stockpile contains prepackaged pharmaceuticals, vaccines, medical supplies, and medical equipment to augment depleted state and local resources in the event of a terrorist attack or other emergency. These packages are stored at strategic locations around the country to ensure rapid delivery anywhere in the United States within 12 hours. Materials will be transported by truck or, in some cases, by air. All transportation protocols have been made in advance.

Following a federal decision to deploy supplies, materials from Strategic National Stockpile will typically arrive by air or ground in two phases. The first-phase shipment will arrive within 12 hours. A state need only ask for help, not for specific items. The program will ship a complete package of medical materials, including a variety of supplies that will be needed in the first hours of operation in response to several anticipated threats. Supplies also are available in separate packages known as *vendor managed inventory.* These packages can be tailored to provide pharmaceuticals, vaccines, medical supplies, and medical products specific to the suspected or confirmed agents.

A Technical Advisory Response Unit accompanies the first shipment of supplies. This unit has five or six Centers for Disease Control and Prevention employees. The unit's pharmacists, emergency responders, and logistics experts will advise local authorities on receiving, distributing, dispensing, replenishing, and recovering Strategic National Stockpile material.

Dispensing medication to the general public during a crisis requires extensive planning and coordination. Local public health agencies cannot accomplish this task alone. Local sites must be designated and set up to receive the public. The time frames for operation are locally established to ensure the public's protection from the biological agent. The most recent Centers for Disease Control and Prevention (2004b) recommendation allocates 10 days to treat an entire population. This can be accomplished by distributing pharmaceuticals through a small number of very large sites or many smaller locations. At each site, members of the general public should be educated, processed, and treated. An important component of processing is calming peoples' fears. Planners must address several important questions. How will the public be educated about the disease? How will they be informed about the location of the site and the treatment that is available? How will the sites be staffed? How will the staff be supported (fed and housed)? How will members of the public be processed and tracked?

If only a small portion of the population requires prophylaxis, only a small number of sites will be put into operation. The prospect of treating an entire population must be addressed in pre-event planning. Most public health agencies have insufficient staff to operate all treatment sites themselves. Volunteers will be required for many operational tasks. Local government employees may provide a ready source of volunteers. During a disaster such as a biological attack, many government services will be curtailed. Volunteers can be recruited from hospitals and other institutions as well as from the general public. All volunteers must be trained, credentialed, and periodically retrained. Volunteers' contact information must be accurately stored and periodically verified and revised as needed. The importance of volunteers who have been trained in advance cannot be overstated.

■ MASS TREATMENT

In the event of a bioterrorism incident, most public health employees will be performing services other than providing direct clinical care. However, their role in processing large segments of the population is critical. Public health workers may be called upon to provide education. A spokesperson must be designated and trained. All of the tasks delineated for preparing for and managing a disaster (see Chapters 26 and 28) also must be performed during a bioterrorism emergency.

Hospitals and their employees must accept the idea that typical levels of hospital care will not be provided during a mass treatment. If surge capacity is reached, resources will be spread thin and a series of difficult decisions will be required. Who will receive care quickly and who must wait? Some persons may not receive any care. Processing surges requires special resources and training. Public health professionals can assist in planning for these contingencies.

Planning for mass treatment must include identifying and securing alternate sites to provide care. These sites may include tents, empty buildings, or open fields. Key community stakeholders should aid in the selection of alternate sites. Planning for alternative sites and securing supplies and other resources are usually expedited when multiple stakeholders can provide input.

■ HOSPITAL COMMUNICATIONS

Reliable communication among hospitals, other sites, and public health leaders is required before, during, and after an event. Relationships must be established prior to an event so that all parties understand what the others provide and need and what communication modality works best for each partner. Simply making a personal introduction to a hospital infectious control practitioner will usually initiate a convenient working relationship.

Questions should provide useful information for both parties. One important goal of creating professional networks is obtaining surveillance data. Questions that require extensive effort (people and resources) to answer may be ignored during an event. Hospitals are understaffed during normal times. This situation is only likely to worsen during a crisis. Reassigning individuals from other jobs to gather data is also unlikely to occur during a bioterrorist attack.

Communication protocols must be established, tested, and evaluated prior to a bioterrorist attack. Even under the best conditions communications will be difficult. Test communication pathways and the ability to communicate under realistic conditions. When threat levels move from yellow to orange, make calls to contacts at local hospitals and test the pathways. At the same time, ask if any unusual events or increased numbers of patients have been seen. During an actual event, all parties will ask questions.

Communication will be a significant problem during a bioterrorism crisis. Channels must be established, secure, and reliable. These issues must be addressed during planning and training.

OTHER ISSUES

Mass Education

One of the most important services that public health can provide is educating the public about health issues. Before and during a biological crisis, public health must use its abilities to educate community members about the potential causes and available treatments for biological agents likely to be used in a bioterrorist attack. Prior to a biological crisis, the public should be educated about biological agents that pose a potential threat to the public's health. Even with extensive education, the public will require more information during a bioterrorism incident. Pathways for disseminating information should be established, tested, and evaluated during planning. Educating the general public can be accomplished in a variety of ways. Some of the typical methods for mass education are media releases, billboards, pamphlets, town hall meetings, and Web sites as well as hotlines for discussing concerns.

Sheltering in Place

Providing medication or treatment is burdensome in the best of times. When considering prophylaxis treatment for large segments of the population, how will the system ensure that the public receives the proper treatment? An important public health concern is that individuals who have been infected with a biological agent may leave the area. If individuals leave, they may spread the disease to other areas. Individuals who leave an area where medication is being dispensed may not receive the proper treatment in a timely manner. Sheltering in place provides a potentially useful solution. If the public is adequately and effectively educated prior to a crisis, they will know why they may need to shelter in place. Then, they can prepare by assembling the necessary food and supplies to accomplish the sheltering. While these actions are necessary, they also are likely to be stressful.

Stress Management

During a crisis, stresses multiply. Post-traumatic stress disorders may appear long after an event has been concluded. Resources for treating stress must be provided for public health workers as well as members of the general public. Remember that stress can be physical, mental, or emotional. It may emerge in a bewildering array of forms. Treatment options include institutional care, outpatient care, and home care. For many, a simple respite at home may be the most useful form of treatment.

Technology

During a disaster, many resources will be required in responding and resolving a biological crisis. Web-based technology will be used extensively, both in the collection and dissemination of information. Web sites that will be used in depicting the biological crisis and in providing appropriate responses should be established in advance. Other Web sites can be used to exchange information among local, state, and federal public health agencies. Some of this information will come from data that have been gathered, processed, and presented in graphical form.

Geographic Information Systems

Computers can translate and display data on maps. Data displayed in this way must contain information such as addresses, zip or area codes, or latitude and longitude coordinates. This type of information must be included when data are added to databases. Such information and displays are useful for tracking the number of sick or deceased individuals during a crisis or determining where they reside. This type of data display is useful in pre-event planning. Data can be stacked in layers. For example, the location of planned treatment centers can be displayed with maps depicting population density. Such an array would highlight areas of potential over- or underservice.

The Food Supply

It is important to remember that biological terrorism also can be directed at crops or farm animals. Unusual diseases or disease clusters in plants or animals should be evaluated by knowledgeable experts. Local governments should ensure that veterinarians and farmers are alerted to this possibility and informed as to where they should report any unusual outbreaks.

Funding

How do public health agencies continue to fund homeland security issues? A more important question is whether allocated funds have been used in the best possible manner. Spending money is relatively easy. Spending it wisely requires work and diligent effort. Building public health infrastructure is a significant challenge. Public health agencies have been underfunded and understaffed for years. Funding requests have been reduced, funds have shifted to other agencies, or funds have simply been misused. Public health must use monies allocated for homeland security to prepare adequate protection for responding to terrorist acts. A current concern of public health and political leaders is building an effective infrastructure that can respond to a bioterrorist attack in a timely and effective manner. Building infrastructure includes having trained people, adequate technology, well-planned responses, and a well-educated public. In the event of a bioterrorist attack, the cost of errors or unwise spending decisions will be measured in human lives and suffering.

CONCLUSION

Bioterrorism preparation requires cooperation from many constituent groups. Planning, exercising, and evaluating remain the hallmarks of preparation. Education of professionals and members of the general public is required.

The high school students decided to break into two-person teams. This would avoid overwhelming interviewees and allow sufficient resources to visit the relevant individuals and organizations. One pair of students visited the local health official. The official provided an overview of planning activities that had taken place since January 2002.

The following is a description of the various activities that have been undertaken. A steering committee has been formed. Members of the steering committee include the local police chief, fire chief, emergency services chief, hospital administrator, health commissioner, National Guard commander, county commissioner, editor of the daily newspaper, and chairs of the medicine and public health departments from a nearby university. The group meets every month.

Each member of the steering committee chairs a subcommittee that is responsible for the planning activities in a particular area. The police chief coordinates all area law enforcement personnel. Communications protocols have been written and tested. Dedicated telephone, facsimile, and computer lines have been developed. Telephone calling lists have been developed. Plans for quarantine have been discussed with the National Guard commander. Containment will be a major problem in the event of an emergency. The fire chief has assumed responsibility for decontamination activities. Arrangements have been made with a local mortuary to use the crematory facility if decontamination is needed. Representatives from the National Guard, the governor's office, and the state health commission have met with the local committee.

The emergency services chief is responsible for triage. Members of the public will be directed to appropriate shelters or treatment centers. This committee is also interested in establishing and maintaining surveillance methods. To date, they rely on personal relationships and communications for data. The group has submitted a grant request for funding to implement a computer-based surveillance system. If funded, it will take five years to implement the system.

The hospital administrator has been making arrangements for alternative locations to treat the public. This involves identifying and securing facilities as well as providing basic treatment and communication equipment at each site. A supervisor has been designated for each alternative treatment site. Personnel, largely volunteers, have been assigned to staff the alternate locations. Support for both volunteers and injured persons at the sites are being discussed at the present time. The first training exercise is scheduled for next month.

The health commissioner receives regular updates from the Centers for Disease Control and Prevention. She is training health department personnel in two other fields so that they can continue with normal services in the event of a bioterrorism emergency. The National Guard commander is meeting with federal officials from the U.S. Departments of Defense, Homeland Security, and Health and Human Services. Other government representatives have attended some meetings. The commander's most pressing problem is quarantine and isolation.

The county commissioner represents local elected officials. He is responsible for securing funds from a variety of sources to ensure that the county is ready for an attack that he hopes never comes. The editor of the daily newspaper is responsible for publicizing information and educating the general public. She works closely with colleagues in radio and television stations that serve the county. Protocols and generic outlines for press releases have been drafted.

The chair of public health from the local university supplies expertise, as needed, to all groups. He involves university students in the evaluation of committee operations. The chair of medicine also provides consultation as needed. He supplied the high school students with basic information on Bolivian hemorrhagic fever, also known as Machupo.

Bolivian hemorrhagic fever is caused by the Machupo virus, a member of the arenavirus family. The virus is carried by rats and spread through aerosols of their droppings. The onset of infection is slow and characterized by fever, malaise, headache, and muscle pains. Bleeding from the nose and gums are observed when the disease progresses to the hemorrhagic phase. Isolation of the virus requires Biosafety Level 4 facilities. The disease has an incubation period of 7 to 16 days. Nosebleeds and vomiting of blood occur in the first week of the disease. Fatality rates range from 3 to 30 percent. As of early 2004, no cases of Bolivian hemorrhagic fever had been linked to terrorism.

References

Centers for Disease Control and Prevention. Emergency preparedness and response. 2004a. Available at www.bt.cdc.gov/emcontact/determine.asp.

Centers for Disease Control and Prevention. 2004b. Bioterrorism information for healthcare. www.cdc.gov/ncidod/hip/Bio/bio.htm.

Centers for Disease Control and Prevention. 2004c. Strategic National Stockpile. Available at www.bt.cdc.gov/stockpile/index.asp.

Purver, R. 1995. Chemical and biological terrorism: The threat according to the open literature. Canadian Security Intelligence Service. Available at www.csis-scrs.gc.ca/eng/miscdocs/tabintre.html.

Resources

Periodicals

Blendon, R.J., Benson, J.M., Desroches, C.M., and Weldon, K.J. 2003. Using opinion surveys to track the public's response to a bioterrorist attack. *Journal of Health Communications* 8(Supplement 1):83–92.

Garcia, E., and Horton, D.A. 2003. Supporting the Federal Emergency Management Agency Rescuers: A variation of critical incident stress management. *Military Medicine* 168(2):87–90.

Guharoy, R., Panzik, R., Noviasky, J.A., Krenzelok, E.P., and Blair, D.C. 2004. Smallpox: Clinical features, prevention, and management. *Annals of Pharmacotherapy* 38(3):440–447.

Jacobs, L.M., Burns, K.J., and Gross, R.I. 2003. Terrorism: A public health threat with a trauma system response. *Journal of Trauma* 55(6):1014–1021.

Jacobs, L.M., Emanuelsen, K., McKay, C., and Burns, K. 2004. Bioterrorism preparedness—Part II. Smallpox vaccination in a hospital setting. *Connecticut Medicine* 68(1):27–35.

May, T., Aulisio, M.P., and Silverman, R.D. 2003. The smallpox vaccination of health care workers: Professional obligations and defense against bioterrorism. *Hastings Center Report* 33(5):26–33.

Mitchell, A.M., Sakraida, T.J., and Kameg, K. 2003. Critical incident stress debriefing: Implications for best practice. *Disaster Management and Response* 1(2):46–51.

O'Connor, M.J., Buckeridge, D.L., Choy, M., Crubezy, M., Pincus, Z., Musen, M.A. 2003. BioSTORM: A system for automated surveillance of diverse data sources. *Proceedings of the American Medical Informatics Association Symposium* 1071–1078.

Ollerton, J.E. 2004. Emergency department response to the deliberate release of biological agents. *Emergency Medical Journal* 21(1):5–8.

Pennington, H. 2003. Smallpox and bioterrorism. *Bulletin of the World Health Organization* 81(10):762–767.

Reich, D.S. 2003. Modernizing local responses to public health emergencies: Bioterrorism, epidemics, and the model state emergency health powers act. *Journal of Contemporary Health Law Policy* 19(2):379–414.

Sandman, P.M. 2003. Bioterrorism risk communication policy. *Journal of Health Communications* 8(Supplement 1):146–151.

Sidel, V.W. 2003. Bioterrorism in the United States: A balanced assessment of risk and response. *Medicine, Conflict, and Survival* 19(4):318–325.

Sinha, G. 2004. Uncertain threat. Does smallpox really spread that easily? *Scientific American* 290(1):18–20.

Books

Clarke, G., and Stillwell, J. 2003. *Applied GIS and Spatial Analysis.* New York: Wiley.

Hillard, R., Zitek, B., and Gebler, B. 2003. *Emergency Psychiatry.* New York: McGraw-Hill.

Lindler, L., Lebeda, F., and Korch, G. 2004. *Biological Weapons Defense: Principles and Mechanisms for Infectious Diseases Counter-Bioterrorism.* Totowa, NJ: Humana Press.

Maantay, J., and Ziegler, J. 2004. *GIS for the Urban Environment.* Redlands, CA: ESRI.

National Institute of Medicine. 1999. *Chemical and Biological Terrorism: Research and Development to Improve Civilian Medical Response.* Washington, D.C.: National Academy Press.

National Institute of Medicine. 2002. *Countering Bioterrorism: The Role of Science and Technology.* Washington, D.C.: National Academy Press.

Ralston, B. 2004. *GIS and Public Data.* Albany, NY: Delmar Learning.

Ursano, R.J., Fullerton, C.S., and Norwood, A.E. 2004. *Bioterrorism: Psychological and Public Health Interventions.* New York: Cambridge University Press.

von Lubitz, D.K. 2003. *Bioterrorism: Field guide to Disease Identification and Initial Patient Management.* Boca Raton, FL: CRC Press.

Von Meyer, N. 2004. *GIS and Land Records.* Redlands, CA: ESRI.

Web Sites

- Health Resources and Services Administration:
  www.hrsa.gov/bioterrorism.htm
- Johns Hopkins University, Center for Civilian Biodefense Studies:
  www.hopkins-biodefense.org
- Laboratory Response Network:
  www.phppo.cdc.gov/nltn/pdf/LRN99.pdf
- National Academy of Science:
  www.nap.edu/firstresponders
- National Center for Post-Traumatic Stress Disorder:
  www.ncptsd.org
- National Institute of Mental Health, Post-Traumatic Stress Disorder:
  www.nimh.nih.gov/anxiety/ptsdri1.cfm
- Occupational Safety and Health Administration:
  www.osha.gov/SLTC/biologicalagents/bioterrorism.html
- St. Louis University, Center for the Study of Bioterrorism:
  www.bioterrorism.slu.edu
- U.S. Department of Justice, Office for State & Local Domestic Preparedness Support:
  www.ojp.usjoj.gov/osldps
- U.S. Food and Drug Administration:
  www.fda.gov/oc/opacom/hottopics/bioterrorism.html

Organizations

Association for Professionals in Infection Control and Epidemiology
1275 K Street, NW, Suite 1000
Washington, D.C. 20005-4006
Phone: 202-789-1890
Fax: 202-789-1899
E-mail: APICinfo@apic.org
Web site: www.apic.org

Centers for Disease Control and Prevention
1600 Clifton Road
Atlanta, GA 30333
Phone: 404-639-3311, 404-639-3534, or 800-311-3435
E-mail: www.cdc.gov/netinfo.htm (Web form)
Web site: www.cdc.gov

Federal Emergency Management Agency
500 C Street, SW
Washington, D.C. 20472
Phone: 202-566-1600
Web site: www.fema.gov

U.S. Department of Homeland Security
Washington, D.C. 20528
Web site: www.dhs.gov/dhspublic/index.jsp

U.S. Environmental Protection Agency
1200 Pennsylvania Ave., NW
Washington, D.C. 20460-0001
Phone: 202-272-0167
Web site: www.epa.gov

U.S. Food and Drug Administration
5600 Fishers Lane
Rockville, MD 20857-0001
Phone: 888-463-6332
Web site: www.fda.gov

PART

VII

The Media

CHAPTER

30

The Media: Cultivating Contacts and Developing Relationships

Jan Larson

Chapter Objectives

After reading this chapter, readers will:

- Understand the importance of not letting members of the media see fear.
- Remember that "public" is an important aspect of public health.
- Know how to avoid making obvious errors when working with the media.
- Recognize the importance of cooperating with members of the media.
- Appreciate that relationships with members of the media can be cordial.
- When speaking publicly, recognize the importance of using words that members of the general public will understand.
- Understand that members of the media have a job to do.
- Recognize the importance of making oneself available to the media.

Chapter Summary

This chapter is about relationships between the public health community and members of the media. The media encompasses newspapers, magazines, television, radio, and the Internet. The format of this chapter differs from that of most of the others in this book. The author of this chapter is a county editor for a daily newspaper serving a population in excess of 100,000. She has been recognized by professional organizations for the quality of her work. The chapter not only provides information, but also serves as an example that exemplifies contemporary standards for writing.

Case Study

A junior member from the local board of health and an assistant health commissioner were talking about an upcoming board meeting. The board member wanted to approach the local newspaper and request that the paper prepare an article about the results of a year-long bicycle safety program. The number of bicycle-related injuries had declined over the year. Further, the number of cyclists seen wearing bike helmets had increased dramatically. The board member recalled seeing another board colleague become embarrassed during a recent interaction with a television reporter. The assistant health commissioner agreed that the success of the bike program was indeed newsworthy, but was worried about adverse publicity from problems encountered during a restaurant inspection during the previous month.

One board of health member said, "I am considering making up an emergency so that I can leave the meeting early."

The assistant health commissioner replied, "That sounds like a good idea. I always get flustered when talking to a reporter."

What advice would you offer to each of these persons?

■ INTRODUCTION

Some in the public health profession view working with the media as a necessary evil. They realize that they need the media to get news out to the most people in the least amount of time. The relationship between public health and the media doesn't have to be an unpleasant and adversarial one. In fact, it can be very rewarding to team up with the media in serving the public. However, it doesn't mean it will be easy. People who have worked in the public health profession often realize very quickly that the media can be their best friend and an effective tool to reach out to citizens or it can be their worst enemy during an already stressful situation. Following are some suggestions on how to establish a good relationship with the media in the first place and how to exercise it to keep it healthy.

DON'T LET THEM SEE YOUR FEAR

Many public health professionals are comfortable with communicable diseases and hazardous chemicals, but put a microphone in their faces and they freeze up with fear. The thought of being quoted in a newspaper or filmed for the six o'clock news is enough to make them forget every bit of training they have mastered over the years.

So the first bit of advice is crucial: Don't wait until a crisis is raging before you meet representatives of the local media. The fact is, if a reporter knows you on a personal basis before a big story breaks, the less likely he or she will be to go for the jugular. The same goes for the media's relationship with public health officials. The more you know them, the more likely you will be to share information with them. And ultimately, that will benefit the public.

Some television stations and newspapers require their staff to introduce themselves to health department staff before a crisis occurs, according to Steve France, assignment manager for the Fox news station in Toledo, Ohio. "The better you know somebody, the more cooperative people are going to be," says France, who has been in the TV news business for 18 years.

AS UNCOMFORTABLE AS YOU MAY FEEL, REMEMBER THAT IT IS "PUBLIC" HEALTH

Working with the media may not show up in most public health classes and textbooks, but it is a necessary part of the job. And good public health officials who establish good working relationships with the media think of themselves as truly public officials. They realize that working with the media, as unpleasant as it may be at times, can actually pay off for the health department and its citizens.

Such officials do not view the media as an enemy, but rather as a valuable partner. Health department board members need to come to the same realization. If they fail to conduct their business as a "public" board, problems will eventually catch up to them. "Use reporters to get health information facts out to the public," suggests Wood County Board of Health member Alice Davis. "Consider reporters as part of the health care team."

Reporters can tell their readers or viewers how to prevent the spread of West Nile virus, list when the next flu vaccines will be offered, calm their fears about a meningitis outbreak, and tell them which local stores were caught selling cigarettes to minors. They can reach vast numbers of people in a 30-second news bite or a few lines of newsprint. Of course, that's in an ideal world.

HORROR STORIES AND HOW TO AVOID THEM

Nearly everyone who has had to deal with the media has at least one horrendous tale to tell—some are embarrassingly funny, others are genuinely hurtful. Though she can laugh at it now, years later, communicable disease nurse Amy Jones in Wood County, Ohio, recalls being the immediate center of attention when some children were infected with Hepatitis A after eating at an elementary school cafeteria. With the microphones thrust into her face, Jones was trying to answer the questions of the impatient reporters. She was horrified that night as she watched the evening news. The one clip that wasn't cut out of the story showed Jones answering the question about where the elementary children and staff were electing to get their shots. "Most of them got it in the butt," Jones responded. This was not exactly the quote she wanted to be remembered by, but Jones turned the embarrassing moment into a learning experience. "I think you need a bad experience to make you think—I shouldn't have said that," she said. "Experience is your best teacher."

But some bad experiences with the media can't be laughed at, even years later. Though nearly two decades have passed, Health Commissioner Larry Sorrells still remembers the sting of negative publicity when his health department in Wood County, Ohio, investigated a possible heightened number of child leukemia cases in the northern portion of the county. To this day, Sorrells can recall the first meeting between public health officials and worried residents. On one side of the table were the health representatives and on the other were the parents holding ill children. And in the middle of it all, of course, was the media. "It was the worst time in my career," Sorrells recalls. "There were implications we were hiding something."

Many public health officials know all too well how it feels to be ambushed by the media.

Brad Espen, director of environmental services at the Wood County Health Department, still remembers one of his first experiences with the media when he was visiting a trailer park with sewer problems. Espen had agreed to an on-camera interview, but was not informed that an angry crowd would be awaiting his arrival at the park. "I walked into it with the cameras rolling," Espen recalls.

HOW TO GET THE MEDIA TO PLAY NICE

No matter how much blame public health officials may place on the media for poor reporting, most will admit that they play a big role in how a story is played.

Above all else, don't say "no comment." Those words ring of one thing—that you as a public health official know something and won't share it with the public, which believes it has the right to share in your knowledge. Don't let those words come out of your mouth.

Next, be honest. "Lay the facts out as you know them," Sorrells advises.

And don't speculate. "If you don't know an answer, say so. Be honest, calm and nonconfrontational," Espen says. If you don't know the answer to a question, try to get the answer as quickly as possible.

Don't use "off the record" unless you understand exactly what it means. You can't blurt something out and then think it will magically not appear on tape or in print by quickly adding "off the record." That guarantee only works if you utter "off the record" before you reveal some information, and only if the reporter agrees to the deal.

According to Espen, the best advice is "If you don't want it printed, don't say it." And before you start talking, be aware of what information you can release and what is confidential. You don't want to be in the middle of a press conference and suddenly realize that you are sharing confidential information. "Try to think hypothetically what the questions may be and how you can answer them," Espen says.

And don't forget, if the news story is big enough, your agency won't be the only one involved. That means you will need to coordinate with other agencies exactly who will be releasing information and what details they will be reporting.

■ IT CAN BE A ROSY RELATIONSHIP

Don't be discouraged; many public health officials do have healthy relationships with the media.

Newspapers and TV news stations can quickly get the word out about critical situations such as rabies cases, SARS prevention, anthrax scares, and sewage leaks. When the crisis is over, if a reporter has found you to be open and honest, he or she will be far more likely to come back to do a feature story on your health department's food inspections, efforts to prevent teen pregnancies, and suggestions on how to keep mosquitoes from populating local properties. And then, if you're lucky, the reporter will come back again when you ask him or her to do a story on your health department levies on the upcoming ballot or your effort to get public comments on a local health assessment. The reporter may even help explain to the public that you are raising the costs for birth and death certificate copies because the state is forcing you to do so.

According to Ned Baker, founder of the National Association of Local Boards of Health, "An effective trustworthy working relationship between the health department and the news media makes the news media a partner in the community's public health system." In addition, according to Espen, "Trust is the big thing."

Don't fall for the false notion that just because you are surrounded by public health programs everyday that everyone else in your community knows what services you provide. So let the media do just that for you—let them tell your citizens through photographs, sound bites, and stories what your personnel do for the public.

And remember, if you play nice, most media will play fair.

HOW TO SPEAK THEIR LANGUAGE

You went through years of higher education so you could speak eloquently using 15-letter medical or environmental terms—but the media has not. And neither have the vast majority of the readers and viewers. So don't bother trying to impress the media or the public with your professional jargon. You won't impress anyone; you will just lose them before you get any important information across to them.

And worse yet, you may even lead to inaccurate information being spread. If the reporter doesn't understand what you are saying, there is no way he or she can relay that information to the public. Resist the temptation to use huge words and jargon that means something to others in your profession, but nobody else.

In addition, remember that not everyone knows what all those acronyms mean that you and your colleagues use in your everyday speech. You will need to spell out exactly what the acronyms mean so your media coverage doesn't look like a confusing bowl of alphabet soup.

That may mean you have to take it down a notch. It's not that the public is dumb, they just want their information in easily digestible bites. "I've always believed in the KISS theory—keep it simple stupid," board member Alice Davis says. This not only refers to the level of information shared, but also the quantity. You may have countless bits of information about smallpox vaccinations or the dangers of secondhand smoke, but stick to the basics. Give the media the most important data—what they absolutely must know. Otherwise, your three most important facts may get lost in the laundry list of other details. "I try to water it down as much as possible," Espen says. That way it may actually be digestible to the average person.

KEEP IN MIND, YOU AREN'T THE ONLY ONE DOING A JOB

OK, you may take your role as a public health official very seriously, but many media people take theirs quite seriously as well. So to get the most accomplished together, you should be ready to meet some of the needs of the media.

If you want reporters to pick up on a story, learn how to type up a simple press release or get used to picking up the phone and calling a reporter. Make your story sound appealing, but stick to the facts. They need to know the five w's and h—who, what, where, when, why and how. Try to cover as many of those as possible in press releases.

And realize that the media doesn't just want the happy stories. They want the bad ones, too. So the best you can do when an issue arises is to get ready for the possible flood of media. "When you see something coming, prepare for it," Sorrells advises.

Be prepared to meet some pretty demanding deadlines. Whereas newspapers have a 24-hour cycle to collect their news, TV reporters are sometimes on a constant treadmill of covering stories. Consequently, they can be quite ruthless at times. "There's a difference with TV reporters," Espen says, "They're awfully aggressive and they just show up." "I'll know right away when I talk to a reporter if I'm going to be open with them or not," he says. "You can tell prior to them turning on the camera what kind of interview it will be."

Be prepared to experience a wide range of news-collecting styles, depending on the type of media covering your agency. Although health department personnel may have a comfort level working with their local newspaper reporters, that may disappear the second a national news story occurs in your area. You will undoubtedly notice a huge difference between working with local and national media.

National journalists tend to attack a story much more aggressively. If your department is at the center of a national story, you should prepare to be swamped by media—very quickly. National media can be at the source of any story within a couple hours, and they want answers when they get there.

Many health departments have predetermined public information officers who handle the bulk of questions from the media. Though that one person is the face that appears in front of the camera, their statements are the result of several people within the health department deciding what information will be released.

AS MUCH AS IT HURTS, MAKE YOURSELF TRULY ACCESSIBLE

Remember, if the media doesn't get answers from you, they will have to go somewhere else to get their questions answered—and that information may not be as accurate as you would like. So make yourself available. Don't dart out after a meeting, a press conference, or an interview. Though your fear and flight instinct may be overwhelming, stick around for questions. "Be perceived as trustworthy, honest, and available to the news media," Baker suggests. And be aware that the media has some pretty tricky deadlines to deal with—especially TV. It only counts if you are available when and where they need you. "They have to be available for live clips," France, of Fox News, says. "Being available is key. In our case, we need it now."

In crisis situations, when you are juggling 50 different duties at once, don't leave the media hanging. Ignoring them will only result in poor coverage of the story. Bite the bullet and talk with them. "Come and talk to us," France says. "As soon as you answer our questions, we will leave."

And don't make the mistake that some agencies make in allowing only one person to speak with the media—and then fail to make sure that person will be available.

"The worst scenario is if you have a head honcho and no one else is allowed to talk," France says. Learn to trust others in your organization to deal with the media in their areas of expertise. They may go through the painful educational process of learning to work with the media, but it will pay off in the end. "Designate and delegate to other key staff the capability of meeting and talking with news media on specific program areas," Baker advises.

■ DON'T JUST SHARE THE GOOD NEWS

Don't expect the media to put the word out about your upcoming health levy if you don't share with them the bad food-inspection reports. And don't expect reporters to rush to publish your influenza vaccine clinics if you won't give them the messy details on the latest meth (methamphetamine) labs found in your jurisdiction. Sharing the good and bad news will not only strengthen your relationship with the media, but also with the public. Your citizens want to know you can be trusted to give them the truth—even when it's not particularly pretty.

Like most relationships, absence does not actually make it stronger; it makes it fade into a distant, perhaps waning, memory. So stay in touch with your media contacts, even when there is no big story looming. Suggest story ideas, but don't push for immediate coverage. Just like you, the media is juggling several different topics at once, and it will get to yours when there is time.

In fact, when you least expect it, your story idea may work its way to the top of the news pile—especially during a slow news day.

This doesn't mean that you should regurgitate every insignificant item discussed during your last board of health meeting in a press release in hopes of getting more media coverage. The reporters won't care, and neither will the public. And don't bury important information that you want the media to notice in a droll press release. It may never get the notice it deserves if you don't present it as something newsworthy to begin with.

And try this—confront an issue with the media before the reporters come knocking on your door. If a story arises that you know the media will want to cover, don't try to bury it. Concealing information often backfires and results in your agency looking as if it is trying to hide information that the public deserves to know. And calling your media contacts about a story will help you earn their trust on this and future stories.

SO LET'S KEEP IT SIMPLE

If you want to make the most out of your relationship with the media, you have to do your part:

- Send clearly worded press releases to your pre-established media contacts or give them a call and explain very plainly what you want.
- Respect the media's deadlines. It may make it tough for you, but news deadlines can be very demanding—especially TV news. They won't wait for you, so if you don't give them accurate information, they will go elsewhere to get whatever information they can get a hold of as their next deadline looms.
- Be very, very aware of the words coming out of your mouth. You don't want to see something horrible show up in a 30-second sound bite.

In exchange, you can reap some wonderful rewards from working side by side with the media:

- Your health department can become a household word—and a positive one at that. The public can actually gain a real understanding of your role in aiding public health.
- A healthy relationship with the media ensures you coverage of a wide range of services provided by your agency. It could bring heartfelt stories about your nurses' visits with new inexperienced mothers or stories of how your sanitarians helped rid a neighborhood of nuisance rodents.
- Realize that you can't get the word out by yourself—at least not as fast or as thoroughly. If you want your public to reduce standing water in their yards to prevent mosquitoes or if you want people to take precautions to avoid an epidemic, you must turn to the media. So learn how to make the most of it.

Remember, it's up to you to make sure your relationship doesn't go sour with the media. That doesn't mean you need to sweet talk reporters. Just give them the truth. Then they will go away . . . and come back again when you need them to get the word out again to your public.

SOURCES

The following people were interviewed during the preparation of this chapter:

- Ned Baker, founder of the National Association of Local Boards of Health
- Alice Davis, member of Wood County Board of Health, Bowling Green, Ohio

- Brad Espen, Director of Environmental Services for Wood County Health Department, Bowling Green, Ohio
- Steve France, Assignment Editor for Fox news station in Toledo, Ohio
- Amy Jones, Communicable Disease Nurse for Wood County Health Department, Bowling Green, Ohio
- Larry Sorrells, Health Commissioner for Wood County Health Department, Bowling Green, Ohio

CONCLUSION

Returning to the conference that preceded the regular health board meeting, the board member and assistant health commissioner sought advice from a colleague who had experience interacting with members of the media. Recalling that reporters are busy, the health department drafted a document package about the bicycle safety program. It contained two versions of a press release, one short and one long. It also had a page of bulleted facts and results for reporters to use in formulating their own reports or in asking questions. A list of individuals and contact information comprised the last sheet of the media package. A computer disk contained electronic copies of the text and several digital photographs for illustration.

The assistant health commissioner invited the reporter who usually attended the health board meeting to meet for coffee. The agenda was simply to get acquainted. They agreed to meet again the next week. At that time, the reporter proposed printing a regular column about the results of all restaurant inspections. Members of the public had a right to know about the food they were consuming. The possibility of adverse publicity should help to promote better food-handling procedures. With approval from the board of health, the column began the next month. Over the next year, the number of food-service inspection violations declined.

The morning coffee meetings became regular events. Over the next few months, the newspaper agreed to co-sponsor the bicycle safety campaign for the next year. The assistant health commissioner had chided the reporter that supporting a safety program decreased the probability of having bad news to report. The newspaper's publisher called this an investment in the community and a way to generate good news that would be reported.

Resources

Periodicals

Emerson, D. 2003. When medicine makes the news. *Minnesota Medicine* 86(4):26–31.

Kertesz, L. 2003. The numbers behind the news. Helping the public understand medical research results. *Healthplan* 44(5):10–18.

Mullin, S. 2003. Getting to know you: Forging relationships between public health and the press. *Journal of Urban Health* 80(1):5–6.
Stewart, C.N. 2003. Press before paper—when media and science collide. *Nature Biotechnology* 21(4):353–354.

Books

Brown, L. 2004. *Media Relations for Public Safety Professionals.* Sudbury, MA: Jones & Bartlett.
Diggs-Brown, B., and Glou, J.L.G. 2003. *Public Relations Style Guide: Formats for Public Relations Practice.* Belmont, CA: Wadsworth.
Henslowe, P. 2003. *Public Relations: A Practical Guide to the Basics.* London: Kogan Page.
Salzman, J. 2003. *Making the News (revised).* Boulder, CO: Perseus Publishing.
Schenkler, I., and Herrling, T. 2003. *Guide to Media Relations.* Upper Saddle River, NJ: Prentice-Hall.

Web Sites

- American Public Health Association, Media Advocacy Manual: www.sph.uth.tmc.edu/cahp/media-advocacy.htm
- Americans for Non-Smoker's Rights, Media Guide: www.no-smoke.org/media.html
- Centers for Disease Control and Prevention, Office of Communication, Media Relations: www.cdc.gov/od/oc/media
- Henry J. Kaiser Family Foundation: www.kff.org/about/publicopinion.cfm
- Institute for Public Strategies: www.healthadvocacy.org
- Massachusetts Public Heath Organization: www.mphaweb.org/advocacy.html

Organizations

American Public Health Association
800 I Street, NW
Washington, D.C. 20001-3710
Phone: 202-777-2742
Fax: 202-777-2534
E-mail: comments@apha.org
Web site: www.apha.org

Annenberg Public Policy Center
3620 Walnut Street
Philadelphia, PA 19104-6220
Phone: 215-898-7041
Fax: 215-898-2024
E-mail: appcdc@appcpenn.org
Web site: www.annenbergpublicpolicycenter.org

Centers for Disease Control and Prevention
1600 Clifton Road
Atlanta, GA 30333
Phone: 404-639-3311, 404-639-3534, or 800-311-3435
E-mail: www.cdc.gov/netinfo.htm (Web form)
Web site: www.cdc.gov

Environmental and Energy Study Institute
122 C Street, NW, Suite 630
Washington, D.C. 20001
Phone: 202-628-1400
Fax: 202-628-1825
E-mail: eesi@eesi.org
Web site: www.eesi.org

CHAPTER

31

Managing the Flow of Information

L. Fleming Fallon, Jr.
Eric Zgodzinski

Chapter Objectives

After reading this chapter, readers will:

- Understand media relations from the perspective of public health.
- Know how to establish working relations with members of the media.
- Appreciate that members of the media should be involved with public health projects and programs early on.
- Know how to identify available media outlets.
- Understand the importance of providing materials to the media in a usable and accessible format.
- Appreciate the value of honesty in relations with members of the media.

Chapter Summary

The media is a diverse collection of formats, outlets, and working professionals. Persons working in public health must understand and learn to work with members of the media. Honesty and integrity provide important foundations for any relationships between people working in either field. Neither field can or should control the other. Both must work in cooperation. Relationships and rules for interacting must be developed and agreed on in advance. Members of the media can become important allies of public health.

Case Study

Hank had been working for the health department for over 30 years. He was convinced that he had witnessed all of the events that public health could deliver. For Hank, there were no more surprises. Tom was a relatively new employee, having joined the health department just over three years ago. Tom had made a point of cultivating friendships with several people who worked in different forms of the media.

"Tom," said Hank, "why do you waste your time talking to those people who work for the newspaper and the radio and television station?"

"They are my friends," replied Tom.

"Friends, huh?" shot back Hank. "Anyone can tell you that friendships are not possible with members of the media. They are just out for a story."

"Hank, you just don't get it," said Tom, starting to walk away.

"Tom, you have a lot to learn. It is you who does not get it," mumbled Hank to no one in particular.

What comments would you offer to Hank or Tom?

INTRODUCTION

The goal of public health departments is to protect the health of the people they serve. Elements of the media are integral partners in this process. Information must be disseminated. By extension, relations with the media are important to the success of a local health department. A professional journalist wrote Chapter 30. It presents the viewpoint of a member of the media. This chapter presents similar material. However, it is written from the perspective of a local health department.

The effectiveness of any agency may be measured in terms of how well it attains its goals. A measure of the effectiveness of a local health department is an evaluation of the success of agency programs. The local board of health and the local health department are public servants. The public must be made aware of the programs provided by a health agency so that individuals may benefit from the services offered. A health agency also has the responsibility to inform and educate its public about health issues and dangers. This responsibility extends to the larger community and can include influencing policy and laws that impact public health.

Board budgets are typically too limited for conducting the entire scope of programs and services that are desired. To try and increase budgetary allocations, local departments of health and their controlling boards may want to enlist the assistance and cooperation of community officials, educators, volunteer organizations, and others who can contribute to successfully meeting relevant goals and objectives. Various forms of the media such as billboards, newspapers, radio, television, and other print outlets are efficient means by which to disseminate information. Media representatives should be courted so that they will cooperate with their local board of health.

It is difficult for any person, let alone a public health official, to view someone in the media as a friend. However, because of information-sharing needs, the pace of information exchange, a more knowledgeable public, and the numerous concerns of public health, it is wise to learn how to befriend and work with members of the media. As with any relationship, both parties must benefit from the partnership. If there is not a sound partnership between public health and the media, public health will usually be the loser.

INCORPORATE THE MEDIA FROM THE BEGINNING

Projects and programs are the means by which a health agency achieves its goals and objectives. Media representatives may be included as advisers early in the planning process. They can be instrumental in suggesting effective media strategies. Their effective communication experience in working with members of the public in the past can help sharpen the focus of a media plan. Members of the media can help identify the best means of reaching the desired target audiences. They may assist in rallying other media outlets by networking within and across the various media formats. They may have information on additional resources for the project, including funds. Editors, reporters, and journalists know local politicians and trends and understand how to be effective within their communities. When politicians and members of the public understand agency goals, media representatives are likely to support the agency's objectives. They will have become highly desired team members.

In most situations, appropriate representatives of the media should be brought in at the beginning of a project or program. A health department or any other public health entity should be prepared and have accurate information assembled before calling upon the media. To minimize chances of misinformation, members of the media should be informed early in a situation and kept abreast of a project or program's development on a regular basis.

The media is a key component to successfully promoting public health. Working relationships must be built for two main reasons. First, when trust exists, there is a greater probability of the media responding to a request for assistance from the public health community. Second, relations based on trust are less likely to be attacked than are nonexistent or antagonistic relationships. The most important beneficiary of a successful working relationship is a community and its people, because they will benefit from the receipt of accurate and timely information.

IDENTIFY AVAILABLE MEDIA OUTLETS

Investigate the scope of media options that are present. Read their publications, newsletters, flyers, or billboards. Watch or listen to regional and local television and radio shows. Become well informed about the policies and politics surrounding each media source. Know who owns, operates, and influences each media form. Determine the methods and style of operation of the different personalities within the various types of media. Identify the industry leaders in each media area. Note which media businesses and individuals are reputable, fair, and unbiased. Identify the audiences of each media source.

Develop a file for each of the locally available media outlets. Determine which ones are effectively reaching the different age, ethnic, culture, occupational, religions, educational, and economic groups in the community. Build and maintain a file of the contact persons, reporters, program technicians, directors, and administrators who work in each organization. Select the format and staff personalities that are best able to facilitate the attainment of departmental objectives. After considering the target audience, time line, and available funds, select the preferred and alternate media outlets to approach for assistance in promoting departmental objectives for the year. Make appointments to meet with lead media people. Schedule meetings in their offices.

Before involving any members of the media, public health must prepare itself. This involves reviewing policy objectives and program goals. Objectives for the media should be established and discussed. Ground rules for interactions between public health and members of the media also must be established and discussed. Involved persons must agree to any ground rules before they can be considered to be binding on all parties.

DEVELOP WORKING RELATIONSHIPS

Expect to take the lead in establishing media relationships. Media employees are always busy with immediate tasks. Current work always has priority. Something else is usually emerging that demands their attention. It is necessary to become a respected, friendly, and familiar name so that you can promote the work of the health department. Media representatives are most receptive to organizations' whose messages they are familiar with and whose purpose is valued. Become a regular attendee at public meetings and community events. When possible, become a supporter or collaborator for community events.

Ground rules are extremely important when dealing with the media. These should be established and agreed on in advance. Discussions about information or materials are always on the record. Requests for discussions to be off the record must be made and agreed upon by all parties in advance of the conversation.

PROVIDE MATERIAL

It is important to remember that the media frequently uses short (10 to 15 second) sound bites. Comments may be reported in a different context than they were originally presented. Careful initial drafting and meticulous revision improves messages and press releases. Material that is distributed at a press conference or with a press release kit should be supplied with supporting explanatory information. Better yet, it should be provided on a computer disk in a format that can be readily used.

The media selected to promote a program objective must be suitable for the target audience. Some types of media target very specific audiences. Some are simply preferred by a specific segment of society. It is estimated that Americans are exposed to 5,000 advertisements each day. There is great competition for people's attention. Regardless of the content, an organization's message must be appealing, timely, relevant, and brief. The role of the media is to get people's attention, to provide information, and to convey a message. Public health uses the media to address public health needs. Offer to provide information on health issues by giving talks to civic organizations. Volunteer to be available for radio and television news interviews and for other programs. Submit text for radio and television news spots. Offer to write occasional health-related news stories. A health agency must be visible in its community. The head of the agency should be a familiar name.

Sharing factual health wellness information and giving inoculations are not the only goals of a health agency. Knowledge of facts alone seldom results in changed health behaviors that lead to improved health. The social and economic environments of community neighborhoods have significant roles in determining health. A local health department has a responsibility to address broad social and economic conditions that contribute to public health problems. Support for improving public health must come from a community-wide base. Media should be viewed as a tool to secure this community base. An established base can then implement and support responsible public health policies in its community. In return, the health agency will be helping the media do its job.

BE HONEST

A health agency cannot be effective if the public's respect and trust have not been earned. One statement that is interpreted or shown to be false or misleading will undermine an agency's integrity and standing in its community. It may take years to repair the damage to an agency's reputation. A health agency has a job to perform and a responsibility to the public it serves.

Share reasonable information that is not misleading. Hold timely new conferences and provide information through periodic press releases. If information is not available, admit it. Never make up facts. More than the reputation of the source is at risk. A health department is a public agency and has a responsibility to the public to be honest and forthright.

CONCLUSION

Members of the media are working professionals just as are people working on behalf of public health. The latter must understand the former to maximize public health–media relationships. Both parties must learn to work together. Honesty and integrity are critical for successful and ongoing interactions. Ground rules and relationships for interacting must be delineated and agreed on in advance. Members of the media and public health can become mutually important allies.

Hank, the older employee in the case study, did not trust members of the media. By avoiding them, Hank had lost some valuable opportunities to promote and improve public health. Members of the community were the real losers. Without the media, they were denied access to Hank's experience and expertise.

Tom, the younger employee, must be careful not to break confidences or divulge information that might lead to panic. On balance, though, his approach was sensible. He had established a rapport with members of the media. Tom's friends regularly sought his opinion on matters pertaining to public health. He was careful to be honest, knowing that his reputation could be permanently tarnished by supplying false information.

Resources

Periodicals

Haugen, M. 2003. When you're the source. *Minnesota Medicine* 86(4):62–63.

Snow, A.A., and Pilson, D. 2003. Clarifying press before paper. *Nature Biotechnology* 21(6):597–598.

Wilner, A.N. 2003. Physicians and the press. What to say, what not to say. *Medical Economics* 80(13):87–88.

Books

Baines, P., Egan, J., and Jefkins, F. 2003. *Public Relations: Contemporary Issues and Techniques*, 3d ed. New York: Butterworth-Heinemann.

Carstarphen, M.G., and Wells, R.A. 2003. *Writing PR: A Multimedia Approach*. Boston: Allyn and Bacon.

Merlis, G. 2003. *How to Make the Most out of Every Media Appearance: Getting Your Message Across on Air, in Print, and Online*. New York: McGraw-Hill.

Stewart, S. 2003. *Media Training 101: A Guide to Meeting the Press*. New York: John Wiley.

Web Sites

- American Public Health Association, Media Advocacy Manual: www.sph.uth.tmc.edu/cahp/media-advocacy.htm
- Centers for Disease Control and Prevention, Office of Communication, Media Relations:
  www.cdc.gov/od/oc/media
- Johns Hopkins University School of Public Health Center for Communication Programs:
  www.jhuccp.org/topics/advocacy.shtml

Organizations

American Public Health Association
800 I Street, NW
Washington, D.C. 20001-3710
Phone: 202-777-2742
Fax: 202-777-2534
E-mail: comments@apha.org
Web site: www.apha.org

Annenberg Public Policy Center
3620 Walnut Street
Philadelphia, PA 19104-6220
Phone: 215-898-7041
Fax: 215-898-2024
E-mail: appcdc@appcpenn.org
Web site: www.annenbergpublicpolicycenter.org

Centers for Disease Control and Prevention
1600 Clifton Road
Atlanta, GA 30333
Phone: 404-639-3311, 404-639-3534, or 800-311-3435
E-mail: www.cdc.gov/netinfo.htm (Web form)
Web site: www.cdc.gov

PART VIII
The General Public

CHAPTER

32

Tax Levies

Kimberly Moss

Chapter Objectives

After reading this chapter, readers will:

- Know how to conduct a tax levy campaign.
- Appreciate legal requirements related to conducting a tax levy campaign.
- Know how to construct and staff a tax levy campaign committee.
- Generalize information in this chapter to any local jurisdiction in the United States.

Chapter Summary

This chapter is about tax levies. Many jurisdictions inadequately fund public health departments. One particularly viable alternative form of funding is a special purpose or dedicated tax levy. A tax levy campaign requires careful planning, oversight, and coordination to be successful. In all jurisdictions, election law rules and regulations govern the conduct of a tax levy campaign. General information is provided and augmented by examples from a county in Ohio.

Case Study

While conducting a strategic planning session, the Mossyvale local health district reviewed the budget for the next 10 years. The Mossyvale board of health has determined that it does not have sufficient funds to conduct mandated programs. Without more income, the district will have to lay off personnel and cut programs. The board has decided to put the issue of need to the voters in the form of a tax levy. Before they proceed, the following questions must be answered:

- How much money should be requested?
- What are the legal requirements for a levy? How does the board proceed?
- Is a tax levy campaign committee necessary? If so, how is it organized?

INTRODUCTION

Money is needed to operate any agency and to provide any type of service. Health-related services are no exception. Methods of funding a health department or health district vary throughout the country. Many such units are supported by money raised through taxation. Operating funds may come from general tax revenues. Alternatively, they may be raised through local tax levies that are established and approved for this purpose.

The process of organizing and conducting a tax levy for health-related services is the subject of this chapter. This chapter provides an expanded case study of a tax levy campaign taken from a single county in Ohio. The referenced statutes are specific to Ohio. Readers are advised to seek assistance from legal counsel when contemplating a tax levy within their own jurisdictions.

TAX LEVIES

Mechanisms and sources of funding for public health programs and initiatives differ from state to state. This is especially true at the local level. Complicating the issue of funding is a wide variety of organizational configurations. Some states have local health districts, whereas others have regional health districts. Some coordinate all local health services at the state level.

Statutory authority for public health can be found in state law. Statutes and ordinances vary from state to state. In many states, a primary role of a local board of health is identifying and providing funding for the health district that it oversees.

Local health districts can receive funds from a variety of sources. These include budgetary funding from local general tax revenues, fees for services, fees for inspections and licenses, state subsidies, grants, and tax levies (Scutchfield and Keck, 2002). A local board has the responsibility to ensure that sufficient funds are available to operate the programs and activities of the health district (Ohio Association of Local Boards of Health, 1991). Accordingly, board members must be well informed about the fiscal aspects of the health district's operations.

Some health districts must obtain operational funding directly from residents. This is most commonly accomplished by a tax levy. The reality of this approach is that voters must periodically approve a tax on themselves. Without such periodic authorization for funding, a health district must curtail programs and services.

Including board members in strategic planning for the health district is paramount to gaining their support for a levy campaign. The decision to request a tax levy begins with the board of health.

How does the health district get to this point? A board must first know the source of its current funding. Funding comes from a variety of sources. In a general health district, townships usually pay part of the budget for the health district using funds received from general tax revenues. Other sources, such as grants and fees, combined with the tax income, constitute the revenue portion of the budget. Sometimes the cost of the programs and services that the health district provides is not covered by the income generated by available revenue sources. At this time, a board may consider a special tax levy.

In the following discussion on tax levies, two assumptions have been made. The first is that existing revenue sources are not sufficient to meet projected operating needs of a health department. The second is that a special tax levy is legal within the jurisdiction served by the health department.

A levy also can be placed on the ballot for the purpose of constructing a building to house the health district. Whether the levy is for operating expenses or for a building, the language of the levy must be specific. You should seek legal counsel with an attorney who has experience in such matters. Such actions usually reduce stress and avoid both procedural errors and personal headaches.

The legal authority that is responsible for funding a health department is the appropriate starting point for a discussion of tax levies. In Ohio, the legal authority for public health activity is the Ohio Revised Code. The taxing authority for general health districts in the State of Ohio is vested with county commissioners. Other states have similar regulations and authorities. Ohio statutes require county commissioners to certify that the revenues needed to operate a health district exceed the taxing limit established by the state's legal code. After such a certification is filed with the appropriate jurisdictional body (in Ohio, this is the board of county commissioners of the county within which the general health district is located), a special taxing authority for the purposes of supporting a health department is established. In essence, boards of health require county commissioners to actually place a tax levy on an election ballot.

Timing is essential for any levy campaign. Many legal requirements and organizational activities must be met prior to voting. Legal filing deadlines exist for most electoral jurisdictions. Tax levies may not be legally placed on ballots in all elections. Jurisdictions that have conducted successful levy campaigns suggest that the health board check with the appropriate electoral board to avoid missing deadlines.

In Ohio, a local health board takes the first legal step. By resolution, that body requests the auditor of the county to certify the current tax valuation (typically real property) to the taxing authority. The resolution further specifies the number of mils required to generate the specific amount of revenue requested by the health board (Ohio Revised Code 5705.03(B)). In a related resolution, the board of health certifies to the county commissioners that the estimated amount of money within the legally allowed taxing limit for the specific period of time will be insufficient (Ohio Revised Code 5705.29).

The county commissioners must then pass a resolution declaring it necessary to place, replace, or renew a levy (Ohio Revised Code 5705.03). The county commissioners must pass another resolution that is parallel to the one passed by the board of health. The county commissioners declare that the amount of taxes raised by the county that are within the legally allowed taxing limit will not be sufficient to provide an adequate amount of money for the board of health to carry out its programs. The second resolution concludes with a declaration that a tax levy in excess of the legal limitation is needed. The board of elections must publish a legal notice in a local newspaper that the proposed levy will appear on the ballot of an upcoming election. While these steps are being taken, a levy campaign committee should be assembled and begin to plan the campaign.

THE LEVY CAMPAIGN COMMITTEE

Levy campaign committees are essential for success on voting day. Although the board of health is responsible for fundraising for the health district, community stakeholders as well as health department employees are usually quite involved and vital to the success of the levy. Board of health members should provide the nucleus around which the committee is formed. Health department staff members often are asked to volunteer their time and participate on the committee. It is important to remember that it is illegal for employees to use their regular paid time to conduct levy campaign activities. Community leaders should be invited to participate in the campaign. As the number of people involved increases, the amount of work for any particular individual decreases. A chairperson, vice chair, secretary, and treasurer are required to head the campaign committee and coordinate its activities.

Chairperson

The campaign chairperson should be a community leader who has experience participating in levy campaigns. The chair is often a board member, staff member, or someone who is well known in the community. Usually this person has connections to resources and can take advantage of those connections. The chairperson coordinates the activities of the levy campaign committee, chairs meetings, and delegates duties.

Vice Chairperson

The vice chair is the right-hand assistant to the chairperson. This individual should be someone with the potential for connections within the community. In communities or districts that rely on repeated tax levies, the vice chair position is often used for training the chair of the next campaign.

Treasurer

Because this person is responsible for money, the treasurer is required to register with the local board of elections. The treasurer often works closely with a legal counsel to ensure that all activities, not just finances, of a levy campaign committee are within the law. The local board of elections can frequently supply material and guidance to a treasurer. In Ohio, the Office of the Secretary of State (1996) has prepared such a document. The treasurer has reporting responsibilities. Most states have reporting requirements related to campaign contributions and committee activities.

Secretary

The secretary has the responsibility to take notes of all full committee meetings. These notes should be kept and archived for future reference and documentation in case any legal problems arise. The secretary also should maintain a permanent chronology of the entire campaign. This record often includes copies of newspaper articles and pictures as well as a timeline of events and committee activities.

SUBCOMMITTEES

If the work of the campaign committee is delegated to subcommittees, the process moves more smoothly and individual volunteers do not become overburdened. Subcommittees are often established to meet a specific need. For example, funds are typically required for publicity and committee activities during the course of a campaign. A fundraising committee is often established to obtain the necessary resources. A sign committee is useful because yard signs are usually placed in strategic areas prior to any election. Advertising is also a necessary committee. Newspaper ads, pamphlets, and radio spots usually contribute to a successful campaign. A speakers committee is useful to coordinate efforts that promote the campaign at service organization meetings and other places. Depending on the type and size of the levy, other committees also may be necessary. Promoting an initial or replacement levy usually requires more effort than does seeking a renewal.

Fundraising

The fundraising committee usually includes board members as well as community members who know which individuals in the community to approach for a contribution to the campaign. Fundraising has legal requirements and restrictions. Money collected for conducting the campaign must be kept separate from health department funds. It is necessary for the treasurer to open a checking account that strictly adheres to applicable local campaign finance rules and regulations. A letter-writing campaign is a good way to begin fundraising. A letter may be written to community leaders and businesses asking for donations to support the levy campaign.

Advertising

The advertising committee has a critical but often enjoyable responsibility, namely, conveying the committee's message to voters in affected communities. An effective campaign slogan is a useful way to focus the campaign and make it easy for people to remember. Campaign slogans can be used for signs, billboards, pamphlets, radio spots, and newspaper ads. A single catchy slogan can be a powerful tool that contributes to the success of a levy campaign. Public service announcements may be available through local media outlets. However, successful levy campaigns do not rely solely on public service announcements. They are willing to pay for advertising time to distribute their message. Health department employees or people who have utilized the department's services are often spokespersons in media advertising. Local cable television companies often have a channel that is available for public service announcements at little or no cost. Local channels may be willing to air public service announcements more often during a levy campaign. Sponsoring poster contests that focus on public health is also very helpful in promoting public health during a levy campaign. This is a way to involve school-aged children in the campaign. Although they may not be able to vote, children often have considerable influence on their parents.

Signs

The sign committee is responsible for designing signs to be put in yards, on major highway intersections, and at other strategically determined locations. The campaign's slogan can be used, but most signs simply tell voters how to vote for the levy. Simplicity is useful because most signs must be read with a glance. Some suggestions include the following examples: "Vote yes for issue 3, your health depends on it," "a yes vote for issue 3 means a yes vote for your health," or "vote yes for good health." Avoid making the message on the sign too long. Fewer words on a sign improves the chances of conveying the committee's message to voters. Use simple color schemes that are easily visible. Be strategic when placing campaign signs. Signs cost money. Placing them along more-traveled routes increases the effectiveness of money spent on advertising. Local ordinances may limit where and when a yard sign can be placed. Local election boards can provide copies of applicable regulations. They should be scrupulously followed. Signs usually must be removed by a certain date. Make sure the committee has a sign-removal plan.

Speakers

The speakers committees should include the health board president, the medical director, and the health commissioner. Other persons in positions of leadership in the health department should also participate. Service organizations and other community groups should receive notices that members of the community are available to speak. Individuals who have been available as speakers at other times should be welcomed during a levy campaign. Material used during levy speaking engagements should be coordinated among the speakers so that the committee's message is uniform and consistent. Keep presentations short and focused. Effective speakers prepare answers to questions that are likely to be asked by members of the audience in advance.

■ AFTER THE VOTE

After the levy vote, the committee should meet to review the outcome and evaluate the committee's activities. Documentation is especially important at this meeting. Remember to promptly remove all signs that are placed in the community during the campaign. When the committee's activities and the voting outcome are understood by all concerned, the committee can disband, but only after all required reports have been filed and accepted by the board of elections.

A truly successful campaign is a continuous process that begins after the first levy is passed. Special care must be taken to document all programs and activities that are supported with tax dollars. Successful departments of health take every opportunity to let the people know how their tax dollars are at work for them. Members of the community should be given ownership in the programs that they are supporting. Township trustees and county commissioners must be kept informed of health district activities.

The health commissioner or health officer must be willing to take every opportunity to provide awareness of public health activities to members of the community. A member of the board of health should consider offering to serve as a member of a township trustee association or a similar body. This provides a continuous presence. It is a mistake to be seen only at an annual district advisory committee meeting or when assistance is needed for another tax levy. Operating an effective public health department requires the cooperation of township trustees and county commissioners. Effective and successful health boards continually and carefully nurture relationships with these bodies. Newsletters can be helpful in sharing a health department's agenda as well as for thanking supporters. Health board members should attend meetings of other community agencies and governing boards. Becoming known and maintaining visibility over time is useful when funding is needed. Members of a community appreciate receiving presentations or reports that include statistics on how the tax levy has assisted the health district fulfilling its duties and operate programs that address public health concerns. A graph depicting how many activities or people assisted in each township during a levy campaign is a powerful method for conveying the message that public health is in everyone's best interest.

CONCLUSION

Revisiting the Mossyvale board of health, the needed funding level was established by a community health assessment that was concluded three months ago. Existing sources of revenue were investigated. The health department receives a small sum (less than 10 percent of the proposed budget) as a line item in the local government's budget. Test and license fees are returned to the health department. These will cover approximately 25 percent of the proposed budget. The difference (65 percent of the budget) must be obtained through other means. Grants provide occasional funds, but the board reserves these for the programs designated in the grant application. Besides, grants are not guaranteed from year to year.

After investigating applicable state, county, and local statutes, the board's legal counsel determined that the local health district could support itself through a direct, dedicated tax. To be legal, such a tax levy has to be approved by voters each time it is to be imposed.

A special tax levy committee was created to assist the board and health department in raising the needed funds. Following the procedures outlined in the chapter, the committee organized a levy campaign. The committee made its case before voters in a variety of venues. In the next general election, voters approved a 12-mil tax on property for the next 10 years. After thanking members of the tax levy committee for their efforts, the committee was disbanded. The board and the health department moved to implement the recommendations of the community health assessment using the funds provided for that purpose by the local citizenry.

References

Office of the Secretary of State. 1996. *Ohio Campaign Finance Reporting Handbook*. Columbus, OH: Office of the Secretary of State.

Ohio Association of Local Boards of Health. 1991. *Board of Health Leadership Guide, A Prescription for Excellence.* Columbus, OH: Ohio Department of Health.

Ohio Revised Code. Available at www.legislature.state.oh.us/laws.cfm.

Scutchfield, F.D., and Keck, C.W. 2002. *Principles of Public Health Practice*, 2d ed. Albany, NY: Delmar.

Resources

Periodicals

Jacobson, M.F., and Brownell, K.D. 2000. Small taxes on soft drinks and snack foods to promote health. *American Journal of Public Health* 90(6):854–857.

Nemes, J. 1990. Tax levy gives hospital chance for survival. *Modern Healthcare* 20(48):41–42.

Pierce, J.R., and Blackburn, C.P. 1998. The transformation of a local health department. *Public Health Reports* 113(2):152–159.

Royse, D., and Hazelton, M.M. 1985. Passing a mental health levy: a successful campaign outline. *Journal of Mental Health Administration* 12(2):18–21.

Books

Amerhein, T.A. 2000. *Newcomer's Guide to Winning Local Elections.* Lincoln, NE: Universe.

Faucheux, R.A. 2002. *Running for Office: How Smart Political Candidates from School Board to President Win Tough Elections by Using the Right Campaign Strategies, Techniques, and Messages.* New York: M. Evans.

Grey, L. 1999. *How to Win a Local Election: A Complete Step-by-Step Guide.* New York: M. Evans.

Shaw, C. 2004. *The Campaign Manager: Running and Winning Local Elections,* 3d ed. Boulder, CO: Westview Press.

Strachan, J.C. 2003. *High-Tech Grass Roots.* Lanham, MD: Rowman & Littlefield.

Web Sites

- *News Gazette* (Champaign, Illinois): www.news-gazette.com/story.cfm?Number=5696
- County Board of DuPage County, Illinois: www.co.dupage.il.us/finance/budget2004/OFI-004-03.pdf
- Ohio Association of County Behavioral Health Authorities: www.oacbha.org/docs/Laws/REVISED%20CODE/Chapter5705_Tax_Levy_Law.htm
- Pima County, Arizona: www.co.pima.az.us/finance/bud9900

Organizations

Ohio Association of County Behavioral Health Authorities
42 East Gay Street, Suite 1600
Columbus, OH 43215

Phone: 614-224-1111
Fax: 614-224-2642
E-mail: cdiaz@oacbha.org
Web site: www.oacbha.org

National Association of County and City Health Officials
1100 17th Street, Second Floor
Washington, D.C. 20036
Phone: 202-783-5550
Fax: 202-783-1583
E-mail: naccho@naccho.org
Web site: www.naccho.org

National Association of Local Boards of Health
1840 East Gypsy Lane Road
Bowling Green, OH 43402
Phone: 419-353-7714
Fax: 419-352-6278
E-mail: nalboh@nalboh.org
Web site: www.nalboh.org

Public Health Foundation
1220 L Street, NW, Suite 350
Washington, D.C. 20005
Phone: 202-898-5600
Fax: 202-898-5609
E-mail: info@phf.org
Web site: www.phf.org

CHAPTER

33

Marketing Public Health and Public Health Departments

Kathy S. Silvestri

Chapter Objectives

After reading this chapter, readers will:

- Identify the key principles of marketing.
- Discuss how the principles of marketing apply in a local health department and public health setting.
- Define the term *social marketing*.
- Compare and contrast the use of the key principles of marketing in social marketing strategies.

Chapter Summary

This chapter discusses the application of marketing strategies in local public health department settings. The key principles of traditional marketing are reviewed and applied to social marketing theories and strategies. These are reinforced with examples of how to apply them in a public health setting.

Case Study

Senior managers of the health department were meeting to discuss programs. "Programs are only part of the problem," complained one manager, "many people in the community simply do not know that we exist."

"Nonsense," interjected a long-time employee. "People still talk about the food poisoning outbreak that we investigated. Thanks to our efforts, no one died."

"Sure," said the first, "that investigation was conducted in 1986."

The Health Officer just listened. Nancy was new to her position and concerned with promoting the department's latest initiative. She realized that traditional announcements in the newspaper were not as effective as they could be. What advice would you offer to Nancy?

■ INTRODUCTION

The health of a community is protected and improved through public health measures, yet how do people define public health? Are their replies influenced by personal experiences, direct knowledge of the services offered by a local health department or district, current events that have affected the health of many, or by the media? A vision of public health in America was presented in *The Future of Public Health* (1988), which placed the definition of public health at the very top of the conceptual elements necessary for the successful coordination of federal, state, and local health improvement efforts. *The Future of Public Health* proposed a three-part definition based on the following questions: What are the common goals of public health that outline its mission? With what areas of need is public health concerned (defining its substance)? How is public health different from the activity of health agencies (identifying an organizational framework)?

Successful marketing strategies promoting products and services in the public and private sectors begin with a clear definition of purpose. They end by satisfying both the public's objectives and the goals of the agency that provides them. An overarching need is to clearly define and market the goals and objectives of public health and a local health department or district. This logically leads to identifying the key principles of marketing and their applications within public health and introducing the concepts of social marketing to address the needs of a community.

Businesses, churches, universities, hospitals, political parties, volunteer organizations, and public health departments perform activities to aid market exchanges. Marketing professionals define a potentially successful exchange as two or more parties that have something that is valued, wanted, or needed by the other party. The exchange is successful when each is willing to give up something of value to receive something of value in exchange (Kotler, 2003). In other words, successful marketers make sure they have something that appeals to people, appears beneficial, and is worth sacrificing something to obtain it.

Currently, the traditional borders of marketing have extended beyond profit-oriented organizations to include not-for-profits operating in both the public and private sectors. Not-for-profits have a very different bottom-line objective. They must generate just enough income to get the job done (Boone and Jurtz, 2004). Local health departments continuously face funding uncertainties. Most depend on multiple sources, including state health agency categorical grants, local funds, the state, direct federal funds, and fees and reimbursements. Thus, they are vulnerable to the ever-changing economic and political climates (Turnock, 2004). In addition, local health departments may face competition from local public and private organizations.

Public health practitioners may directly provide services to the community or contract them out to others, including local colleges and universities, health centers, hospitals, churches, and state health agencies. Many local health departments provide resources such as education materials, health and environmental testing kits, and clinical services and personnel (Turnock, 2004). To succeed, health departments must clearly identify goals and objectives and strive to find the most cost-effective ways to provide their services. Marketing provides a planning process to create and maintain relationships that will satisfy the objectives of both individuals and an organization (Boone and Jurtz, 2004).

State and local health departments may consider several nontraditional marketing categories, including person, place, cause, event, and organization marketing. **Person marketing** uses a celebrity or authority figure to attract the attentions of a target market. A retired athlete may be used to promote physical fitness and healthy nutrition; police officers may be effective in speaking to teens about drug and alcohol abuse. **Place marketing** attempts to attract visitors to a particular area; to improve the images of towns, cities, or states; or to attract new business. Positive relationships cultivated between the local health department and the community enhance place marketing efforts. If a social issue, cause, or idea must be identified and marketed to a selected target market, **cause marketing** will be used. The "Drive safe, drive sober" slogan of the National Commission Against Drunk Driving promotes holiday drinking safety. In 2003, the Centers for Disease Control and Prevention helped state and local health departments combat the spread of the West Nile Virus through its health promotion and education campaign "Fight the bite!" The American Cancer Society promotes "Relay for Life" events to target markets through **event marketing.** This is one of the most common marketing strategies used by local health departments. The final nontraditional marketing category is **organization marketing,** which may be used by churches, labor unions, and political parties or by service and government organizations to persuade others to receive their services, recognize and accept their goals, or make contributions. Health commissioners use organization marketing when they report to their boards of health, make presentations at a state conference, or speak to potential fund sources.

Whether traditional or nontraditional, marketing is designed to plan, price, promote, and distribute the products and services capable of satisfying the needs and desires of consumers (Kotler, 2003). The key principles of marketing include knowing one's consumers, creating products or services that they want or need, finding ways to get the products or services to consumers, and making a commitment to continue to change and adapt the products or services to meet the consumers' ever-changing desires, needs, and preferences.

KNOW THE CONSUMERS

Successful marketing strategies focus on consumers from beginning to end. Marketers sell products and services. To do so, they must know as much as they can about their target audience. Marketing companies conduct surveys and sponsor research to determine the age, gender, race or ethnicity, income, specific geographic location, and how much of a product or service individuals, groups, or organizations will consume within a potential market. These characteristics are closely related to the client's needs, uses, or behavior toward a product or service (Kotler, 2003).

For a group of people to be considered a **market**, they must want or need the product and be willing and able to acquire it. The next step in a marketing strategy is to determine if the product or service should be offered to an entire audience, or **total market**. Alternatively, it may be advantageous to divide potential consumers into **market segments** based on the characteristics they have in common as groups, individuals, or organizations (Kotler, 2003). Teen magazines have a total market audience ranging in age from preteens through young adults. Some goods, such as hair styling products and acne control preparations, may have value and benefits for this entire market. In contrast, ads featuring alcoholic beverage products should be restricted to the market segment of young persons who can legally make such purchases.

Local health departments or districts have the responsibility to serve all members of the community and to provide a mix of programs that address the core essential services. The problem is that everyone doesn't necessarily want or need each program or service offered. Further, the demand for services is constantly changing. Because funding and human resources are often scarce, it is extremely difficult to serve all the people all of the time. Community health assessments are a valuable tool (see Chapter 4) to quantitatively identify the age, gender, race, ethnicity, and geographic location of specific target populations or specific health concerns. Health departments can use this objective information to tailor and focus their inventories of products and services to address the key health concerns within a community. Focus groups and town meetings can also provide insights to the desires and needs of a community. A commitment to a systematic health assessment process greatly reduces the guesswork of health planning and marketing strategies.

CREATING PRODUCTS THAT ARE WANTED OR NEEDED

A **product** can be an idea, a service, a good, or any combination of the three. Consumers don't just purchase products. In reality, consumers buy the benefits and satisfaction they believe the products will provide. Members of a potential market have needs and desires that must be identified. This assessment drives the product research and development process, which results in a **product mix.** The product mix is composed of all the products and services that an organization makes available. If programs or services within the product mix are related, they represent a **product line**. The product line may include a particular program or service that is unique and appeals to a very specialized market (Kotler, 2003). As an example, the product mix of a weight loss company may include counseling services, special foods, and exercise classes. Varied types of exercise programs constitute a product line within the mix; exercise classes specifically designed for pregnant women are an example of a product item within the product line.

The product mix of a local health department is diverse and is mandated by the 10 Essential Public Health Services written by the Public Health Steering Committee of the Public Health Service (Public Health Foundation, 2004). The product mix of programs and services often targets several distinct markets or market segments. General categories of services may include immunization programs for adult influenza and childhood diseases, communicable disease control programs, and epidemiological surveillance. Other commonly offered products include prenatal and early childhood care, including Women, Infants, and Children services, health screenings, sexually transmitted disease counseling and testing, and family planning services. Environment-related products include food, milk, and restaurant inspections and solid waste management programs. Community health educational efforts are features of many programs (Turnock, 2004).

Research is conducted to determine which products are relevant for a given population. Companies that produce consumer goods label such activity *market research.* Health departments use an analogous process and call it *community health assessment.* Additional details on community health assessment can be found in Chapter 4. Disaster preparations are a recent addition to the product mix of public health agencies. Additional details on these activities are available in Chapters 26 through 29. See Chapter 34 for additional information about departments that provide primary health care services.

LINKING PRODUCTS AND CONSUMERS

Marketing strategies depend on delivery systems and effective promotional campaigns to get products into the hands of consumers. **Marketing channels**, or distribution systems, connect products and services with consumers who want or need them. They help to make product acquisition as simple as possible by eliminating any unnecessary marketplace contact. Print ads often provide toll-free phone numbers to help potential consumers obtain additional information or locate a local supplier for a desired product or service. Local health departments may become the marketing channel between a manufacturer of child protective car seats and parents who have a need for them within a community. Another effective and proven distribution system involves health departments, physicians' offices, local hospitals, and other outlets that distribute vaccines received from pharmaceutical companies to persons needing such protection.

Promotion campaigns inform, persuade, and influence a consumer's decision towards a product or service. The attention–interest–desire–action concept describes the steps consumers take when reaching such decisions. For a promotional message to be effective, it must first get the attention of potential consumers and then engage their interest in a particular product or service. The message must also convince potential consumers that they want or need the product being promoted. Once potential consumers' needs or desires have been established, the result should be the action of acquiring the product or service. At the very least, it should create a positive attitude toward acquiring a product or using a service at some time in the future (Boone and Jurtz, 2004).

Promotional campaigns utilize a mix of personal and nonpersonal techniques to achieve specific marketing objectives. **Personal promotion** is conducted between two people over the telephone, during videoconferencing, or through interactive computer links. **Nonpersonal promotions** include advertising, direct marketing, public relations, and other techniques. Advertising strategies feature paid communications in newspapers, television, radio, magazines, and billboards. They also may include electronic and computerized forms of communication such as the Internet and advertisements. Electronic ads often appear on video screens at sporting events and in other public locations. Direct marketing techniques include direct mail, product and service catalogs or brochures, telemarketing, direct-response ads on television or radio, and the use of electronic media. Many local health departments publish newsletters and special event calendars to promote their programs and services. Others are turning to the electronic media by developing Web sites with links to local organizations and services and to state and national health resources (Boone and Jurtz, 2004).

MAKING A COMMITMENT TO CHANGE AND ADAPTING PRODUCTS

A product's **life cycle** moves through several phases. The first phase is the **introduction stage**, which is when the product is first presented to the market. **Growth** occurs as the product increases in popularity. During **maturity**, a product reaches its peak and begins a downward trend over time. The end stage is **decline**, which is when product purchase and use begins to fall at a rapid rate. Different elements within the product mix will ultimately have varying life cycles. The difficulty is managing, changing, or adapting products, programs, and services to meet the ever-changing needs and desires of people within the market or accepting that the market itself has been altered (Boone and Jurtz, 2004). The rising Latino population in the United States presents an example of how the public health marketplace is changing. Ads and education efforts aimed at reducing or eliminating smoking designed for the general public have been relatively ineffective in Latino communities. After studying the Latino culture, tobacco control efforts are being redesigned to incorporate changes in language, visual presentation, and content.

How is the product mix of a local health district determined? Local, state, and federal laws mandate certain programs and services. If funded by local levies, community leaders also influence the mix. Programs must be periodically evaluated and adapted to effectively respond and meet the ever-changing wants and needs within a community. The restaurant inspection duties of an environmental services department may change if a local clean indoor air ordinance is passed. If the evaluation of an immunization program reveals a decrease in the percentage of two-year-olds that are fully immunized, a health department administration plan must be adapted to include changes in dates, times, and locations as needed.

MARKETING AND LOCAL HEALTH DEPARTMENTS

Marketing the programs and services of a local health department results in social exposure. Social exposure is a state of awareness in which community residents can readily identify and describe the benefits, programs, and services provided by their local health department. Local health department leaders may be reluctant to allocate funds for marketing activities if the trade-off is a decrease in direct services to consumers. Grant opportunities may support targeted promotion campaigns for selected programs or services. For the most part, cost-efficient measures must be utilized to promote the day-to-day activities of a health department.

Start small with on-hold telephone messages that promote health department services, upcoming public health programs, special events, and service schedules. Next, consider updating or designing a department logo. A well-designed logo becomes a trademark that is synonymous with the organization it represents. This symbol serves to establish a visual link between the local health department and the community it serves. Graphic art companies may be hired to do the job. Another option is to purchase computer software and plan the logo in-house. An effective design is simple and colorful with clean lines and easy-to-read fonts. When colors are chosen, determine how they will appear if reproduced in gray scale. Traditionally reserved for letterhead and envelopes, contemporary health department logos appear on posters, flyers, bulletins, staff uniforms, shirts, hats, and many other items.

Public service announcements promote social causes or address social concerns. Advertising and national health agencies, such as the Centers for Disease Control and Prevention, often donate their expertise and prepare public service announcements for use by state and local health agencies. Quarterly newsletters produced by local health departments help to build relationships with a community. They can communicate and reinforce organizational missions and objectives while providing up-to-date service schedules, fees, locations, and contact information. In addition, they can provide information concerning public health issues and concerns.

Local newspapers and television and radio stations can be partners to cost-effectively market for local health departments. Newspapers may come to depend on the health information and expertise of local health departments and other health care providers to produce periodic health improvement columns and feature articles. Radio stations may invite the health commissioner and other staff to participate in interviews to discuss or debate health issues and concerns. Television and radio stations providing media coverage for special events and programs may effectively increase the level of community response and participation (Boone and Jurtz, 2004). Effective local media partnerships can be invaluable marketing assets.

Many local health departments are budgeting to develop and maintain their own Web sites. Building an effective Web site involves several key steps. First, establish a mission for the site by creating a statement that explains the overall goals of the organization. Next, identify the purpose for the site. Is the site's purpose to introduce the health department to the community, promote its services, or provide public health education? Finally, design a site that is colorful and inviting, provides information that is clear and concise, maintains consumer privacy and security, and above all, is easy to navigate (Boone and Jurtz, 2004). Once the Web site is up and running, it must be maintained by frequently updating its information and appearance. The first thought may be to reduce costs by delegating this responsibility to existing health department staff members who may be familiar with or have an interest in Web page design. The chosen staff members will most likely be asked to assume these duties in addition to their normal responsibilities. Work overload may keep them from attending to the Web page in a timely manner. Assuming that funding is available, an alternative is to contract this service out.

Web pages provide a marketing channel to make local health department products readily available to the community. Products that may be featured include local health assessment reports, health information pamphlets and brochures, local health information data sets, and schedules of upcoming events.

Advertising is often the target of criticism, but promotion provides information and education that are necessary for health improvement and personal well-being in contemporary society. Each year, the emphasis on health promotion strategies increases as nonbusiness organizations allocate more funds to prevention activities. In today's competitive and unstable economic environment, long-term survival may depend on promotion and the incorporation of marketing strategies into the planning processes of local health departments. Public health has the unique challenge of trying to change unhealthy, but well-established, social norms. Social marketing incorporates the basic principles of marketing to modify individual behavior, improve social and economic conditions, and reform social policy (Glanz et al., 2002).

SOCIAL MARKETING AND PUBLIC HEALTH

Public health continues to face its most daunting challenge, persuading and encouraging people to change behaviors that are negatively impacting their health. High-fat and high-carbohydrate diets, lack of a regular exercise routine, smoking, binge drinking, and other unhealthy behaviors are contributing to the increased prevalence of diabetes, cancer, and cardiovascular disease. Years of public awareness campaigns and health education have alerted people to the negative consequences of their day-to-day choices. For some, these choices have even resulted in a decline in their health. Yet many seem unwilling or unable to break those old, familiar bad habits. People often resent public health interventions, stating that they interfere with their individual rights. Others protest and resist public health initiatives that appear to mandate how businesses should conduct their day-to-day operations (Glanz et al., 2002). Attempts to limit smoking in public places invite spirited debates. Nonsmokers believe they have the right to breathe smoke-free air, whereas smokers believe this is the first step in limiting many of their personal rights and behaviors.

Another challenge for public health practitioners is that the effects or outcomes of successful public health programs are not immediately apparent. Significant changes in chronic disease mortality and prevalence rates will not occur for several years, and changes in individual behaviors may not be visible to the general public and local policymakers. For these reasons, communities and organizations often make the choice to finance established medical treatments that satisfy identified health needs versus making an investment in health and disease prevention. In spite of the challenges, public health practitioners have a job to do and they are turning to social marketing to help them succeed. Social marketing is a process that markets social change (Glanz et al., 2002).

What motivates people to make permanent changes in behaviors that are comfortable and satisfying? In reality, public health practitioners and local health departments are in the business of marketing health improvement. Local health departments want to facilitate exchanges so that their consumers get the measure of health services they want and need to live independent and full lives. In return, local health departments fulfill their mission, goals, and objectives to help people improve their health. The ultimate product to market is optimum health. The product mix includes unlimited support and assistance to change unhealthy lifestyles and behaviors. Each exchange has an associated cost or price that must be paid.

To achieve better health, a consumer must be willing and able to give up something of value. This can be using free time to exercise or to prepare healthy meals, spending money to join an exercise program or local gym, or foregoing the pleasure received from smoking cigarettes or relaxing on the couch after work or school. It is not always convenient to adopt healthy lifestyles, but the rewards are great. Social marketing is a continuous health-improvement cycle that begins with gathering information to determine the health-related needs of community populations. It then progresses through the planning, implementation, and evaluation of programs designed to influence or change individual behaviors. The ultimate goal is to change the social norms of a community (Glanz et al., 2002).

Social marketing incorporates the key principles of marketing. Public health practitioners must first learn everything they can about the public they serve. The goal of social marketing is to influence individual behaviors versus the traditional public health goals of increasing their knowledge or changing their personal attitudes. Social marketers then design programs specifically for target audiences and those most in need of the services that may help them to change their behaviors. Finally, to be effective, health practitioners must be willing to review, refine, and change the programs as needed (Glanz et al., 2002).

Public health departments and staff must be able to get people to believe that the long-term and immediate benefits of changing individual behaviors outweigh their personal sacrifices. Studying health behavior models and theories is useful to help public health practitioners understand change and the maintenance of health behavior. The Health Belief Model proposes that people who acknowledge the beneficial effects of health information are likely to make choices that will improve their health. The Theory of Reasoned Action proposes a relationship between an individual's beliefs, attitudes, intentions, and a resulting behavior. The Transactional Model of Stress and Coping addresses how people respond and cope with stressors. The Transtheoretical Model discusses how to reach individuals who may be at various stages of readiness to change. Taken together, these theories of health behavior identify the reasons and methods that influence peoples' decisions to choose healthy behaviors (Siegel and Doner, 1998).

As public health practitioners become familiar with the individuals and groups that they serve, these models and theories of health behavior help them to identify existing negative behaviors and the pros, cons, benefits, and costs related to continuing and maintaining them. This information is used to customize a program or service (time, place, location, messages, starting points, and the like) to encourage individuals to consider, plan, or adopt changes in behavior. Finally, health practitioners must effectively promote the program or service to convince individuals that the benefits outweigh the costs of changing the behavior. Over time, changes in the individual behaviors of many people translate into a change in community social norms (Siegel and Doner, 1998).

At times, it is the job of public health to convince policy makers rather than individuals to change their behaviors. Policy makers usually adopt one of three positions on public health policy or programs. They may support them, oppose them, or remain neutral. Improving the public's health may mean drafting new local regulations or changing a voting position on bills sponsored at the state level (Siegel and Doner, 1998). It is important for local and state health departments to keep legislators and local policymakers informed of current health status information. To gain their support early, successful local health leaders involve members of this influential group at all levels of health assessment, program planning, and promotion.

The most difficult social changes to market may be those that will improve the social and economic conditions within a community. An ideal community provides education, employment, and housing opportunities so that all can live healthy, independent, and productive lives. The need and desire to change negative social and economic conditions may not match the political demands of the public or policy makers. Welfare and public assistance benefits are decreasing, yet homelessness and poverty persist for families, children, and individuals. Social marketers monitor policymakers and proposed changes, advocating for those in need.

Successful social marketing strategies translate into improved health for individuals and the communities in which they live. Changing social norms requires the efforts of community partners working together with common goals and objectives. Local health departments can benefit from partnering with other public agencies, health volunteers, professional organizations, foundations, the media, consumer organizations, local businesses, and individual for-profit manufacturers in the challenge to change individual and community behaviors.

CONCLUSION

Marketing public health and local health departments is important and necessary for survival of both local health departments and the field of public health in general in modern society. The public often ignores the need for public health services until there is a crisis. Marketing strategies help public health practitioners shift from being reactive to being proactive. The ultimate goal of a local health department is to improve the health and well-being of the community it serves. There is no better time than the present to market local health department products, services, and health solutions.

Returning to the initial case study, Nancy decided to contact the director of a Master of Public Health degree program in a local university. During their meeting, the program director agreed to assign three students from a social marketing class to help the health department.

The first order of business was to inventory available programs and read a copy of the health department's most recent assessment of community needs. One student coordinated the effort to align needs and programs in order of importance.

Another student created a logo, or identity, for the health department. The logo would appear on all departmental materials and communications. The goal was to have members of the community associate the logo with the programs that are provided by the health department. The student convened several focus groups to gather perceptions of community members and solicit ideas from them.

The third student contacted media outlets in the community to solicit their ideas and possible assistance. Representatives offered suggestions and agreed to help design brochures and other promotional materials.

The community and academic public health department have entered into a long-term affiliation. The school provides students and the health department provides opportunities to apply their skills and many of the concepts discussed in this chapter.

References

Boone, L.E., and Jurtz, D.L. 2004. *Contemporary Marketing*, 11th ed. Mason, OH: Thompson South-Western.

Glanz, K., Rimer, B.K., and Lewis, F.M. 2002. *Health Behavior and Health Education: Theory, Research, and Practice*, 3d ed. San Francisco, CA: Jossey-Bass.

Kotler, P., and Armstrong, G. 2003. *Principles of Marketing*, 10th ed. Upper Saddle River, NJ: Prentice Hall.

National Institute of Medicine. 1988. *The Future of Public Health*. Washington, D.C.: National Academy Press.

Public Health Foundation. 2004. Ten Essential Public Health Services. Available at www.phf.org/essential.htm.

Siegel, M., and Doner, L. 1998. *Marketing Public Health: Strategies to Promote Social Change*. Gaithersburg, MD: Aspen Publishers.

Turnock, B.J. 2004. *Public Health: What It Is and How It Works*, 3d ed. Sudbury, MA: Jones & Bartlett.

Resources

Periodicals

Burayidi, M.A. 2003. The use of electronic messages to promote seat belt use. Report of a pilot study in Wisconsin. *Injury Control and Safety Promotion* 10(4):257–260.

Dutta-Bergman, M.J. 2003. A descriptive narrative of healthy eating: A social marketing approach using psychographics in conjunction with interpersonal, community, mass media, and new media activities. *Health Marketing Quarterly* 20(3):81–101.

Konradi, A., and DeBruin, P.L. 2003. Using a social marketing approach to advertise Sexual Assault Nurse Examination (SANE) services to college students. *Journal of American College Health* 52(1):33–39.

Kreuter, M.W., and Wray, R.J. 2003. Tailored and targeted health communication: Strategies for enhancing information relevance. *American Journal of Health Behavior* 27(Suppl 3):S227–S232.

Niederdeppe, J., Farrelly, M.C., and Haviland, M.L. 2004. Confirming "truth": More evidence of a successful tobacco countermarketing campaign in Florida. *American Journal of Public Health* 94(2):255–257.

Stephenson, M.T. 2003. Mass media strategies targeting high sensation seekers: What works and why. *American Journal of Health Behavior* 27 (Suppl 3):S233–S238.

Books

Applebaum, K. 2004. *Marketing Era: From Professional Practice to Global Provisioning*. New York: Routledge.

Davidson, D.K. 2003. *Selling Sin: The Marketing of Socially Unacceptable Products*, 2d ed. Westport, CT: Greenwood Publishing Group.

National Institute of Medicine. 2003. *The Future of the Public's Health in the 21st Century*. Washington, D.C.: National Academy Press.

Simmons, J., and Clifton, R. 2004. *Brands and Branding*. New York: Bloomberg Press.

Web Sites

- American Marketing Association: www.marketingpower.com
- Food Safety Training & Education Alliance: www.fstea.org/resources/socialmark/NewSocMkt
- Health Marketing Quarterly: www.haworthpressinc.com/store/product.asp?sku=J026
- Population Services International: www.psi.org
- Social Marketing.com: www.social-marketing.com

Organizations

American Public Health Association
800 I Street, NW
Washington, D.C. 20001-3710
Phone: 202-777-2742
Fax: 202-777-2534
E-mail: comments@apha.org
Web site: www.apha.org

Centers for Disease Control and Prevention
1600 Clifton Road
Atlanta, GA 30333
Phone: 404-639-3311, 404-639-3534, or 800-311-3435
E-mail: www.cdc.gov/netinfo.htm (Web form)
Web site: www.cdc.gov

National Association of County and City Health Officials
1100 17th Street, Second Floor
Washington, D.C. 20036
Phone: 202-783-5550
Fax: 202-783-1583
E-mail: naccho@naccho.org
Web site: www.naccho.org

National Association of Local Boards of Health
1840 East Gypsy Lane Road
Bowling Green, OH 43402
Phone: 419-353-7714
Fax: 419-352-6278
E-mail: nalboh@nalboh.org
Web site: www.nalboh.org

Public Health Foundation
1220 L Street, NW, Suite 350
Washington, D.C. 20005
Phone: 202-898-5600
Fax: 202-898-5609
E-mail: info@phf.org
Web site: www.phf.org

CHAPTER

34

Organizing and Operating Clinics

Adam Kinninger
L. Fleming Fallon, Jr.

Chapter Objectives

After reading this chapter, readers will:

- Appreciate the need for clinics operated by local health departments.
- Understand that access is an important aspect of planning and operating community clinics.
- Recognize that cultural sensitivity is needed when operating clinics.
- Know the federal guidelines for health department clinics.
- Understand funding issues related to local clinics.
- Recognize the need for cultural sensitivity by clinic staff.
- Appreciate the importance of marketing to the success of a clinic.

Chapter Summary

Significant portions of the population lack health care insurance. Increasingly, people without health care insurance are relying on clinics operated by local health departments for medical services. Access is an important consideration when planning and operating a clinic. Marketing and promotion are important but must be accomplished with sensitivity to the cultures of projected groups of users. Clinic staff members must be well trained in their areas of professional expertise. Funding must be planned and secured.

Case Study

The twins wanted to compete on athletic teams at their high school. Amanda was a runner. She had been running in a local park in the evenings all summer. Both her speed and endurance were steadily improving. Her brother Ben loved soccer. He could run for hours without becoming tired. He seemed to be a natural at defense, having a knack for reading plays as they evolved, often arriving in time to break up the opponent's momentum. School rules required medical clearance before either could participate in athletic activities.

Their widowed mother had a steady job as a bookkeeper for a small construction firm in town. As was the case with many people in the community, she appreciated the job and did not complain about the relatively low rate of pay. She did not really miss the health benefits because she and her two children were generally healthy. When the local economy improved, she would look for a better job with benefits. The problem was the need to obtain the medical clearance for Amanda and Ben so that they could play on their high school teams. What options were available to Amanda and Ben's mother?

■ INTRODUCTION

As of 2001, more than 41 million Americans were without health insurance (U.S. Census Bureau, 2002). This figure represents an increase of 1.4 million people over the number of uninsured in 2000. These statistics are disturbing, but they reflect a continuing trend. Access to health care is critical to the well-being of individuals and society as a whole. Health care professionals have the responsibility to ensure that their communities maintain maximum productivity by providing access to health care services to those without health insurance. One successful model for delivering this care is through health care clinics that are operated by local health departments.

When organizing a health care clinic, it is essential to understand the cultural aspects of the population that will be served. Initiating and developing relationships with people in the community that lack adequate health insurance coverage is instrumental in understanding who constitutes the target constituency. After determining the needs of the community, a health department will be able to organize its clinic to meet the needs of the community.

In America, minorities are more likely to be uninsured than Caucasians. Only 69 percent of Hispanics, 81 percent of Blacks, and 82 percent of Asians and Pacific Islanders are insured. Their Caucasian peers are insured at a rate of 90 percent (U.S. Census Bureau, 2002). In addition, among those between the ages of 18 and 64 years of age, both full-time and part-time workers are more likely to have health insurance (83 percent) than nonworkers (75 percent). Among the poor, workers were less likely to be covered (51.3 percent) than nonworkers (63.2 percent) (U.S. Census Bureau, 2002). Many persons erroneously believe that most people who lack insurance are nonworkers. In reality, most people who lack insurance are employed in low-income jobs. Many small business owners do not generate sufficient revenue to provide health insurance coverage for their employees. At the same time, they do not pay large enough salaries for these employees to purchase insurance on their own.

ACCESS TO HEALTH CARE SERVICES

Traditionally, hospitals have been the health care providers of last resort. In previous decades, hospitals shifted costs to private insurers by raising fees for services to cover unreimbursed expenses. As fee structures became more tightly controlled, hospitals shifted the burden to government-sponsored programs such as Medicaid. Recent regulations have limited such cost shifting. Although hospitals are required to provide care, they have tried to find legal ways to minimize their expenses for nonpaying customers. The result has been a growing number of consumers who lack access to basic, nonemergency health care services.

A growing number of local health departments are choosing to establish clinics to deliver basic health care services to persons living within their areas of jurisdiction. Such clinics are replacing hospitals in their communities as the health care providers of last resort. The impetus for such actions is often similar. Results from community needs assessments identify significant portions of local populations as having no health care insurance. A second reason for establishing local clinics is that the community in general is medically underserved. Local boards of health identify a need in their communities and decide to address it in a direct manner.

It is important to understand the inequities that exist within the American health care system. The ability to effectively organize and operate a health care clinic rests on a community's ability to understand, communicate, and connect with its target population. The demographics about the uninsured in the country provide insight as to who will be likely to seek service from a health department clinic. It is important to understand the issues that target populations are confronted with that may prevent them from receiving quality health care services. An in-depth knowledge of the demographics of your community should be the primary focus once a board of health has decided to establish and operate a health care clinic. For a clinic to be as effective as possible, a health department must maximize its resources. Important details on which to focus are location, cultural competence, and the average age of the target group.

The location of a clinic is critically important. Choose a location that will be easily accessible by public and private transportation. It is important to identify and locate the nucleus of the target community. This will help to narrow a list of potential locations for a clinic. Visibility and ease of access are basic requirements. Location may be a greater concern in small communities than in larger metropolitan areas where public transit is available. The importance of location will be magnified in those communities that lack public transportation. If many in the target populations lack the resources to travel to the clinic, then its effectiveness will be dramatically reduced.

Cultural competence also should be an organizational priority. In order to maximize the interaction with users of clinic services, it is essential that clinic employees be able to communicate with them in a way that will make them feel welcomed and understood. For example, when establishing a clinic in a location with a large population of people who have limited English language skills, it will be important to include signs, literature, employees, and clinicians that incorporate their native language in the clinic.

Another important demographic is the age of the members of the target population. Paying special attention to the age of projected constituents can help determine the types and mix of procedures that are likely to be required. Once the types of procedures and services that will be offered are determined, the health department should consider aggressively advertising the benefits derived from them. For example, if the community has a large number of middle-age people who are genetically prone to hypertension, the clinic may decide to promote blood pressure screenings and distribute brochures on the problem. Another example is to aggressively distribute information about the importance of receiving prenatal health services in a community that has an abnormal neonatal mortality rate. By focusing campaigns and tailoring the program and services of a clinic to address the greatest needs of the residents in a community, the health department increases the potential impact of its clinic operations.

Healthy people are more productive than persons who are ill. Health department clinics contribute to healthy workers in a community. By extension, they contribute to societal well-being. Knowledge of a service area's demographic characteristics ensures that a clinic addresses the issues of those with the greatest needs. An administrator's top goal should be to increase access to health care services. Clinic administrators and local departments must be concerned with addressing inequities that exist for specific, underserved populations.

OPERATIONAL GUIDELINES

When organizing and operating a clinic, it is important for administrators to have an in-depth knowledge of operational guidelines. Administrators must be familiar with accrediting bodies and their requirements, funding sources, and staffing regulations. Some guidelines will be in the form of local policies, whereas others will come from state and federal mandates. Each state has guidelines to which all health and human services must adhere. Another option is to seek accreditation through an organization such as the Joint Commission on Accreditation of Healthcare Organizations.

In less-populated areas, federal regulations governing rural health clinics may be applicable. In most circumstances, these are mobile clinics that provide health care in an area with a shortage of personal health service providers. These qualifications can be found in the Public Health Service Act regulations (PHSA 5330(b)(3) or 1302(7)). Criteria for areas that qualify as having a health professional shortage are defined in section 5332(a)(1)(A) of the Public Health Service Act. Further information about migrant qualifications and other related issues can be found in the Interpretive Guidelines—Rural Health Clinics (National Rural Health Association, 2004). Areas of personnel shortage are found in urban as well as rural localities. Locations that qualify as having a health care personnel shortage may also qualify for financial aid. Consult the Department of Health and Human Services for information on qualification guidelines and standards (bhpr.hrsa.gov/shortage/hpsacrit.htm).

FUNDING

Funding for health clinics can come from many different sources. Most states have special funds set aside to provide grants for starting and operating such facilities and services. The federal government also has special funding set aside to assist health clinics. Information about funding through these grants can be obtained from the U.S. Department of Health and Human Services and from each state health department.

Grants from these organizations may not be sufficient to cover the costs of daily operations and treatments rendered by a facility to the local community. To bridge the gap between funding and operating expenses, it may be necessary to seek funding from private sources or through local tax referendums. Donor campaigns may be one way to successfully supplement the funding of a clinic. This is especially true in areas with a significant corporate presence. Corporations may be willing to donate larger sums of money in exchange for advertisements and publicity. Municipalities may choose to supplement funding for their clinics through local health tax referendums.

Tax support is usually needed for a health department clinic. A local needs assessment often supplies the impetus to provide funding for services at a clinic. A local needs assessment helps to pinpoint the services for which the community has the greatest need. Much of the funding that is normally available through government sources will only support clinic programs that provide services to children and young mothers. If the board wishes to provide services to the adults in the community, it may be necessary to secure funding from additional sources to meet operating expenses.

Other sources of financial support for health clinics are Medicaid and Medicare. Many clinic visitors may qualify for assistance through these two programs. Medicare is the nation's largest health insurance program, covering nearly 40 million Americans at a cost of just under $200 billion (Department of Health and Human Services, 2004a). Persons aged 65 and older, some persons with disabilities who are under age 65, and individuals with permanent kidney failure requiring dialysis or a transplant are eligible for Medicare. Medicare has two parts: Hospital Insurance (Part A) and Medical Insurance (Part B). Care provided within a health clinic is supported by Part B of the Medicare insurance plan. Additional information on Medicare benefits is available online (www.medicare.gov).

Medicaid is a health insurance program for certain low-income people. It is funded and administered through state–federal partnerships (Department of Health and Human Services, 2004b). States are responsible for establishing the criteria by which funds will be distributed within broad guidelines established by the federal government. Currently, about 36 million people are eligible for Medicaid. This includes persons with low incomes, high medical bills, and disabilities.

Medicaid benefits vary from state to state, but they must include inpatient and outpatient hospital services, doctors' surgical and medical services, laboratory and X-ray services, and well-baby and childcare services, including immunizations. Many of these are services that can be provided by local health clinics. It is essential to take advantage of these funds when providing quality care to your community. Be sure to be familiar with all the state regulations and finding opportunities that apply to a community clinic.

CLINIC STAFF

Staffing for a health clinic is essential to the day-to-day success of the operation. Before determining the mix of employees that is appropriate for a clinic, it is important to consider applicable state laws and regulations, the people that will be served, and the services that will be offered. Some states may require that a physician oversee all medical care being performed at a clinic. Other states may allow a physician to write standing orders that are then carried out by physician assistants or nurse practitioners. Thus, it is important to have a complete understanding of applicable state guidelines when considering the staffing requirements of a proposed facility.

Many states will now allow for standing orders to be written by physicians, with nurse practitioners and physician assistants handling most patient care responsibilities. Guidelines usually require physicians to make periodic visits to review charts and practices. A physician must also be available for consultation during all hours that the clinic is in operation. It is very important for clinic staff to establish a trusting relationship with the physician who serves as the clinic's medical director. The communication lines between clinic staff and the medical director must be maintained to ensure success. Bi-weekly or monthly meetings with all clinical staff will help to maintain a climate of positive communications in a health clinic.

It is important that members of the clinical staff establish relationships with several area physicians. In this way, they will become familiar with the strengths and weaknesses of particular physicians and practitioners with regards to consultations and information requests. They will also be able to approach physicians based on their areas of specialization. For example, if the clinic needs a consultation about a mother who is having a particularly difficult pregnancy, it is advantageous for the clinic to have an established relationship with a local obstetrician. Advice or case management assistance can be obtained over the phone. Similar situations exist for children and pediatricians or older adults and cardiologists. Some essential lifelines may come from area doctors and their support.

Drug companies often provide another important link in the public health system. Pharmaceuticals are costly. Even people who have health insurance often lack the ability to pay for all of their prescription drugs. One way that clinicians can help reduce costs for their patients is to provide drug samples. Creating a positive working relationship with area pharmaceutical representatives is one way for a clinic to obtain drug samples. Samples are often important contributions to a clinic. Another source of samples may be local physicians' offices. Once again, it is important to establish working relationships with local physicians. The ability to ask for samples is an important skill for clinic staff. Make sure that area physicians know what types of samples are most often used. Always express appreciation for their support. This should be done in writing. Consider providing recognition for physicians and pharmaceutical companies. Always ask permission before making public recognition. Some persons prefer to donate in an anonymous manner. Never turn down any assistance. Local physicians and drug companies can be major advocates if proper appreciation is shown to them.

It is important for the health clinic staff to have up-to-date information about available drug treatments. However, they may be able to prescribe effective drugs that are older and less costly than those that are currently under patent protection. Generic drugs often provide effective treatment, but pharmaceutical companies may not actively market them because they are available from many sources and do not generate as much revenue as nongenerics. Encourage clinic staff to be informed providers and use generic drugs that are effective in managing some conditions. However, medications should not be prescribed solely based on cost. Personal well-being must always be the first consideration. However, it is important to remember that higher costs do not always equate with more effective treatment.

Another important community contact may be a local hospital that receives state funding. State-funded hospitals are an important element in the public health infrastructure. Such hospitals can help local clinics when they encounter people that require care beyond the capabilities of local clinical staff. Establishing a relationship with such a facility will provide access to advanced technology and care. State-funded hospitals are often located in large urban areas and may be linked to medical schools.

Other important services that may be obtained from local hospitals are radiology and laboratory services. These types of assistance can potentially save clinics substantial amounts of money. Talking with local hospitals and radiologists may yield partnerships to provide assistance at reduced cost.

MARKETING

Once a local health clinic has been created, funding has been secured, and clinical staff hired, marketing efforts must be undertaken. Analyzing the constituents, the contributors, and the community should yield leads for effectively marketing a health clinic. Marketing can increase the volume of services provided to an area by creating awareness about the available programs and capabilities of a clinic.

First, analyze the prospective users of the clinic. What are the demographics of the community? Marketing programs must be targeted at these demographic factors. If there are many non-English-speaking people in the target population, then marketing efforts must use their language. Large populations of single mothers will be interested in well-baby clinics and other related services that can assist them. It is important to keep the goals and mission statement of a clinic facility at the forefront of marketing strategies. If the mission is to serve a community and create a healthy climate, then advertise the services that will provide the greatest help to the community in achieving these goals.

Marketing to contributors is also important. Send local physicians and other medical workers information on how they can become involved with the clinic. Provide them information on the types of services offered by the clinic and the impact of the clinic on the local community. If the positive aspects of the clinic are demonstrated to area medical workers, the number of supporters is likely to increase.

Finally, market the clinic's goals for community health to members of the community. Make the clinic a service and a facility that the community can be proud of and support. Market community service opportunities to high school students and college students in the area. Young adults are one of the largest groups of supporters of community service available. They may also become users of clinic services. If the health department can get the community to believe that the clinic plays a positive role in the community, and if the population accepts the goals of the clinic, then more than enough support will be obtained to successfully operate the clinic. The clinic's success will have a positive impact on the community.

CONCLUSION

Many local health departments open clinics after conducting needs assessments of their communities. Access to a community-run clinic is an important consideration. Sensitivity to the cultures of targeted populations increases utilization. Local health clinics must follow state and federal guidelines. Funding is available from state and federal resources. Continued funding for community clinics is often challenging. Clinic staff must be carefully selected and trained. Marketing clinic programs and services in appropriate and sensitive ways helps to build user volume.

Returning to the opening case study, cost and access are negative factors that contribute to inadequate health care. Giving up their desire to compete was not an option for Amanda and Ben. An emergency room visit was a poor option; the twins were too healthy to justify the expense of an emergency room consultation. Instead, the twins were taken to a clinic operated by the local health department.

The local clinic is staffed by a physician assistant and a nurse midwife. Two physicians are on call to provide consultations and advice. Three nurses coordinate the flow of sick and well persons. They also administer immunizations and other routine injections. The clinic has a sliding scale of fees based on income.

The health department budget makes up any shortfalls in operating revenues. The board of health looks upon the clinic as a long-term investment in the health of the community. The board knows that the amount of money spent on prevention and wellness is usually far less than that spent on disease treatment. The board has saved the cost of treatment many times over by providing basic and routine health care services at a cost that is affordable to citizens of the community.

References

National Rural Health Association. 2004. Rural Health Clinics—Rules and Guidelines. Available at www.nrharural.org/pagefile/RHCGuidelines.html.

U.S. Census Bureau. 2002. Health Insurance Coverage: 2001. Available at http://www.sipp.census.gov/sipp/workpapr/wp243.pdf

U.S. Department of Health and Human Services. 2004a. Centers for Medicare and Medicaid Services. Available at www.cms.hhs.gov/medicare.

U.S. Department of Health and Human Services. 2004b. Centers for Medicare and Medicaid Services. Available at www.cms.hhs.gov/medicaid.

Resources

Periodicals

Clifton, G.D., Byer, H., Heaton, K., Haberman, D.J., and Gill, H. 2003. Provision of pharmacy services to underserved populations via remote dispensing and two-way videoconferencing. *American Journal of Health System Pharmacy* 60(24):2577–2582.

Hajat, A., Stewart, K., and Hayes, K.L. 2003. The local public health workforce in rural communities. *Journal of Public Health Management and Practice* 9(6):481–488.

Heller, B.R., and Goldwater, M.R. 2004. The Governor's Wellmobile: Maryland's mobile primary care clinic. *Journal of Nursing Education* 43(2):92–94.

O'Toole, T.P., Conde-Martel, A., Gibbon, J.L., Hanusa, B.H., and Fine, M.J. 2003. Health care of homeless veterans. *Journal of General Internal Medicine* 18(11):929–933.

Parsons, R.J., Murray, B.P., and Dwore, R.B. 2003. Trends in rural healthcare delivery in the United States, 1990–1999. *Journal of Hospital Marketing and Public Relations* 14(2):23–36.

Scala, M. 2003. Developing rural information and assistance programs. *Issue Brief—Center for Medicare Education* 4(7):1–4.

Books

Aguirre-Molina, M., and Molina, C. 2003. *Latina Health in the United States: A Public Health Reader.* New York: Wiley.

Baer, D.L. 2003. *Doctors in a Strange Land: The Place of International Medical Graduates in Rural America.* Lanham, MD: Rowman & Littlefield.

Loue, S., and Quill, B.E. 2001. *Handbook of Rural Health.* New York: Kluwer.

National Institute of Medicine. 2003. *The Future of the Public's Health in the 21st Century.* Washington, D.C.: National Academy Press.

Stamm, B.H. 2003. *Rural Behavioral Health Care: An Interdisciplinary Guide.* Chicago: American Psychological Association.

Web Sites

- American Medical Student Association: www.amsa.org/programs/gpit/ruralurban.cfm
- Kansas City Free Health Clinic: www.kcfree.org
- National Association of Rural Health Clinics: www.narhc.org/about_us/about_us.php
- Nemours Health Clinic: www.nemours.org/no/nhc
- Rural Assistance Center—Rural Health Clinics: www.raconline.org/info_guides/clinics/rhc.php

- Scripps—Community Health Clinics: www.scrippshealth.org/71.asp

Organizations

American College of Healthcare Executives
One North Franklin, Suite 1700
Chicago, IL 60606-4425
Phone: 312-424-2800
Fax: 312-424-0023
E-mail: geninfo@ache.org
Web site: www.ache.org

American Medical Association
515 N. State Street
Chicago, IL 60610
Phone: 800-621-8335
Web site: www.ama-assn.org

American Public Health Association
800 I Street, NW
Washington, D.C. 20001-3710
Phone: 202-777-2742
Fax: 202-777-2534
E-mail: comments@apha.org
Web site: www.apha.org

Centers for Medicare & Medicaid Services
7500 Security Boulevard
Baltimore, MD 21244-1850
Phone: 877-267-2323 or 410-786-3000
Web site: www.cms.hhs.gov

Joint Commission on Accreditation of Healthcare Organizations
One Renaissance Blvd.
Oakbrook Terrace, IL 60181
Phone: 630-792-5000
Fax: 630-792-5005
E-mail: customerservice@jcaho.org
Web site: www.jcaho.org

National Association of Local Boards of Health
1840 East Gypsy Lane Road
Bowling Green, OH 43402
Phone: 419-353-7714
Fax: 419-352-6278
E-mail: nalboh@nalboh.org
Web site: www.nalboh.org

National Rural Health Association
One West Armour Blvd., Suite 203
Kansas City, MO 64111-2087
Phone: 816-756-3140
E-mail: mail@nrharural.org
Web site: www.nrharural.org

PART

IX

Other Health Departments and Jurisdictions

CHAPTER

35

State Health Departments

Gary Crum

Chapter Objectives

After reading this chapter, readers will:

- Have an understanding of the interrelationships that exist between local and state health departments.
- Understand the variety of roles undertaken by state health departments.
- Know how local health department administrators can maximize their relationships with state health department officials.

Chapter Summary

This chapter reviews the wide variety of interrelationships between state and local health departments. Some states have complete control over local health department operations, whereas other local health departments are autonomous. This chapter outlines the general roles of state health departments and the special policy-setting role the state assumes in the federal–state–local mix of public health duties. Finally, mechanisms for viewing and reducing potential tensions between state and local health departments are offered.

Case Study

The administrator of a frugal rural county health department has concluded that a state regulation affecting fees for restaurant inspections should be revised. The agency's costs for such inspections are running about 18 percent higher than the maximum fees permitted by the state health department. This can be tolerated for the rest of the current fiscal year, but it cannot be sustained for much longer without cutting services in another area of local operations. The local health department's money-saving action will be to lay off a long-time employee. The area that will be cut is health education, an area with fewer state mandates. What steps should be taken and what allies should be recruited to bring about a change in state regulations? What arguments might be used with state health department officials and state legislators to bring about the policy change? Should the state health department's director be expected to assist with the proposed change? What potential opponents would you expect to such a proposal and how might they be recruited or neutralized?

INTRODUCTION

State health departments are key players in the national public health effort. The federal government plays a key role, too, especially with regards to funding. Federal money comes in the form of categorical programs such as family planning (Title X) or as large block grants such as Maternal and Child Health (Title V). These funds often flow through the state before they reach local health departments. Therefore, although people actually receive the vast majority of public health services from local health departments, state statutes regarding public health duties largely determine how federal funds and political and regulatory power is shared with local health departments.

State health departments, which have various names in different states, usually oversee local health department activities for regulating environmental health concerns such as inspecting restaurants and public swimming pools, investigating animal bites, and abating sewage nuisances. The state also generally sets the fees for such local activities or sets a process by which the fees can be set by local health departments.

Vaccination programs, a major outreach effort of most local health departments, are often dependent on state vaccine contracts for group purchasing. They also depend on state nursing-practice protocols that tell local health department nurses how to practice nursing. Even large federal block grants for preventive health services and maternal and child health services are adapted, with federal oversight, by each state. The adaptations are all different and are based on decisions made by state health officials. Some state health departments funnel generous amounts of federal dollars to local health departments, whereas others retain a large share of federal dollars at the state capital.

State–local health department relationships vary. Each state is different. In some states, the state health department staffs some local health departments. A convenient example is provided by the state of Virginia. The State of Virginia hires and pays the salaries of employees who are assigned to work for local health agencies. At the other extreme are local health departments that are largely financially autonomous from the state. Ohio, for example, has 88 counties and over 140 local health departments that receive very little state funding. However, next door in Kentucky there are 120 counties and fewer than 60 local health departments. Some counties have combined into district health departments. They receive large amounts of funding from the state in the form of a state block grant system to local health departments. **Figure 35-1** summarizes state–local relationships in the 50 states.

The variety of state–local relationships is a function of the fact that state health laws establish the infrastructure for delivery of federal funds and for enforcing public health regulations. Thus, the federal government has little say in how each state decides to share power with local governments and local boards of health. It is up to state governments to decide if there will even be a local public health apparatus in addition to

Centralized	**Decentralized**	**Centralized and Decentralized**	**Joint / Shared**	**None**
States where local health departments operate under strict state health department control.	States where local health departments are operated by local governments rather than state governments.	States where only some local health departments (e.g., large cities) are largely autonomous of the state.	States where states and local governments/boards have a dual responsibility for local health department operations.	States with no local health departments.
Arkansas	Arizona	Alaska	Alabama	Rhode Island
Delaware	Colorado	California	Florida	
Louisiana	Connecticut	Hawaii	Georgia	
Mississippi	Idaho	Illinois	Kentucky	
New Mexico	Indiana	Maine	Maryland	
Vermont	Iowa	Massachusetts	Minnesota	
Virginia	Kansas	Nevada	North Carolina	
	Michigan	New Hampshire	Ohio	
	Missouri	New York	Washington	
	Montana	Oklahoma	West Virginia	
	Nebraska	Pennsylvania		
	New Jersey	South Dakota		
	North Dakota	Tennessee		
	Oregon	Texas		
	South Carolina	Wyoming		
	Utah			
	Wisconsin			

Figure 35-1 State–Local Health Department Relationships

Source: Bureau of Health Professions (2000).

the statewide agency. For example, Rhode Island has no local health departments.

States differ in how they structure their local health departments. States also differ with regards to the functions that are administered by the state health department and those that are delegated to local jurisdictions. For example, the top state public health official may or may not hold a cabinet-level appointment. In some states, the senior public health executive reports to a cabinet-level appointee of the governor. Some states do not require the head of the state health department to be a physician. Titles also vary.

Continuing with Kentucky and Ohio as examples, the head of the Ohio Department of Health has the title of *director* and is a member of the governor's cabinet. In Kentucky, the health department director carries the title of *health commissioner* and reports to a minister in the governor's cabinet who oversees a broad array of human services departments, including Medicaid, aging, public health, and developmental disabilities. In Ohio, the title of *health commissioner* is reserved for leaders of local health departments.

Some state health departments have massive responsibilities and large numbers of staff. They may oversee the operation of health care delivery services such as hospitals. Others have largely regulatory and funding responsibilities, rendering few or no services directly to the populace of their states. In those states, the local health departments provide programs and services.

In all states, the state health department plays a key role in setting regulations for public health bills passed by the state legislature. State health officials also interact with a wide variety of public health stakeholders who themselves have potentially powerful allies in the legislative, judicial, and executive branches of government. Local health departments are often disappointed to find that when seeking power or policy relief from the state health department, they have no ally. Their expected natural ally often has a different agenda than the local health departments might expect.

The state health department director may also be called the *state health commissioner*, depending on the state. In the past, this person was invariably a physician. However, more and more states are allowing local and state health directors to be nonphysicians. An advanced degree is still generally required, especially the Master of Public Health or its equivalent.

A state health director reaches that post through a variety of career pathways. Two such avenues are to be appointed by the governor or appointed by a statewide board of health. The statewide board of health is usually composed of health experts appointed by the governor to lengthy terms to give it some protection from being swayed by the political winds. It takes time for a new governor to change the direction of a health department, because it can take years to restructure the state board of health membership. Thus, many in public health circles think that local and state public health administrators should be appointed by a board of some kind rather than by a single elected official. Public health, more so than most other areas, is a field that requires both expertise and autonomy.

Some of the strongest government powers in the Western world reside in health departments, in particular, the power of quarantine. In many jurisdictions, the top public health official has the authority to take persons off the street and incarcerate them without a court order or the approval of local law enforcement officials. Restaurants, grocery stores, and swimming pools can be padlocked on a moment's notice in many jurisdictions if the local health director or local board of health decides that they pose an imminent risk to the public's health.

Quarantine has been seldom used in recent decades. It was originally developed to prevent movement of people infected with communicable diseases such as scarlet fever, cholera, and plague. However, in the current environment in which governments are increasingly concerned with the possibility that the next epidemic might be purposeful or due to an act of bioterrorism, health directors have been revisiting the quarantine policies in each state. All state health departments have developed new bioterrorism plans, and staffs are increasingly revisiting the role of quarantine powers.

■ STATE HEALTH DEPARTMENT STRUCTURE

The state health director and a small number of political appointees generally head a state health department. They often share power with several long-time civil servants, merit system employees who have job protections not available to political appointees. Political appointees serve at the will of the governor or state board of health and can be dismissed for any reason. Civil servants cannot be removed from their posts very easily, especially if they have seniority based on many years of service.

In reality, new health directors arriving at a state health department can make some changes, but seldom as many as they envisioned prior to their arrival. The budget of the state health department is set by legislative mandates as many as two years earlier in states that have a biennial budget process. Also, mandated services must be provided until lengthy policy changes can be crafted.

For example, family planning and abortion are often part of a health department's scope of operations and may be two of the most controversial policies in state government. New governors may come in with a strong pro-life or pro-choice mandate, but find that they must faithfully operate a federally funded family planning program or a sexual abstinence program. It can take years before either can be altered. Failure to faithfully operate these programs until the changes can be approved at the various levels of government can result in political or legal sanctions being brought against state policy makers and the governor. Legal sanctions may be brought as a result of judicial review.

As mentioned earlier, a state may have a statewide board of health composed of people appointed for lengthy terms by previous governors or legislative groups. This process is expressly designed to prevent any quick policy changes in the crucial area of public health protection. Such a board and its policies may be at odds with the current governor's policy desires.

Generally, there are three health-related units of state government: environmental health programs, health education and promotion programs, and clinical services.

Environmental Programs

Environmental programs vary greatly from state to state. Generally, they include such functions as food safety, home sewage disposal (septic field layouts), radon control, vector control (rats, mice, mosquitoes, and flies), rabies control (animal bite investigations), and other programs. Some of these other programs may include a far-ranging set of responsibilities for environmental health policies affecting milk producers, trailer parks, marinas, hazardous waste disposal, solid waste disposal, public water system standards, air and water pollution, tattoo parlor inspections, brothel inspections (in Nevada), plumbing standards, building codes, and radiation safety (e.g., X-ray machine inspections). Actual inspections relating to such programs are often not performed by state employees, but may take place in the local health departments under the scrutiny of state officials. If local health officials do not report directly to the state but rather to an autonomous local board of health, any failure by a local health department to meet the state's expectations may result in local health funds being cut off. Under the laws of some states, the state health director can assume the local health department's functions if the local health department is determined to be putting the local population at risk.

Health Education and Promotion

The area of health education and promotion has traditionally been relatively small, but it is becoming increasingly important in addressing chronic diseases such as heart disease, cancer, and stroke that are attributable to lifestyle choices. Tobacco use, obesity, sedentary lifestyles, unsafe workplaces, malnutrition, risky sexual behaviors, inadequate parenting skills, undetected illnesses, and a variety of other problems fall into the realm of a health education. In the past, public health did not offer vaccines or screening tests. A common result was a door-to-door effort by nurses who brought needed health understanding to affected families in an area. Home visitation services are being re-created in many states. A common goal is meeting the needs of new parents who require additional assistance to ensure that children are screened early for health problems. At the same time, parents are given data and help to get their children off to a healthy start in life. Nurses, social workers, and paraprofessionals assume health education roles in homes, mirroring the earlier model of public health delivery.

Clinical Services

A registered nurse, followed by a registered sanitarian or an environmental worker, is likely to be the most frequently encountered public health professional. State health department workers design and oversee the services that are provided to people. Such services are usually delivered by local employees in local health department buildings, not in state health department facilities.

Among the commonly encountered areas of state health department clinical program oversight are vaccination protocol development and enforcement, infectious disease surveillance, tuberculosis and sexually transmitted disease screening (including AIDS), cancer screening, family planning, and well-child clinics. Depending on the state, clinical oversight by state health departments may also impact other tasks. Such tasks include health education and promotion, school health services, home-delivered skilled nursing services to sick elderly patients, migrant health clinics, and full-service primary care clinics staffed by physicians, nurse practitioners, and physician assistants. Registered dietitians often work with nurses and other professionals to provide services often overseen by state policy makers, including the Women, Infants, and Children (WIC) program funded by the U.S. Department of Agriculture. This large-budget program provides food vouchers for needy pregnant women and young children.

Other State Health Department Functions

State health departments may be intimately involved in other service programs such as state Medicaid programs for residents who cannot afford health care, environmental protection, services for the aged, mental health services, oral health care programs, occupational health protection, violence and suicide prevention, youth-related services, women's health services, migrant/immigrant health programs, prison health programs, alcohol and drug abuse prevention, newborn screening services, hospital and nursing home regulations, child welfare promotion, grocery inspections, and ambulatory clinic inspections.

Vital statistics are an important area of state involvement. State offices collect mortality and morbidity statistics from around the state. Many states manage death records and birth certificate protocols. Some states maintain cancer registries.

Some state health departments, such as Hawaii and Texas, provide complex hospital services. Those responsibilities mirror the difficult management challenges facing acute care facilities throughout the nation, such as maintaining services in a competitive environment with inflation and complicated third-party payer, legal, and regulatory demands.

Finally, state health departments have been mandated by the federal government to improve bioterrorism readiness. The federal government has provided funds for bioterrorism readiness activities. Virtually every person on the globe is vulnerable to bioterrorism threats (Smolinski et al., 2003). This presents an important new demand for health department staff training and deployment at both the state and local levels.

STATE–LOCAL RELATIONSHIP TENSIONS AND OPPORTUNITIES

In the eyes of a local health department administrator, the state health apparatus may be seen as the power base for decision making. This is especially true when local health department personnel are actually frontline state employees. In most states, local health department staff are not state employees. The state often becomes a policy setter that local departments often dislike, but without which they cannot survive.

In states where the local health department is not staffed by state employees, several commonly heard complaints arise. Local jurisdictions complain that the state health department does not adequately champion frontline public health needs in the legislature. Local health departments often think that states provide insufficient funds to local public health and keep too great a share of federal funding for themselves. State governments are accused of micromanaging local health departments that have special regional or health status challenges atypical to the rest of their state.

Local and state views of reality differ. Each complains that the other's view of political reality is erroneous. From time to time, states tend to complain about the disorganization of local health departments. States decry the lack of performance standards relative to what a local health department should be and the services it should provide. States complain about the variety of local responses, and misresponses, to state inquiries and directives. Some states' legislators and administrators comment about the inadequacy of community contributions in funding some local health departments.

State health departments uniformly complain that the federal government sends them new mandates that are not accompanied by adequate funds. Local health departments likewise accuse states of enacting regulations that create the same unfunded mandate hardships for them.

How to cope with these tensions? One successful strategy is to develop state–local initiatives. A good way to accomplish this kind of teamwork is to select an issue that is already high on the agendas of both the governor and state legislators (Akter, 2001). As long as the issue is a legitimate public health matter of some importance, this approach will bear public health advances in the state. Such an approach is less adversarial and wastes less time. Another approach is to increase communications. The states do not always understand all of the local factors that prevent some local health departments from quickly responding to state initiatives. By sharing problems with the state rather than complaining that they should know about them, an increased sensitivity can be achieved and more reasonable timeframes adopted by the state. By the same token, if states share more information about some of the federal and state political pressures under which they operate, local departments might be more tolerant of state dictates.

Having each level dwell on the best aspects of their respective and different roles is productive. The typical advantages of being a state health department staff person usually include a better salary, a strong union or protection via civil service, and the opportunity to contribute to broad public policies affecting large numbers of persons. The major advantage of being a staff person in a local health department is actually delivering the services.

■ CONCLUSION

State and local health departments operate under a variety of complex models that vary from state to state. Their respective staffs must cooperate closely and put their differences aside whenever possible to make the division of labor work. In the end, the people being served must be the main consideration. Local public health administrators that fail to reach a functional working arrangement with state and federal officials will often end up short-changing those they are trying to serve.

This does not mean that local health departments must eschew any autonomy they have been given in their state. It does mean that that autonomy must be exercised in accordance with the division of labor established for that state, in conjunction with a commitment to healthy collaboration and cooperation. Anything else will result in state–local tensions that will reduce the quality and quantity of services delivered to the state's citizens, many of whom depend on the health department for essential, life-sustaining services.

Returning to the county health administrator in the case study, after receiving approval from the local board of health to pursue a change in the regulations to permit higher fees, he wisely sought support for this state policy change from other health departments in similar straits. He knew that without widespread support from other health departments for increased fees, his effort might be doomed. Increasing fees is often equated by politicians as increased taxes. Even then, the state might be unwilling to bow to pressure unless the local health departments are able to generate some legislative momentum for changing the underlying fee-setting statutes.

If possible, friendly state health officials and state legislators, not necessarily those from the legislative district where the administrator works, should be recruited. University experts and lobbyists with health connections may also be brought in, but this will require funds not usually available to local health departments. An exception to this trend would be to seek funding from the state health department or the state public health association.

Five main strategies were developed for changing the fee structure. Fee structures were compared with adjoining states, where inspections are funded at different levels. Fee levels were correlated with the number of outbreaks of food-borne illness. State executive and legislative branch officials were reminded that their children eat in the pizzerias and other restaurants where inspections must be conducted often and carefully to protect the public. The administrator reviewed the detailed steps in each inspection and the types of problems encountered that require expertise. He listed numerous unfunded mandates sent to local agencies by state policy makers interested in appeasing constituents but not interested in raising taxes or fees. Delicately, a group of health administrators from all parts of the state reminded the legislature that it passed a law requiring local health departments to conduct an annual review of local child fatalities, but allocated no additional funding to undertake this new task. Data was collected to support the argument that the fees being charged are indeed inadequate and were originally based on a conservative cost analysis.

Unless prohibited by a legal or ethical conflict, the state health director should be called upon to assist in developing a new regulation. The state health director may be willing to have staff members work with specific legislators to restructure the statutes affecting the state's right to set such fees. Statewide regulation changes are much easier to obtain if a statute does not have to be revised. Some states allow the state health department to unilaterally revise fees. In some states, local health departments can set some of their own fees.

Working closely with key potential opponents to try and neutralize strong opposition is useful when seeking statewide regulatory policy changes. Potential opponents of this type of fee change include restaurant owner associations, taxpayer associations, food service workers unions, and the Chambers of Commerce. Letters of endorsement from any local restaurant owners who appreciate the efforts of local and state health department workers in helping them provide safer services should be obtained. Large restaurant chains are generally more likely to provide such support for new fees and higher inspection standards, because they sometimes already hold their stores to more expensive cleanliness standards than their local competition.

References

Akter, M. 2001. *Public Health in the Political Arena.* Jefferson City, MO: Missouri Department of Health and Senior Services.

Bureau of Health Professions. 2000. *The Public Health Workforce: Enumeration 2000.* New York: Center for Health Policy, Columbia University School of Nursing.

Smolinski, M.S., Hamburg, M.A., and Lederberg, J. 2003. *Microbial Threats to Health: Emergence, Detection, and Response.* Washington, D.C.: National Academy Press.

Resources

Periodicals

Coid, D.R., Williams, B., and Crombie, I.K. 2003. Partnerships with health and private voluntary organizations: What are the issues for health authorities and boards? *Public Health* 117(5):317–322.

Weil, T.P. 2003. Governance in a period of strategic change in U.S. healthcare. *International Journal Health Planning Management* 18(3):247–265.

Books

Centers for Disease Control and Prevention. 2003. *The National Public Health Performance Standards.* Atlanta, GA: Public Health Practice Program Office, Centers for Disease Control and Prevention.

Web Sites

Each state and the District of Columbia department of health has a Web site. Five representative examples follow.

- Arizona Department of Health Services:
  http://www.hs.state.az.us/
- New Jersey Department of Health and Senior Services:
  http://www.state.nj.us/health/
- North Carolina Department of Health and Human Services:
  http://www.dhhs.state.nc.us/
- Ohio Department of Health:
  http://www.odh.state.oh.us/index.asp
- Utah Department of Health:
  http://www.health.utah.gov/

Organizations

American Public Health Association
800 I Street, NW
Washington, D.C. 20001-3710
Phone: 202-777-2742
Fax: 202-777-2534
E-mail: comments@apha.org
Web site: www.apha.org

Association of State and Territorial Health Officials
1275 K Street NW, Suite 800
Washington, D.C. 20005-4006
Phone: 202-371-9090
Fax: 202-371-9797
Web site: www.astho.org

Centers for Disease Control and Prevention
1600 Clifton Road
Atlanta, GA 30333
Phone: 404-639-3311, 404-639-3534, or 800-311-3435
E-mail: www.cdc.gov/netinfo.htm (Web form)
Web site: www.cdc.gov>

National Association of Local Boards of Health
1840 East Gypsy Lane Road
Bowling Green, OH 43402
Phone: 419-353-7714
Fax: 419-352-6278
E-mail: nalboh@nalboh.org
Web site: www.nalboh.org

National Environmental Health Association
720 S. Colorado Blvd., Suite 970-S
Denver, CO 80246-1925
Phone: 303-756-9090
Fax: 303-691-9490
E-mail: staff@neha.org
Web site: www.neha.org

Public Health Foundation
1220 L Street, NW, Suite 350
Washington, D.C. 20005
Phone: 202-898-5600
Fax: 202-898-5609
E-mail: info@phf.org
Web site: www.phf.org

CHAPTER

36

Federal Departments and Agencies

Marie M. Fallon
Vonna J. Henry
Anthony J. Santarsiero

Chapter Objectives

After reading this chapter, readers will:

- Identify the federal role and mission in public health.
- Identify resources available from the federal government.
- Describe the protocols for requesting assistance from the federal government.
- Understand the expectations the federal government has of local public health agencies as well as what local public health agencies can expect from the federal government.

Chapter Summary

This chapter describes the role and mission of the federal government as it relates to local public health agencies. Resources that are available from the federal government and methods for accessing those resources for local public health will be identified. The chapter also discusses the federal government's expectations of local public health agencies and what local public health agencies can expect from the federal government. Web sites are provided to direct readers to additional sources of information. These are provided in the body of the chapter.

Case Study

Aloma County serves a diverse population of approximately 75,000 people and is located about an hour's drive from a large metropolitan area. Recently, the local health department implemented the Mobilizing for Action through Planning and Partnerships (MAPP) process, a community-wide strategic planning tool for involving members of a community in a partnership with public health officials to improve the health and quality of life in a community. (National Association of City and County Health Officers, 2004).

Three strategic issues were identified as priorities during the MAPP process. First, the county is becoming more diverse and has experienced an influx of immigrants who have significant health problems, including tuberculosis. Second, problems with adult obesity in the county are increasing. Third, the health department has concluded that during a bioterrorism incident, an outbreak of an infectious disease, a public health threat, or an emergency, the county's resources would be severely stretched. Complicating these issues is the fact that only a few professional staff members understand epidemiology and terrorism preparedness. Even fewer are trained in emergency response.

As a result of the MAPP process, the health officer, with full involvement from the Aloma County board of health, has begun to identify resources and develop programs to address these strategic issues. Several questions have been asked. What is the federal government's role and mission? How do these interface with the local or state government's role and mission? What resources are available from the federal government? Which federal agencies can provide assistance on the best practices of public health? How can assistance be obtained from the federal government? How can federal resources be requested and used in an emergency? What expectations does the federal government have of local public health agencies, and conversely, what can local public health agencies expect from the federal government?

INTRODUCTION

In the event of an emergency, the federal government can provide extensive resources to states and local municipalities. However, these resources must be specifically requested. The federal government can provide resources and assistance in other instances as well. Again, such resources and assistance must be requested. This chapter describes the departments and agencies of the federal government that support public health. It discusses the forms of assistance that are available and delineates procedures to request help during an emergency and protocols to use when applying for aid and resources during normal times.

Some of the text contained in this chapter was obtained from official federal government web sites. Such text has been included without being changed. Finally, the content of this chapter has been reviewed for accuracy by the Centers for Disease Control and Prevention.

THE ROLE AND MISSION OF THE FEDERAL GOVERNMENT

The Department of Health and Human Services (DHHS) is the U.S. government's principal agency for protecting the health of all Americans and providing essential human services, especially for those who are least able to help themselves. DHHS works closely with state, local, and tribal governments. Many DHHS-funded services are provided at the local level by state, county, or tribal agencies or through private sector grantees. The department's programs are administered by 11 DHHS operating divisions, including 8 agencies in the U.S. Public Health Service and 3 human services agencies. In addition to the services they deliver, the DHHS programs provide for equitable treatment of beneficiaries nationwide, and they enable the collection of national health and other data (Department of Health and Human Services, 2004a).

The DHHS strategic goals for fiscal years 2003–2008 are contained in **Figure 36-1.**

U.S. Public Health Service Agencies

The Centers for Disease Control and Prevention (CDC) is recognized as the lead federal agency in protecting the public's health and safety. This responsibility includes providing credible information to enhance health decisions and promoting health through strong partnerships, both home and abroad. The CDC develops and applies disease prevention and control, environmental health, and health promotion and education activities designed to improve the health of the people of the United States.

Goal 1:	Reduce the major threats to the health and well-being of Americans.
Goal 2:	Enhance the ability of the Nation's healthcare system to effectively respond to bioterrorism and other public health challenges.
Goal 3:	Increase the percentage of the Nation's children and adults who have access to healthcare services, and expand consumer choices.
Goal 4:	Enhance the capacity and productivity of the Nation's health science research enterprise.
Goal 5:	Improve the quality of healthcare services.
Goal 6:	Improve the economic and social well-being of individuals, families and communities, especially those most in need.
Goal 7:	Improve the stability and healthy development of our Nation's children and youth.
Goal 8:	Achieve excellence in management practices.

Figure 36-1 Department of Health and Human Services Strategic Goals

Source: Department of Health and Human Services, 2004b.

The CDC's vision for the twenty-first century is *Healthy People in a Healthy World—Through Prevention.* The CDC's mission is to promote health and quality of life by preventing and controlling disease, injury, and disability. The CDC is composed of the following:

- The **National Center on Birth Defects and Developmental Disabilities** (NCBDDD) provides national leadership for preventing birth defects and developmental disabilities and for improving the health and wellness of people with disabilities.
- The **National Center for Chronic Disease Prevention and Health Promotion** (NCCDPHP) prevents premature death and disability from chronic diseases and promotes healthy personal behaviors.
- The **National Center for Environmental Health** (NCEH) provides national leadership in preventing and controlling disease and death resulting from the interactions between people and their environment.
- The **National Center for Health Statistics** (NCHS) provides statistical information that will guide actions and policies to improve the health of the American people.
- The **National Center for HIV, STD and TB Prevention** (NCHSTP) provides national leadership in preventing and controlling HIV infection, sexually transmitted diseases, and tuberculosis.
- The **National Center for Infectious Diseases** (NCID) prevents illness, disability, and death caused by infectious diseases in the United States and around the world.
- The **National Center for Injury Prevention and Control** (NCIPC) prevents death and disability from nonoccupational injuries, including those that are unintentional and those that result from violence.
- The **National Immunization Program** (NIP) prevents disease, disability, and death from vaccine-preventable diseases in children and adults.
- The **National Institute for Occupational Safety and Health** (NIOSH) ensures safety and health for all people in the workplace through research and prevention.
- The **Epidemiology Program Office** (EPO) strengthens the public health system by coordinating public health surveillance; providing support in scientific communications, statistics, and epidemiology; and training in surveillance, epidemiology, and prevention effectiveness.
- The **Public Health Practice Program Office** (PHPPO) strengthens community practice of public health by creating an effective workforce, building information networks, conducting practice research, and ensuring laboratory quality.
- The **Office of the Director** (CDC/OD) manages and directs the activities of the CDC; provides overall direction to, and coordination of, the scientific/medical programs of CDC; and provides leadership, coordination, and assessment of administrative management activities.

The CDC performs many of the administrative functions for the **Agency for Toxic Substances and Disease Registry (ATSDR)**, a sister agency of CDC and one of the other eight Federal public health agencies within DHHS. The director of CDC also serves as the administrator of ATSDR (Centers for Disease Control and Prevention, 2004a). The mission of ATSDR is to serve the public by using the best science, taking responsive public health actions, and providing trusted health information to prevent harmful exposures and disease related to toxic substances (Centers for Disease Control and Prevention, 2004a).

The mission of the **Health Resources and Services Administration (HRSA)** is to improve and expand access to quality health care for all. The goal of HRSA is moving toward 100 percent access to health care and zero health disparities for all Americans. As *The Access Agency* of the Department of Health and Human Services, HRSA assures the availability of quality health care to low income, uninsured, isolated, vulnerable, and special needs populations and meets their unique health care needs. The strategies of HRSA are to eliminate barriers to care, eliminate health disparities, assure quality of care, and improve public health and healthcare systems (Centers for Disease Control and Prevention, 2004a).

The **National Institutes of Health (NIH)** today comprises one of the world's foremost medical research centers. NIH is the Federal focal point for health research and the steward of medical and behavioral research for the Nation. The mission of NIH is science in pursuit of fundamental knowledge about the nature and behavior of living systems and the application of that knowledge to extend healthy life and reduce the burdens of illness and disability. The goals of NIH are: (1) to foster fundamental creative discoveries, innovative research strategies, and their applications as a basis to advance significantly the Nation's capacity to protect and improve health; (2) develop, maintain, and renew scientific human and physical resources that will assure the Nation's capability to prevent disease; (3) expand the knowledge base in medical and associated sciences in order to enhance the Nation's economic well-being and ensure a continued high return on the public investment in research; and (4) exemplify and promote the highest level of scientific integrity, public accountability, and social responsibility in the conduct of science (National Institutes of Health, 2004).

The **Food and Drug Administration (FDA)** is responsible for protecting the public health by assuring the safety, efficacy and security of human and veterinary drugs, biological products, medical devices, our Nation's food supply, cosmetics, and products that emit radiation. The FDA is also responsible for advancing the public health by helping to speed innovations that make medicines and foods more effective, safer and more affordable; and helping the public get the accurate, science-based information they need to use medicines and foods to improve their health (Food and Drug Administration, 2004).

The mission of the **Indian Health Service (IHS)** is to raise the physical, mental, social, and spiritual health of American Indians and Alaska Natives to the highest level. The goal of the IHS is to assure that comprehensive, culturally acceptable personal and public health services are available and accessible to American Indian and Alaska Native people. The foundation of the IHS is to uphold the Federal government's obligation to promote healthy American Indian and Alaska Native people, communities and cultures and to honor and protect the inherent sovereign rights of Tribes (Indian Health Service, 2004).

The **Substance Abuse and Mental Health Services Administration (SAMHSA)** is the DHHS agency charged with improving the quality and availability of prevention, treatment, and rehabilitative services in order to reduce illness, death, disability, and cost to society resulting from substance abuse and mental illnesses (Department of Health and Human Services, 2004c).

The mission of the **Agency for Healthcare Research and Quality (AHRQ)** is to support research designed to improve the outcomes and quality of health care, reduce its costs, address patient safety and medical errors and broaden access to effective services. The research sponsored, conducted, and disseminated by the AHRQ provides information that helps people make better decisions about health care (Agency for Healthcare Research and Quality, 2004).

Human Services Agencies

The mission of the **Centers for Medicare and Medicaid Services (CMS)** is to assure healthcare security for beneficiaries. The vision of CMS is that in serving beneficiaries, CMS will open its programs to full partnership with the entire health community to improve quality and efficiency in an evolving health care system (Centers for Medicare and Medicaid Services, 2004).

The **Administration for Children and Families (ACF)** is responsible for Federal programs that promote the economic and social well-being of families, children, individuals and communities (Administration for Children and Families, 2004).

The mission of the **Administration on Aging (AoA)** is to promote the dignity and independence of older people, and to help society prepare for an aging population (Administration on Aging, 2004).

FEDERAL RESOURCES

Funding Resources

Included among the resources the federal government has available to local public health agencies is extramural grant and cooperative agreement funding. The DHHS has approximately 300 grant and cooperative agreement programs, most of which are administered in a decentralized manner by several DHHS agencies. DHHS does not have a single publication that describes all grant programs. Instead, DHHS uses the **Catalog of Federal Domestic Assistance (CFDA)**.

The CFDA, which is compiled and maintained by the General Services Administration, profiles all federal grant programs, including DHHS programs, and lists a specific contact for obtaining additional information and application forms. The CFDA also includes a helpful section on writing grant applications. Local public health agencies should consult the CFDA to find the federal programs of interest to their organization (Department of Health and Human Services, 2004d).

Another federal resource available to local public health agencies is the **Federal Register**. Published by the Office of the Federal Register, National Archives and Records Administration (NARA), the Federal Register is the official daily publication for rules, proposed rules, and notices of federal agencies and organizations, as well as executive orders and other presidential documents (Government Printing Office, 2004). A local health officer should monitor the Federal Register on a frequent basis, daily if possible. All federal grants and cooperative agreements are listed in the Federal Register with the applicable guidelines. Frequently, federal agencies will provide a workshop on the grant application intent and process, with information typically to be found at the applicable federal agency's Web site.

Other DHHS funding opportunities are included on the respective Web sites of the various DHHS agencies (Department of Health and Human Services, 2004e). As an example, the CDC and the HRSA are two of the extramural funding agencies within DHHS directly serving local public health agencies. Several CDC Centers, Institute, or Program Offices (C/I/Os) offer grants and/or cooperative agreements related to their program areas. See the respective CDC C/I/O Web sites for additional information. Within the CDC, the organization responsible for administering funding opportunities for all C/I/Os is the Procurement and Grants Office (PGO). PGO is responsible for: (1) the awarding and administration of CDC's grants and cooperative agreements and those of ATSDR; (2) the acquisition of program-related health studies, professional services, and research and development; and (3) the procurement of services, equipment, commodities, construction, and architectural and engineering services for CDC programs (Centers for Disease Control and Prevention, 2004b).

A unique CDC funding resource is the **Public Health Prevention Service (PHPS)**. In response to the need for a well-developed and highly skilled workforce, CDC established the PHPS in 1997. The primary goal of this three-year service and training program is to develop a workforce that is skilled in planning, implementing, and evaluating prevention programs. This goal is accomplished through a combination of structured and on-the-job training (Centers for Disease Control and Prevention, 2004c). A local public health agency can apply to be a public health agency field site. The local public health agency must first submit a letter of intent and then a completed application.

The HRSA awards grants and cooperative agreements that expand and improve the following areas: primary healthcare for medically underserved people, health and related services for people with HIV/AIDS, maternal and child health, health professions training and education, rural health, telemedicine and organ donation (Health Resources and Services Administration, 2004a). To facilitate the electronic application process for HRSA grants and/or cooperative agreements, local public health agencies must register with the Central Contractor Registry (Health Resources and Services Administration, 2004b).

In addition to the respective DHHS agency funding resources, DHHS is the lead department within the federal government and managing partner for the Federal E-Grants initiative. This is one of 24 initiatives of the overall E-Government program for improving access to federal government services via the Internet. Eleven departments and agencies have been designated as supporting partners for this initiative, which calls for the development of a one-stop electronic grant portal where potential grant recipients will receive full service electronic grant administration. DHHS has established a Web portal that enables local public health agencies to find information on every grant offered by the federal government on one Web site—www.grants.gov. The search for grant opportunities can be completed by a simple full-text search in active or archived documents, by funding opportunity, date, CFDA number, funding activity category, funding instrument type, and/or agency. Local public health agencies can also sign up to automatically receive new grant program announcements and modifications of existing announcements.

Funding opportunities are available to local public health agencies from other federal government departments and agencies. A directory of key contacts with these other organizations can be found at www.hhs.gov/grantsnet/whoswho.htm.

The newest federal department is the Department of Homeland Security (DHS). DHS has three primary missions: preventing terrorist attacks within the United States, reducing America's vulnerability to terrorism, and minimizing the damage from potential attacks and natural disasters. More information about DHS funding and other resources can be found at www.dhs.gov/dhspublic/display?theme=10&content=429.

Other grant and cooperative agreement opportunities can be found at www.hhs.gov/grantsnet/otherresources/index.htm. In addition, another resource available to local public health agencies is the National Grants Management Association (NGMA). More information about the NGMA can be found at www.hhs.gov/grantsnet/otherresources/oresour/ngmares.htm.

Preparation of Grant Applications

Although a wealth of federal resources are available to local public health agencies, insufficient attention is often devoted to preparing applications. This section recommends practical tips to improve a local public health agency's probability of being approved and funded.

A local public health agency should carefully read the guidance provided with the program announcement and review the evaluation criteria specific to how the application will be scored. Also, the application should be organized according to the program announcement and specifications such as page length, printing, margins, font type and size, paper size, pagination, number of copies, and binding should be followed to the letter.

Comprehensive, concise project objectives with realistic and achievable target dates and measurable quantitative results should be developed. These project objectives will establish the basis of the evaluation plan for the project, including both process and outcome measures.

A complete, detailed and fully justified budget should be clearly presented. The Office of Management and Budget has created a common budget information form for nonconstruction programs, known informally as the SF 424A. Use of tables in the budget are encouraged, and budget category line items from the SF 424A should be used and organized with subtotals. Also, the indirect rate (the amount allowed for overhead and support of the institution requesting the grant) should be calculated according to the existing agreement on file with the requesting organization. Finally, a narrative that supports and fully justifies the budget should be included.

Before it is submitted, the application should be reviewed according to an application checklist. One individual should format and prepare the final application and then an external editor should review the final application package. As needed, both programmatic and business assistance should be requested, as provided for in the program announcement. Virtually all successful recipients of grants meet or beat published application deadlines.

CDC Terrorism Preparedness and Emergency Response and Other Resources

The CDC has emergency response resources available to local public health agencies in the event of a bioterrorism incident, outbreak of infectious disease, or public health threat and emergency. Terrorism preparedness and emergency response information can be found at www.bt.cdc.gov. Although not limited to the following CDC resources, specific information about selected resources can be found in several government publications. The following can be downloaded from the Internet at no cost.

The *Biosafety in Microbiological and Biomedical Laboratories, 4th Edition*, describes the combinations of standard and special microbiological practices, safety equipment, and facilities constituting Biosafety Levels 1–4 that are recommended for work with a variety of infectious agents in various laboratory settings (Centers for Disease Control and Prevention, 2004d).

The *Case Definitions for Infectious Conditions under Public Health Surveillance* provides updated uniform criteria for state health agency personnel to use when reporting notifiable diseases to CDC (Centers for Disease Control and Prevention, 2004e).

The *CDC Recommends: The Prevention Guidelines System* contains CDC recommendations for the prevention, control, treatment, and detection of infectious and chronic diseases, environmental hazards, natural or human-generated disasters, occupational diseases and injuries, intentional and unintentional injuries and disabilities, and other public health conditions. This compendium of documents allows public health practitioners and others to quickly access the CDC recommendations from a single point, regardless of where they were originally published (Public Health Practice Program Office, 2004a).

The *Journal of Emerging and Infectious Diseases* is a peer-reviewed publication that tracks and analyzes disease trends. More information can be found at www.cdc.gov/ncidod/EID/index.htm.

The Health Alert Network links the CDC with local public health agencies and to other organizations critical for terrorism preparedness and emergency response. More information can be found at www.phppo.cdc.gov/han.

The *Morbidity and Mortality Weekly Report* contains data on specific diseases as reported by state and territorial health agencies and reports on infectious and chronic diseases, environmental hazards, natural or human-generated disasters, occupational diseases and injuries, and intentional and unintentional injuries. Also included are reports on topics of international interest and notices of events of interest to the public health community (Centers for Disease Control and Prevention, 2004f).

The National Laboratory Training Network is dedicated to improving laboratory practice of public health significance through quality continuing education. It is a training system sponsored by the Association of Public Health Laboratories and the CDC (Public Health Practice Program Office, 2004b).

The Public Health Training Network is a CDC distance-learning system that takes training to the learner. The network uses a variety of instructional media ranging from print-based to videotape and multimedia to meet the training needs of the public health workforce nationwide (Public Health Practice Program Office, 2004c).

The Public Health Law Program leads the CDC's efforts to improve scientific understanding of the interaction between law and public health and to strengthen the legal foundation for public health practice. The Public Health Law Program is a resource for local public health agencies that are interested in strengthening public health practice through better understanding and use of public health law (Public Health Practice Program Office, 2004d). Public health laws are related to the police power reserved to the states. Most local public health agencies and the laws to which they relate are state laws. In the case of an emergency, the resources of the federal government are accessed through the state health agency. State health agency information can be found at www.astho.org/?template=regional_links.php&PHPSESSID=d692262f5067af3f9395fcc1f6195582.

Other resources available to the local public health agencies can be found at www.cdc.gov/other.htm#states. The protocols for requesting federal assistance from the CDC are included in the next section.

PROTOCOLS FOR REQUESTING FEDERAL ASSISTANCE

CDC Protocol for Federal Assistance During a Bioterrorist Incident, Other Outbreak of Infectious Disease, or Public Health Threat and Emergency

The following protocol (**Figure 36-2**) is meant for use by local public health leaders who identify or suspect a bioterrorism incident, other outbreak of infectious disease, public health threat, or emergency in their community. It should be incorporated into a local communications plan for bioterrorism. For simplicity, the term local health officer is used in this discussion. However, depending on the structure, size, and complexity of a local public health agency, this person might be the health commissioner, health administrator, environmental health director, chief epidemiologist, or some other professional in an officially designated leadership role (www.bt.cdc.gov/emcontact/background.asp).

Emergency response contact information for local public health agencies to report a bioterrorism incident, other outbreak of infectious disease, public health threat, or emergency in their community is included in **Figure 36-3**. This figure also provides hotline information for use by local public health agencies.

Other CDC Requests for Federal Assistance

Requests for federal assistance that do not involve a bioterrorism incident, other outbreak of infectious disease, public health threat, or emergency are routinely made of several of the CDC C/I/Os. Often, these requests arrive in the form of seeking technical assistance that can be provided by a CDC grant or cooperative agreement project officers, as well as subject matter experts. This type of federal assistance typically is

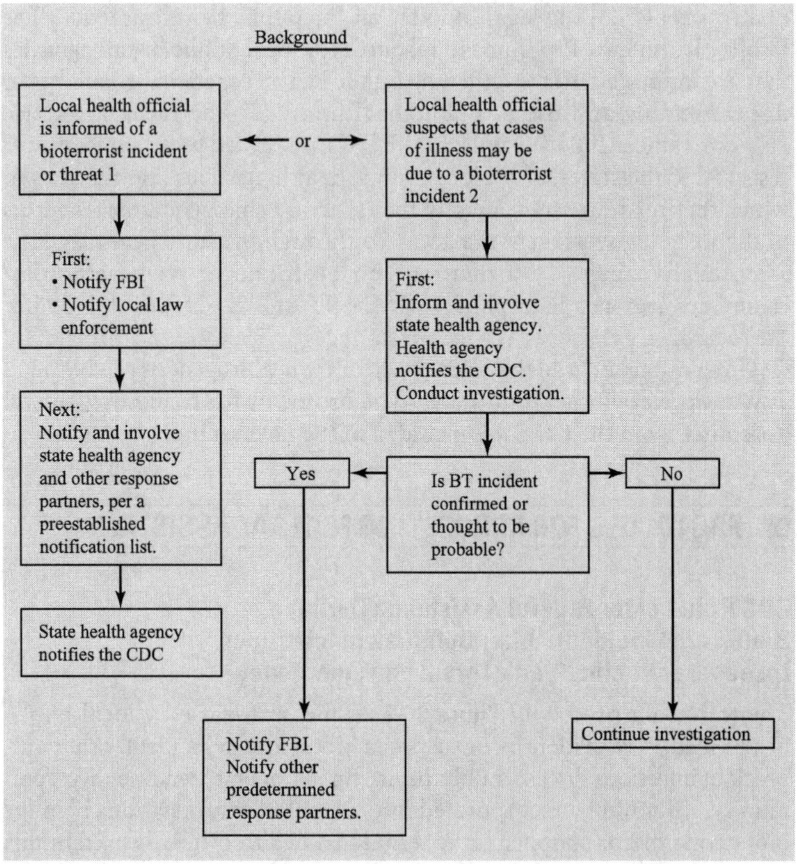

Figure 36-2 Protocols: Interim Recommended Notification Procedures for Local and State Public Health Agency Leaders in the Event of a Bioterrorist Incident

Source: Centers for Disease Control and Prevention, 2004g.

- CDC Emergency Response Hotline (24 hours)
  770-488-7100
  Program questions: 404-639-0385
- Hotline managed by:
- Bioterrorism Preparedness and Response Program
  Program questions: 404-639-0385
- Emergency Preparedness and Response Branch
  National Center for Environmental Health

Figure 36-3 Contacts for Use by State and Local Health Officials, Healthcare Providers

Source: Centers for Disease Control and Prevention, 2004h.

less formalized and structured than during a bioterrorism incident. CDC's major organizational components (C/I/Os) respond individually in their areas of expertise and pool their resources and expertise on cross-cutting issues and specific health threats.

Federal Expectations

As has been described, the federal government has a wealth of resources available to local public health agencies. However, associated with these resources are expectations that the federal government has of local public health agencies utilizing these resources. Similarly, local public health agencies have expectations of the federal government in providing these resources.

All federal grants and cooperative agreements are listed in the Federal Register with their applicable guidelines. Many federal grants and cooperative agreements require that a local public health agency apply within their own state or have a letter of support from their state public health agency. The local health officer must follow the grant or cooperative agreement instructions and complete all application materials.

Local public health agencies are expected to comply with the guidance and requirements for grants and cooperative agreements. Evaluation of the requirements of the grant or cooperative agreement should be completed using quantifiable process and outcome measures described in the application for the grant or cooperative agreement.

In addition to completing evaluation plans, local public health agencies are expected to complete a detailed, justified budget to accompany their applications for a grant or cooperative agreement. Guidance is available for the preparation of a budget request. Following this guidance will facilitate the review and approval of a requested budget (Centers for Disease Control and Prevention, 2004i).

In addition to completing applications in accordance with published guidance for federal grants and cooperative agreements, there are other program announcement additional requirements (AR). A complete list containing full descriptions of these additional requirements can be found at www.cdc.gov/od/pgo/funding/ARs.htm. Examples include, but are not limited to, requirements for human subjects review, inclusion of women and racial and ethnic minorities in research, and humane treatment of animal subjects.

In addition to these requirements and expectations, there are certain restrictions on the use of DHHS funds for lobbying of federal or state legislative bodies and for advocating or promoting gun control (Centers for Disease Control and Prevention, 2004j). Furthermore, every application for a new federal grant or cooperative agreement or renewal of an award submitted on or after October 1, 2003, must include a Dun and Bradstreet Data Universal Numbering System number (Centers for Disease Control and Prevention, 2004k).

Local public health agencies in turn have expectations of the federal government in providing resources. From the federal perspective, the CDC cannot enter a state or local jurisdiction unless it has been asked to assist or an interstate issue is involved. Federal functions are related to international issues, interstate issues, or federal funding and assistance. In the case of a bioterrorism incident, other outbreak of infectious disease, or public health threat and emergency, the resources of the federal government are accessed through the state health agency.

CONCLUSION

Many departments, agencies, and other units within the federal government have been created to provide resources and assistance related to public health needs. The government requires that organizations request assistance using protocols that it has developed. The mission of the federal government is straightforward: protecting the health and well-being of the population of the United States. The mission of the Centers for Disease Control and Prevention is to promote health and quality of life by preventing and controlling disease, injury, and disability.

This chapter has described the federal resources available to the Aloma County health officer. These resources also could be used to resolve some of the local public health agency's challenges and strategic issues that were initially described. Certainly during a bioterrorism incident, other outbreak of infectious disease, or public health threat and emergency, federal assets are available to local public health agencies. During more routine public health challenges, the federal resources available to local public health agencies can also ease the local financial burden and facilitate strengthening of public health infrastructure to support daily public health practice.

The Aloma County health officer has now identified the resources and programs that can be used to address these strategic issues. The health officer and the board of health now understand the federal government's role and mission, including how it interfaces with the local or state government's role and mission. The resources available from the federal government have been described, and additional information has been referenced. Various departments and agencies of the federal government have been included that can provide information or assistance on the best practices of public health. The protocols for requesting assistance from the federal government have been delineated, both during a public health threat and emergency and during less-exigent circumstances. Moreover, the resources of the federal government that can be utilized in an emergency response have been identified. Finally, both federal government and local public health agency expectations have been described.

As the next step, the Aloma County health officer should start developing strategies to fully utilize these resources. Full involvement of the Aloma County board of health is anticipated.

References

Administration for Children and Families. 2004. About ACF. Available at www.acf.hhs.gov/acf_about.html#mission. Accessed February 22, 2004.

Administration on Aging. 2004. Welcome. Available at www.aoa.gov/about/over/over_mission.asp. Accessed February 22, 2004.

Agency for Healthcare Research and Quality. 2004. AHRQ Profile: Advancing Excellence in Health Care. Available at www.ahrq.gov/about/profile.htm. Accessed February 19, 2004.

Centers for Disease Control and Prevention. 2004a. About CDC. Available at www.cdc.gov/aboutcdc.htm. Accessed February 22, 2004.

Centers for Disease Control and Prevention. 2004b. Funding opportunities. Available at www.cdc.gov/funding.htm. Accessed February 19, 2004.

Centers for Disease Control and Prevention. 2004c. Public Health Prevention Service background information. Available at www.cdc.gov/epo/dapht/phps/background.htm. Accessed February 18, 2004.

Centers for Disease Control and Prevention. 2004d. Biosafety in Microbiological and Biomedical Laboratories (BMBL) 4th Edition. Available at www.cdc.gov/od/ohs/biosfty/bmbl4/bmbl4toc.htm. Accessed February 18, 2004.

Centers for Disease Control and Prevention. 2004e. Case Definitions for Infectious Conditions Under Public Health Surveillance. Available at www.cdc.gov/epo/dphsi/casedef/index.htm. Accessed February 17, 2004.

Centers for Disease Control and Prevention. 2004f. Morbidity and Mortality Weekly Report. Available at www.cdc.gov/mmwr/mmwr_wk.html. Accessed February 20, 2004.

Centers for Disease Control and Prevention. 2004g. Interim Recommended Notification Procedures for Local and State Public Health Agency Leaders in the Event of a Bioterrorist Incident. Available at http://www.bt.cdc.gov/emcontact/background.asp. Accessed February 20, 2004.

Centers for Disease Control and Prevention. 2004h. What to do in an emergency. Available at http://www.bt.cdc.gov/emcontact/index.asp. Accessed February 18, 2004.

Centers for Disease Control and Prevention. 2004i. Budgeting guide. Available at www.cdc.gov/od/pgo/funding/budgetguide.htm. Accessed February 17, 2004.

Centers for Disease Control and Prevention. 2004j. Restrictions on the use of DHHS funds. Available at www.cdc.gov/od/pgo/funding/lobbying.pdf. Accessed February 21, 2004.

Centers for Disease Control and Prevention. 2004k. DUNS number requirement. Available at www.cdc.gov/od/pgo/funding/duns.pdf. Accessed February 20, 2004.

Centers for Medicare and Medicaid Services. 2004. Mission, vision, goals, and objectives. Available at www.cms.hhs.gov/about/mission.asp. Accessed February 22, 2004.

Department of Health and Human Services. 2004a. HHS: What we do. Available at www.hhs.gov/news/press/2002pres/profile.html. Accessed February 22, 2004.

Department of Health and Human Services. 2004b. HHS Strategic Plan FY 2004–2009. Available at aspe.hhs.gov/hhsplan. Accessed February 22, 2004.

Department of Health and Human Services. 2004c. Substance Abuse and Mental Health Service Administration. Available at www.samhsa.gov/about/about.html. Accessed February 19, 2004.

Department of Health and Human Services. 2004d. How to find information about HHS Grant Programs. Available at www.hhs.gov/grantsnet/grantinfo.htm. Accessed February 19, 2004.

Department of Health and Human Services. 2004e. Other HHS Agency funding opportunities. Available at www.hhs.gov/grantsnet/otherops.htm. Accessed February 19, 2004.

Food and Drug Administration. 2004. FDA's mission statement. Available at www.fda.gov/opacom/morechoices/mission.html. Accessed February 21, 2004.

Government Printing Office. 2004. The Federal Register (FR): Main Page. Available at www.gpoaccess.gov/fr/index.html. Accessed February 16, 2004.

Health Resources and Services Administration. 2004a. Funding opportunities. Available at www.hrsa.gov/grants/default.htm. Accessed February 21, 2004.

Health Resources and Services Administration. 2004b. Funding opportunities registry. Available at www.hrsa.gov/grants/ccr.htm. Accessed February 20, 2004.

Indian Health Service. 2004. Indian Health Service introduction. Available at www.ihs.gov/PublicInfo/PublicAffairs/Welcome_Info/IHSintro.asp. Accessed February 22, 2004.

National Association of City and County Health Officers. 2004. MAPP. Available at mapp.naccho.org/MAPP_Home.asp. Accessed on February 24, 2004.

National Institutes of Health. 2004. The NIH Almanac. Available at www.nih.gov/about/almanac/index.html. Accessed February 21, 2004.

Public Health Practice Program Office. 2004a. Prevention guidelines system. Available at www.phppo.cdc.gov/CDCRecommends/AboutV.asp. Accessed February 21, 2004.

Public Health Practice Program Office. 2004b. National Laboratory Training Network. Available at www.phppo.cdc.gov/nltn/default.asp. Accessed February 18, 2004.

Public Health Practice Program Office. 2004c. What is the Public Health Training Network? Available at www.phppo.cdc.gov/PHTN/whatis.asp. Accessed February 17, 2004.

Public Health Practice Program Office. 2004d. About the Public Health Law program. Available at www.phppo.cdc.gov/od/phlp/about.asp. Accessed February 21, 2004.

Resources

Books

Cahill, K.M. 2002. *Emergency Relief Operations.* New York: Fordham University Press.

Web Sites

See Web site references throughout the chapter.

Organizations

Centers for Disease Control and Prevention
1600 Clifton Road
Atlanta, GA 30333
Phone: 404-639-3311, 404-639-3534, or 800-311-3435
E-mail: www.cdc.gov/netinfo.htm
Web site: www.cdc.gov

Federal Emergency Management Agency
500 C Street, SW
Washington, D.C. 20472
Phone: 202-566-1600
Web site: www.fema.gov

Health Resources and Services Administration
Parklawn Building
Rockville, MD 20857
Phone: 301-443-3376
E-mail: ask@hrsa.gov or comments@hrsa.gov
Web site: www.hrsa.gov

U.S. Department of Health & Human Services
200 Independence Avenue, SW
Washington, D.C. 20201
Phone: 202-619-0257 or 877-696-6775 (toll free)
Web site: www.hhs.gov

U.S. Department of Homeland Security
Washington, D.C. 20528
Web page: www.dhs.gov/dhspublic/index.jsp

INDEX

N